Understanding Anatomy & Physiology in Nursing

Sara Miller McCune founded SAGE Publishing in 1965 to support the dissemination of usable knowledge and educate a global community. SAGE publishes more than 1000 journals and over 800 new books each year, spanning a wide range of subject areas. Our growing selection of library products includes archives, data, case studies and video. SAGE remains majority owned by our founder and after her lifetime will become owned by a charitable trust that secures the company's continued independence.

Los Angeles | London | New Delhi | Singapore | Washington DC | Melbourne

Understanding Anatomy & Physiology in Nursing

John Knight
Yamni Nigam
Jayne Cutter

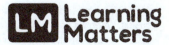

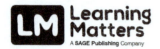

Learning Matters
A SAGE Publishing Company
1 Oliver's Yard
55 City Road
London EC1Y 1SP

SAGE Publications Inc.
2455 Teller Road
Thousand Oaks, California 91320

SAGE Publications India Pvt Ltd
B 1/l 1 Mohan Cooperative Industrial Area
Mathura Road
New Delhi 110 044

SAGE Publications Asia-Pacific Pte Ltd
3 Church Street
#10-04 Samsung Hub
Singapore 049483

Editor: Laura Walmsley
Development editor: Eleanor Rivers
Senior project editor: Chris Marke
Project management: Swales & Willis Ltd, Exeter, Devon
Marketing manager: George Kimble
Cover design: Wendy Scott
Typeset by: C&M
Printed in the UK

Library of Congress Control Number: 2020933766

British Library Cataloguing in Publication data

A catalogue record for this book is available from the British Library

ISBN 978-1-5264-7455-1
ISBN 978-1-5264-7454-4 (pbk)

At SAGE we take sustainability seriously. Most of our products are printed in the UK using FSC papers and boards. When we print overseas we ensure sustainable papers are used as measured by the PREPS grading system. We undertake an annual audit to monitor our sustainability.

Contents

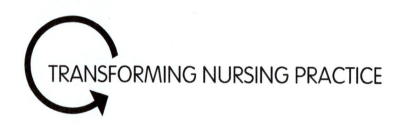

TRANSFORMING NURSING PRACTICE

Transforming Nursing Practice is a series tailor made for pre-registration students nurses. Each book in the series is:

 Affordable

 Full of active learning features

 Mapped to the NMC Standards of proficiency for registered nurses

 Focused on applying theory to practice

Each book addresses a core topic and has been carefully developed to be simple to use, quick to read and written in clear language.

An invaluable series of books that explicitly relates to the NMC standards. Each book covers a different topic that students need to explore in order to develop into a qualified nurse... I would recommend this series to all Pre-Registered nursing students whatever their field or year of study.

LINDA ROBSON,
Senior Lecturer at Edge Hill University

Many titles in the series are on our recommended reading list and for good reason - the content is up to date and easy to read. These are the books that actually get used beyond training and into your nursing career.

EMMA LYDON,
Adult Student Nursing

ABOUT THE SERIES EDITORS

DR MOOI STANDING is an Independent Academic Nursing Consultant (UK and international) responsible for the core knowledge, personal and professional learning skills titles. She has invaluable experience as an NMC Quality Assurance Reviewer of educational programmes, and as a Professional Regulator Panellist on the NMC Practice Committee. Mooi is also a Board member of Special Olympics Malaysia.

DR SANDRA WALKER is a Clinical Academic in Mental Health working between North Bristol Trust and Southern Health Trust. She is series editor for the mental health nursing titles. She is a Qualified Mental Health Nurse with a wide range of clinical experience spanning 30 years and spent several years working as a mental health lecturer at Southampton University.

BESTSELLING TEXTBOOKS

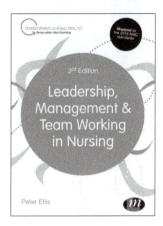

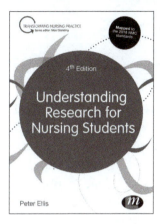

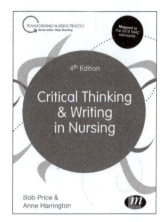

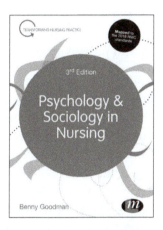

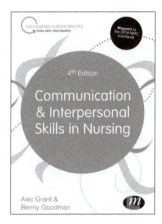

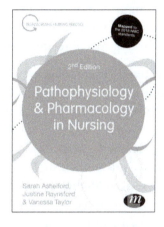

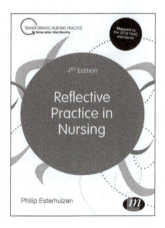

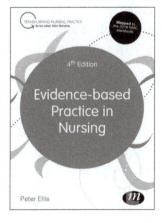

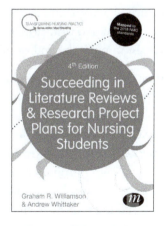

You can find a full list of textbooks in the
Transforming Nursing Practice series at
https://uk.sagepub.com

About the authors

Dr John Knight is Associate Professor in Biomedical Science within the College of Human and Health Sciences at Swansea University. For the last 20 years he has taught anatomy, physiology and pathophysiology on a wide variety of professional degree and diploma programmes including: health and social care, paramedic science, nursing and midwifery. John's first degree is in microbiology; additionally he holds a PhD in immunology and has over 50 published articles in peer-reviewed journals. His teaching at Swansea University has recently been recognised by the presentation of a Distinguished Teaching Award. John has a variety of research interests including the evolution of immune responses, the physiological effects of ageing and immobility and the use of virtual reality simulations in the teaching of anatomy and physiology.

Professor Yamni Nigam is a Professor in Biomedical Science (anatomy, physiology and pathophysiology) and a Fellow of the Higher Education Academy, teaching a wide range of health professionals including nurses and paramedics. Her specialist subjects include digestion, blood, immunology, microbiology, parasitology, wounds (infection and healing) and maggot therapy. Yamni graduated from King's College London and undertook a Master's degree in Applied Parasitology and Medical Entomology at the Liverpool School of Tropical Medicine. After successful completion of her doctorate, Yamni was offered a lectureship teaching anatomy and physiology at Swansea University. In 2001, she set up the Swansea University Maggot Research Group, focusing on scientific investigations of the medicinal maggot and its role in wound healing. Her love of human A&P has persisted and she continues to write articles to support the learning of these subjects for all health professionals. Yamni is the author of over 75 peer-reviewed articles, book chapters and papers.

After qualifying as a nurse, **Professor Jayne Cutter** worked in surgery and intensive care before becoming a Clinical Nurse Specialist in Infection Control. She spent 15 years in this post before leaving the NHS and joining Swansea University as a lecturer. Jayne's research interests include infection control and pedagogy. Although interested in all aspects of infection prevention and control, Jayne has a particular interest in factors influencing compliance. In 2009 she gained a PhD following a study titled 'Factors influencing sustaining and reporting inoculation injuries in healthcare professionals undertaking exposure prone procedures'. In April 2015, Jayne was appointed as the Head of the Department of Nursing at Swansea University and became a professor in 2019. She has been closely involved in developing the new curriculum at Swansea to meet the new NMC Standards for pre-registration nursing programmes. Jayne currently chairs the all-Wales Pre-Registration Nursing and Midwifery Group and has contributed to the development of all-Wales documentation to support the new NMC Standards.

Introduction

Nursing is a profession that continually evolves to meet the ever-changing demands of modern healthcare. As a result, the education of student nurses must also evolve so that registrants are equipped to deal with the challenges of being a qualified nurse.

The Nursing and Midwifery Council (NMC) regulates nurses and midwives in the UK, and nursing associates in England. The role of the NMC is to protect the public. To that end, all student nurses enrolled on a programme leading to registration with the NMC have to complete a programme of study informed by the NMC Standards for pre-registration nursing programmes (2018b). According to Article 5 (2) of the Nursing and Midwifery Order (2001) (legislation.gov.uk, 2002), the NMC must identify standards of proficiency required to enter the register. These standards of proficiency are grouped together under seven platforms and two annexes.

The platforms are:

1. Being an accountable professional
2. Promoting health and preventing ill health
3. Assessing needs and planning care
4. Providing and evaluating care
5. Leading and managing nursing care and working in teams
6. Improving safety and quality of care
7. Coordinating care.

(NMC, 2018b, page 6)

Annexe A focuses on communication and relationship management while Annexe B identifies nursing skills and procedures required of a nurse at the point of registration (NMC, 2018b).

The NMC recognises that nurses require a

comprehensive knowledge of the sciences on which general nursing is based, including sufficient understanding of the structure, physiological functions and behaviour of healthy and sick persons, and of the relationship between the state of health and the physical and social environment of the human being.

(NMC, 2018b, page 50)

It is not enough to learn how to undertake tasks by rote. Nurses must be able to understand what is happening within the body so that when a patient develops a high temperature during a blood transfusion (Chapter 9) or a person with asthma becomes breathless when exposed to pollen (Chapter 4), for example, they can make an informed decision on the appropriate action to take. In short, unless we understand what is 'normal', we can never truly understand how the disease process affects our minds and bodies, and without this understanding, we cannot deliver appropriate care.

We have specifically written this book to ensure that its readers have the requisite underpinning knowledge and understanding of anatomy and physiology to equip them to assess, plan and deliver safe and effective nursing care. Within each chapter, you will find case studies and activities to encourage you to test and apply your newfound knowledge in relation to 'real-world' situations. We have mapped each chapter against the relevant platforms and the procedures in Annexe B to ensure that you have the required knowledge and understanding of anatomy and physiology to meet the NMC Standards for pre-registration nursing programmes (2018a) and achieve proficiency in these standards; see Table 0.1.

Table 0.1   Contents mapped to NMC proficiencies (NMC 2019b, pages 7–18, 32–6)

Platform/annexe	Proficiency	Chapter
Platform 1 Being an accountable professional	1.20 safely demonstrate evidence-based practice in all skills and procedures stated in Annexes A and B	1, 2, 3, 4, 5, 6, 7, 8, 9, 10, 11, 12
Platform 2 Promoting health and preventing ill health	2.2 demonstrate knowledge of epidemiology, demography, genomics and the wider determinants of health, illness and wellbeing and apply this to an understanding of global patterns of health and wellbeing outcomes	1, 2, 5, 6, 13
	2.4 identify and use all appropriate opportunities, making reasonable adjustments when required, to discuss the impact of smoking, substance and alcohol use, sexual behaviours, diet and exercise on mental, physical and behavioural health and wellbeing, in the context of people's individual circumstances	3, 4, 5, 7, 8, 12
	2.5 promote and improve mental, physical, behavioural and other health related outcomes by understanding and explaining the principles, practice and evidence-base for health screening programmes	1, 2, 3, 4, 5, 12

	2.11 promote health and prevent ill health by understanding and explaining to people the principles of pathogenesis, immunology and the evidence-base for immunisation, vaccination and herd immunity	1, 2, 9
	2.12 protect health through understanding and applying the principles of infection prevention and control, including communicable disease surveillance and antimicrobial stewardship and resistance	1, 7, 8, 9, 10
Platform 3 Assessing needs and planning care	3.2 demonstrate and apply knowledge of body systems and homeostasis, human anatomy and physiology, biology, genomics, pharmacology and social and behavioural sciences when undertaking full and accurate person-centred nursing assessments and developing appropriate care plans	1, 2, 3, 4, 5, 6, 7, 8, 9, 10, 11, 12, 13
	3.5 demonstrate the ability to accurately process all information gathered during the assessment process to identify needs for individualised nursing care and develop person-centred evidence-based plans for nursing interventions with agreed goals	1, 2, 3, 4, 5, 6, 7, 8, 9, 10, 11, 12, 13
	3.11 undertake routine investigations, interpreting and sharing findings as appropriate	1, 2, 3, 4, 5, 6, 9, 10, 11
	3.12 interpret results from routine investigations, taking prompt action when required by implementing appropriate interventions, requesting additional investigations or escalating to others	1, 2, 3, 4, 5, 6, 9, 10, 11
Platform 4 Providing and evaluating care	4.8 demonstrate the knowledge and skills required to identify and initiate appropriate interventions to support people with commonly encountered symptoms including anxiety, confusion, discomfort and pain	1, 2, 3, 4, 5, 6, 7, 8, 9, 10, 11, 12
	4.10 demonstrate the knowledge and ability to respond proactively and promptly to signs of deterioration or distress in mental, physical, cognitive and behavioural health and use this knowledge to make sound clinical decisions	1, 2, 3, 4, 5, 6, 7, 8, 9, 10, 11, 12

(Continued)

Table 0.1   (Continued)

Annexe B 1. Use evidence-based, best practice approaches to take a history, observe, recognise and accurately assess people of all ages	1.2 physical health and wellbeing	1, 2, 3, 4, 5, 6, 7, 8, 9, 10, 11, 12
	1.2.1 symptoms and signs of physical ill health	1, 2, 3, 4, 5, 6, 7, 8, 9, 10, 11, 12
	1.2.2 symptoms and signs of physical distress	1, 2, 3, 4, 5, 6, 7, 8, 9, 10, 11, 12
	1.2.3 symptoms and signs of deterioration and sepsis	1, 2, 3 ,4, 5, 6, 7, 12
Annexe B 2. Use evidence-based, best practice approaches to undertake the following procedures:	2.1 take, record and interpret vital signs manually and via technological devices	1, 2, 3, 4
	2.2 undertake venepuncture and cannulation and blood sampling, interpreting normal and common abnormal blood profiles and venous blood gases	1, 2, 3, 4, 5, 9, 10, 11
	2.3 set up and manage routine electrocardiogram (ECG) investigations and interpret normal and commonly encountered abnormal traces	3
	2.4 manage and monitor blood component transfusions	9
	2.6 accurately measure weight and height, calculate body mass index and recognise healthy ranges and clinically significant low/high readings	10
	2.7 undertake a whole body systems assessment including respiratory, circulatory, neurological, musculoskeletal, cardiovascular and skin status	3, 4, 5, 6, 7, 8, 11
	2.8 undertake chest auscultation and interpret findings	3, 4
	2.9 collect and observe sputum, urine, stool and vomit specimens, undertaking routine analysis and interpreting findings	3, 9, 10, 11
	2.10 measure and interpret blood glucose levels	5, 9, 11
	2.12 undertake, respond to and interpret neurological observations and assessments	6
	2.13 identify and respond to signs of deterioration and sepsis	1, 2, 3, 4, 5, 9

4. Use evidence-based, best practice approaches for meeting the needs for care and support with hygiene and the maintenance of skin integrity, accurately assessing the person's capacity for independence and self-care and initiating appropriate interventions	4.1 observe, assess and optimise skin and hygiene status and determine the need for support and intervention	7
	4.8 assess, respond and effectively manage pyrexia and hypothermia	2, 7
5. Use evidence-based, best practice approaches for meeting needs for care and support with nutrition and hydration, accurately assessing the person's capacity for independence and self-care and initiating appropriate interventions	5.1 observe, assess and optimise nutrition and hydration status and determine the need for intervention and support	10
	5.4 record fluid intake and output and identify, respond to and manage dehydration or fluid retention	10
8. Use evidence-based, best practice approaches for meeting needs for respiratory care and support, accurately assessing the person's capacity for independence and self-care and initiating appropriate interventions	8.1 observe and assess the need for intervention and respond to restlessness, agitation and breathlessness using appropriate interventions	4
	8.2 manage the administration of oxygen using a range of routes and best practice approaches	4
	8.3 take and interpret peak flow and oximetry measurements	4

We are confident that you will find this book invaluable as you navigate your way through your nursing degree. One you have qualified as a nurse, this book will continue to provide a useful source of reference as you develop your nursing skills even further on the journey from being a novice to an expert (Benner, 1984).

We sincerely hope you enjoy reading this book and wish you every success in your nursing career.

John Knight
Yamni Nigam
Jayne Cutter

Chapter 1 Cellular physiology and histology

Chapter aims

After reading this chapter, you will be able to:

- describe the structure of a typical human cell;
- describe the movement of materials into and out of cells;
- explain how cells can be used to screen for disease;
- provide a description of the major types of human tissue;
- explain the difference between eukaryotic and prokaryotic cells.

Introduction

Case study: Josie – breast cancer

Josie was showering when she noticed a small but hard lump in her right breast. Josie was quickly referred to the local breast screening clinic for further investigation where ultrasound sonography revealed a dense mass around the size of a large garden pea. The consultant immediately recommended a needle biopsy which was carried out the same day under local anaesthetic. The tissue collected was sent for histological examination and a week later Josie was diagnosed with breast cancer and her treatment options were discussed.

The collection of a tissue sample from a patient is termed a biopsy. There are many types of biopsy ranging from the collection of a peripheral blood sample from a finger prick to a more invasive needle or surgical biopsy. As we have seen in Josie's case, study biopsies may be carried out to look for characteristic tissue changes that may be indicative of diseases such as cancer. Biopsies can also be used to check for infection or to monitor a variety of biochemical parameters in patients.

An average adult body is thought to be constructed from around 50 trillion (50 million million) cells, the majority of which have a finite lifespan, and are continually being replaced as they die. This means that most of the tissues and organs of the human body are not static but in a continual state of flux as senescent, aged cells are replaced.

This chapter will begin by examining the internal structure of a human cell. We will explore how deoxyribonucleic acid (DNA) is organised in the nucleus and the nature of human chromosomes and their use in screening for genetic disease. The individual components of the cytoplasm and structure of the plasma (cell) membrane will be described and mechanisms of transporting materials into and out of cells explored. Once you have a good grasp of cell structure, we will examine how cells are organised into the tissues which are used to construct the human body. Since microbes greatly outnumber human cells, we will examine the nature of bacterial cells which are found colonising the body as part of the microbial biome. To reinforce the key points we will explore the use of cells in detecting disease and examine how certain drugs can target specific cell types to treat disease.

Regions of a cell

Human cells are traditionally split into three distinct regions: the nucleus, the cytoplasm and the plasma (cell) membrane (Figure 1.1).

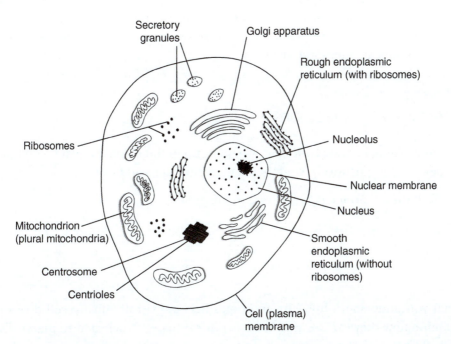

Figure 1.1   Cell structure

The nucleus

In most cells the nucleus is a centrally located structure that is separated from the cyto-plasm by the nuclear membrane (nuclear envelope). The region inside the nuclear membrane is called the nucleoplasm and usually has a granular appearance with a denser inner region called the nucleolus. This granular appearance is due to the pres-ence of condensed chromatin which consists of DNA molecules and histone proteins. The histones function as physical spools around which the DNA is wound and stored in a very compact form (Figure 1.2). This spooling of DNA is essential since each cell, which on average is only around 12 µm in diameter (12 1/000th mm), has to store around 3 metres (10 feet) of DNA.

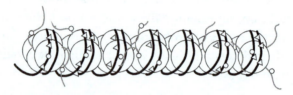

Figure 1.2   Chromatin and the spooling and storage of DNA

Appearance of chromosomes during cell division

When a cell is preparing to divide, the DNA is progressively wound up tighter and tighter so that it begins to fold up upon itself into tight coils; this tightly wound-up DNA is much denser and thicker and condenses in the nucleus in the form of thread-like structures which are referred to as chromosomes. To help you visualise how chromosomes appear, attempt Activity 1.1.

Activity 1.1   Reflection

Find a rubber elastic band and two pens. Loop the elastic band around both pens and progressively wind up the elastic tighter and tighter.

What do you notice is happening to the elastic?

There are some possible answers to all activities at the end of the chapter, unless otherwise indicated.

Now that you understand how chromosomes become visible during cell division, we can examine how they can be used to screen for diseases. Nucleated human cells usu-ally have 23 pairs of chromosomes, giving a total of 46, which is referred to as the diploid number (the normal expected number). The only major exceptions to this rule are the sperm and egg cells (ova) which by necessity must have half the diploid number of chromosomes. Half the diploid number in humans is 23 and this is referred to as the haploid number. Having haploid sperm and ova ensures that during fertilisation the diploid number of 46 is restored and the number of chromosomes remains constant down the generations (Chapter 13). Photographs of human chromosomes can be taken during cell division and placed into their ordered pairs according to size; these photographs are called karyographs and reveal the individual's chromosomal make-up, which is referred to as their karyotype.

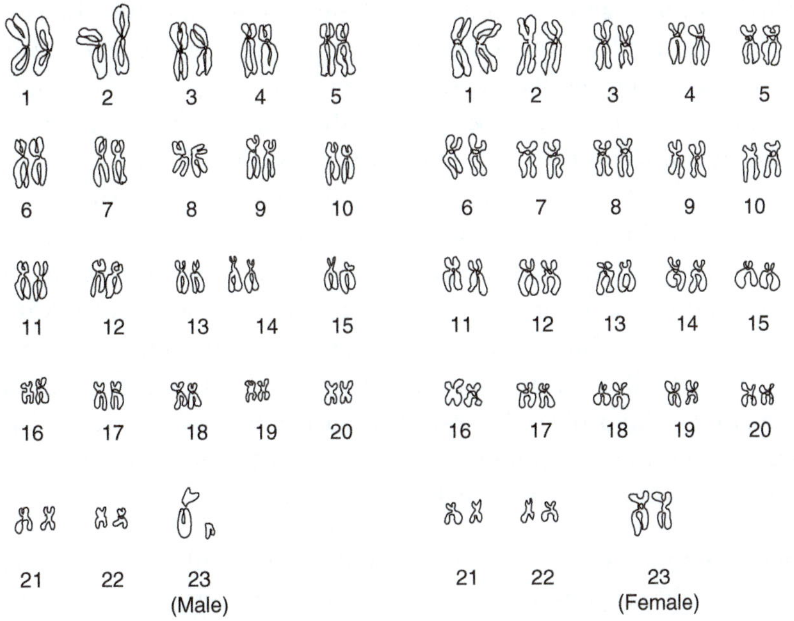

Figure 1.3   Chromosomes and karyotypes

The first 22 pairs of human chromosomes are referred to as autosomes and these appear structurally the same in both males and females (Figure 1.3). The final 23rd pair determines the physical gender of the individual and for this reason these are referred to as the sex chromosomes. Females usually have two XX chromosomes (XX) and males usually have an X and a Y chromosome (XY). However, as we will see in Chapter 13, there are frequently variations in the patterns of sex chromosomes and for this reason not all females are XX and not all males are XY. The sex chromosomes only determine the physical gender of the individual and it is recognised that gender identity can be very fluid; frequently the gender that someone feels aligned to may not necessarily reflect their inherited sex chromosomes.

Examining an individual's chromosomes is most frequently carried out before they are born. During pregnancy foetal cells may be collected by procedures such as amniocentesis or chorionic villus sampling. During amniocentesis the amniotic fluid that surrounds the developing foetus is collected; this will contain cells that have become detached from the foetus as it moves. Since the foetus is continually growing, a large number of the cells harvested will be dividing and therefore have chromosomes visible. The process of karyotyping that follows commonly reveals chromosomal abnormalities such as Down's syndrome and Turner's syndrome (Chapter 14).

The cytoplasm and cytoplasmic organelles

The cytoplasm is the region between the plasma membrane and the nuclear membrane. It is predominantly composed of the endoplasmic reticulum (ER) which consists of a system of interconnected flattened membranes. In diagrams of the cell (see Figure 1.1) only small portions of the ER are usually shown, but in reality this complex labyrinth-like system occupies a large proportion of the cell. The ER is split into two distinct types: the rough ER has a multitude of tiny specialised organelles termed ribosomes embedded within its membranes, which are responsible for its characteristic rough, uneven appearance. Ribosomes are the organelles where amino acids are linked together to form proteins according to the instructions encoded in DNA (Chapter 14); for this reason the rough ER is referred to as a region of protein synthesis within cells. The second type of ER is termed smooth ER since it lacks ribosomes; smooth ER is primarily involved in lipid (fat) synthesis. Fats have a multitude of functions within the body including: synthesis of cell membranes, storage of energy, insulation and cushioning and protecting fragile organs such as the kidneys.

The cytoplasm is an aqueous environment and is filled with a watery fluid called the cytosol. The cytosol functions as a transport medium within cells containing dissolved sugars for energy, amino acids for protein synthesis and a variety of intracellular chemical signals and growth factors which are involved in coordinating the internal biochemistry and physical activities of the cell.

The Golgi apparatus

The Golgi apparatus is a specialised region of smooth ER resembling a series of crescent-shaped stacked membranes (Figure 1.1). The Golgi is frequently referred to as the cell's 'packaging and export' region since it is involved in preparing material for release from cells. Its key role is refining proteins from the rough ER; this usually involves adding sugar residues to the crude amino acid sequences via a process termed glycosylation. The refined proteins may be used within the cell or may leave the Golgi in membranous sacs called secretory vesicles which travel to the cell membrane before their contents are discharged out of the cell. Cells that have a secretory role such as those within endocrine glands may each have several well-developed regions of Golgi apparatus; a good example would be the insulin-producing beta cells of the pancreas.

The Golgi is also responsible for packaging digestive enzymes required for intracellular digestion into small membrane-bound sacs called lysosomes (see below).

Mitochondria

Mitochondria are small bean-/boat-shaped cellular organelles (Figure 1.1) responsible for releasing energy within cells. Each mitochondrion consists of an outer smooth membrane and a highly folded inner membrane. The prominent folds of the inner membrane are termed cristae and associated with these folds are the enzymes responsible for cellular respiration. Within the mitochondria, glucose, which is derived from carbohydrate-rich foods, is reacted with oxygen acquired by our respiratory system to release energy. This energy is then used to synthesise the energy storage molecule adenosine triphosphate (ATP) from adenosine diphosphate (ADP) and free phosphate. This process results in the production of water and carbon dioxide as waste products. Since these biochemical reactions occur in the presence of oxygen, the process is referred to as aerobic respiration.

Glucose $(C_6H_{12}O_6)$ + Oxygen (O_2) → Carbon dioxide (CO_2) + Water (H_2O) + Energy (38ATP)

In theory each molecule of glucose can yield 38 molecules of ATP but in reality this is never achieved, and a yield of around 30 ATPs per glucose molecule is typical. From a nursing point of view the simple equation above tells us something essential about human physiology: to generate the energy necessary to keep us alive we must eat (glucose) and breathe (oxygen). Indeed, a key role that nurses play is in ensuring that their patients receive adequate nutrition and that oxygenation of the blood is maintained.

If the supply of oxygen is significantly reduced then aerobic respiration becomes impossible and the cell is forced into anaerobic respiration. This is a far less efficient process that results in only 2 ATP molecules being produced per molecule of glucose. The incomplete breakdown of glucose also leads to the accumulation of the metabolic waste product lactic acid (lactate). Many people experience the effects of anaerobic respiration when they participate in hard manual labour or when lifting weights in a gym. When muscles are forced into anaerobic respiration the accumulation of lactic acid is usually experienced as soreness, fatigue and sometimes pain.

The plasma (cell) membrane

All human cells are surrounded by an outer membrane referred to as the plasma membrane. This has a multitude of functions including: holding the cell together as a discrete intact unit, regulating the movement of materials into and out of the cell and communication and recognition between cells.

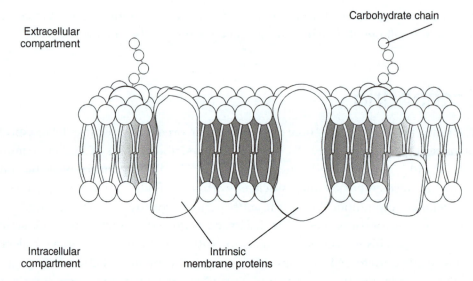

Figure 1.4 Structure of the plasma membrane

The plasma membrane is predominantly composed of a phospholipid bilayer within which are located a variety of proteins (Figure 1.4). Since phospholipid is a fluid, with a similar consistency to vegetable oil, and the denser proteins are positioned throughout its structure, under a microscope it has a mosaic-like appearance, hence the plasma membrane is frequently referred to as having a fluid-mosaic structure. The phospholipid molecules originate from the smooth ER while the integral proteins initially are synthesised by ribosomes, and refined in the Golgi before being transferred to and inserted into the membrane.

The plasma membrane is not a static structure; phospholipid and protein molecules are continually being added and removed depending on the current needs of the cell. The phospholipid bilayer is often referred to as being self-forming. Each phospholipid molecule consists of a hydrophilic (water-loving) head portion and two hydrophobic (water-hating) tails. Since the intracellular compartment of the cell is full of the water-based cytosol and the outside of the cell is surrounded by watery interstitial fluid, the phospholipid molecules naturally form a bilayer as the hydrophobic tails orientate themselves away from the aqueous environments of both the intracellular and extracellular compartments (Figure 1.4).

There are many different types of protein molecules within the phospholipid bilayer, including channel proteins which span the entire width of the membrane and form pores through which materials can enter and leave (see below), and receptor proteins which form three-dimensional pockets into which chemical signals such as hormones can fit.

The glycocalyx

Most of the proteins that are found embedded in the plasma membranes are actually glycoproteins since they have been refined by the addition of sugar (glyco) residues within the Golgi. Some of these sugar residues extend away from the outer surface of the plasma membrane in the form of large polysaccharides and these collectively form a thin shell of sugar around each cell called the glycocalyx (Figure 1.4). The glycocalyx includes a key set of human glycoproteins referred to as the major histocompatibility complex (MHC). These MHC proteins play a key role in cellular recognition. With the exception of genetically identical siblings, every person has their own set of MHC proteins which uniquely identify their cells as belonging within their body. MHC proteins can cause problems when organs are transplanted since the immune system of the recipient will immediately recognise the cells of the donor organ such as a kidney or heart as being foreign and begin to attack the transplant.

For this reason, most organ transplant patients will require immunosuppressive drugs to help reduce the speed of rejection. Unfortunately, because these medications reduce the patient's natural immune responses, they can increase the risk of opportunistic infections. Even with immunosuppressive drugs, gradually the donated organ is usually rejected and some younger transplant patients may have to undergo several transplants during their lifetime. The only major cells that do not have MHC proteins on their surface are erythrocytes (red blood cells); this is fortunate because it allows for routine blood transfusions of cross-matched blood without the risk of transplant reactions and rejection. To help you understand the potential of transplanted organs to be rejected, explore Jack's case study.

Case study: Jack – organ transplant rejection

Jack is a 32-year-old male who received a donor kidney following several years of renal dialysis. Five months after the transplant, he began to experience flu-like symptoms and was unusually tired. His temperature was slightly raised at approximately 38 °C and he noticed that he was passing less urine than normal. Despite making a good recovery in the immediate post-operative period, Jack began to feel some tenderness over the transplant area. His wife made an appointment for Jack to see his GP who suspected that Jack may be rejecting the transplanted kidney. She contacted the transplant team who admitted Jack to hospital where a renal biopsy confirmed the GP's suspicions. A high-dose steroid drug called methylprednisolone was given for three days and fortunately the rejection process was suppressed. After reviewing Jack's medication and reminding him of the importance of taking his medication as prescribed, the team discharged him home.

Jack's case study highlights the importance of patient vigilance following organ transplants; luckily the rejection of Jack's transplanted kidney was suppressed before major damage to the transplanted organ could occur.

Membrane transport

To stay alive and function optimally, each cell has to take up useful molecules (such as oxygen, water, salts, sugars and amino acids), and eliminate waste products such as carbon dioxide, urea and uric acid. Movement of materials across the plasma membrane is called membrane transport.

Simple diffusion

Since the plasma membrane is a fluid structure consisting predominantly of phospholipid, molecules that are fat-soluble are able to dissolve in the phospholipid bilayer and pass rapidly across by a process called simple diffusion.

Simple diffusion can be defined as:

> The passive movement of molecules from a region of high concentration to a region of low concentration until an even distribution of molecules (equilibrium) is achieved.

Gases such as oxygen and carbon dioxide and lipid-based hormones such as steroids including testosterone and oestrogen are highly soluble in the fluid phospholipid bilayer and pass readily into and out of cells via simple diffusion. Simple diffusion also occurs rapidly in the lungs with oxygen inspired at high concentration from the atmosphere before diffusing rapidly across the alveolar air sacs into the blood. Conversely, carbon dioxide is at high concentration in the blood and passes across into the alveoli by simple diffusion before being eliminated during expiration. Concepts such as diffusion are often very abstract in nature, so to help consolidate your understanding of this process, attempt Activity 1.2.

Activity 1.2   Team working

Add a small amount of perfume, aftershave or nail varnish remover (acetone) to a piece of tissue and place it in the centre of the room.

What do you notice?

Now that you have had the opportunity of exploring simple diffusion via the diffusion of odours, we can examine a variant of diffusion.

Facilitated diffusion

Since many of the molecules required by cells are water soluble and not particularly soluble in lipid, they cannot pass across the plasma membrane by simple diffusion. Facilitated diffusion makes use of channel proteins which function as physical passage-ways to carry molecules across the plasma membrane.

Facilitated diffusion can be defined as:

> The passive movement of molecules across the plasma membrane from a region of high concentration to a region of low concentration aided (facilitated) by membrane channel proteins.

Facilitated diffusion is particularly important for getting water-soluble molecules such as sugars, e.g. glucose, into cells. Indeed, as we will see in Chapter 5, when we consume sugar, the hormone insulin is released which increases the number of channel proteins in our plasma cell membranes, facilitating the movement of sugar from the blood into our cells where it can be used to release energy in the mitochondria.

Active transport

Diffusion only allows movement of molecules from a high to low concentration; some-times it is necessary to move molecules against their natural concentration gradients, from a low to a high concentration. Moving material against a concentration gradi-ent requires energy. Fortunately, as we have seen above, cells hold a steady stockpile of energy in the form of the energy storage molecule ATP. Many molecules are con-tinually transported across membranes against their natural concentration gradients, including electrolytes such as sodium (Na^+) and potassium (K^+) and amino acids. Since this process utilises channel proteins, it can be regarded as an ATP-powered form of facilitated diffusion and is termed active transport.

Active transport can be defined as:

> The active movement of molecules against their natural concentration gradients using channel proteins and powered by the energy storage molecule ATP.

Good examples of active transport are the dedicated ion pumps that maintain the cor-rect balance of ions across cell membranes (Figure 1.5). These pumps play a key role in generating electrical signals termed action potentials which are essential to the func-tioning of the nervous system (Chapter 6).

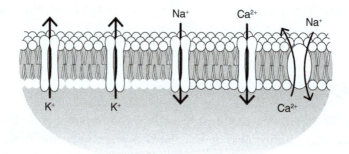

Figure 1.5   Active transport: sodium, potassium and calcium ion pumps

Osmosis

Osmosis is the process by which water passes passively across the plasma membrane.

The classic experiment to help explain osmosis involves taking a vessel such as a beaker and dividing it into two using a semi-permeable material such as cellophane. Into one side of the beaker a solution of sugared water is added, and to the other side pure water is added. If the experiment is left at room temperature for an hour or so then the pure water will gradually move across the selectively permeable cellophane into the side of the beaker containing the sugared water, and the water level on this side of the beaker will begin to rise (Figure 1.6). The cellophane is referred to as being selectively permeable since it has pores that are just large enough to allow the water molecules to pass through but too small to allow the larger sugar molecules through. All human plasma membranes are selectively permeable and behave like the cellophane in this experiment.

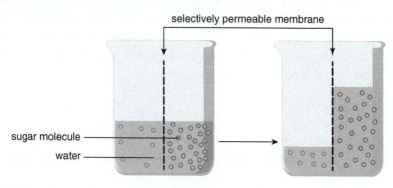

Figure 1.6   The process of osmosis

Source: OpenStax (2013) *Anatomy and Physiology*. Rice University. Available at: https://openstax.org/books/anatomy-and-physiology/pages/preface

Of all the mechanisms of membrane transport, osmosis causes most confusion among students. The reason much of this confusion arises is because there are two common definitions provided for osmosis in textbooks. Although these definitions are worded differently, they are effectively saying the same thing.

Osmosis can be defined as:

> The movement of water from a region of low-solute concentration to a region of high-solute concentration across a selectively (semi-) permeable membrane.

Osmosis is also frequently defined as:

> The movement of water from a region of high water concentration to a region of low water concentration across a selectively (semi-) permeable membrane.

While both definitions are accurate, the second definition is preferable since it highlights that osmosis is actually the diffusion of water through a selectively permeable membrane.

A nice, simple rule to help remember osmosis is that 'water follows solutes', or in plain English, 'water follows sugar, salt or other dissolved material'.

Knowledge of osmosis is essential for nurses to understand how the kidneys function and to understand water balance. Now that you have an understanding of osmosis and diffusion, read through the therapeutic clinical application to develop your understanding of how this knowledge can be applied to a patient with significant kidney disease.

Therapeutic clinical application

Patients with renal failure may undergo peritoneal dialysis in which a catheter is implanted into the abdomen and glucose-rich fluid (known as the dialysate) is infused via the catheter into the peritoneal cavity. The peritoneum acts as a selectively permeable membrane through which excess fluid (and electrolytes and waste products) are drawn out of the blood and into the dialysis fluid. Peritoneal dialysis may be continuous ambulatory peritoneal dialysis (CAPD) in which the dialysate is infused into the abdomen and retained there for approximately eight hours before being allowed to drain. The process is then repeated two or three times a day. Alternatively, automated peritoneal dialysis (APD) may be used in which a machine is used to cycle the fluid into and out of the abdomen. This is usually done overnight.

Isotonic, hypertonic and hypotonic

The term isotonic has become more familiar to the general public with the introduction of isotonic sports drinks. Isotonic solutions are at the same or close to the same concentration as the fluid found in human cells. Nurses routinely use isotonic saline solutions to help keep patients hydrated, particularly when they are confined to bed, unconscious or unable to drink fluids normally. To help you understand the nature and composition of isotonic saline when you are on your next hospital placement, attempt Activity 1.3.

Activity 1.3   Evidence-based practice and research

On your next placement take a few minutes to examine the saline drip bags at the side of your patients' beds; pay close attention to the chemical composition specified.

What do you notice?

Now that you have an understanding of the composition of isotonic saline, we can explore why these are routinely used in clinical practice.

Human cells are stable in isotonic solutions because the concentrations of dissolved materials (solutes) are equal on both sides of the plasma membrane and so no net movement of water is occurring.

In health, the blood is a near-perfect isotonic medium kept at the same concentration as the cytosol of our cells by a multitude of homeostatic mechanisms. However, in certain diseases human cells can be taken out of their isotonic comfort zone, which can cause damage and in some circumstances become life-threatening.

Dehydration

In patients with diabetes the presence of large amounts of sugar (hyperglycaemia) results in the blood becoming too concentrated. Highly concentrated blood is referred to as being hypertonic (too concentrated) to human cells. In hypertonic solutions water will leave the cells of the body by osmosis and move into the blood, and this can lead to progressive dehydration which is a common presenting symptom in patients with undiagnosed or poorly controlled diabetes.

Dehydration caused by not drinking enough fluids or by severe vomiting or diarrhoea will similarly lead to hypertonic blood and loss of water from cells. As cells lose water, their cell membranes become loose and flaccid and may take on a crinkled appearance;

this phenomenon is referred to as crenation. Progressive loss of water from the intra-cellular compartments can lead to tissues of the body such as the skin becoming noticeably looser, and this can be detected in patients using skin-pinch tests. As well as being a sign of shock, prolonged capillary refill time may also indicate dehydration.

Dehydration is also characterised by the mucous membranes of the body drying out which is why many people wake up with a dry mouth after drinking too much alcohol, which is known to cause dehydration by promoting diuresis (increased urination). A common cause of dehydration in hospital patients is infection with norovirus. To help develop your knowledge of this problem, attempt Activity 1.4.

Activity 1.4   Evidence-based practice and research

An outbreak of norovirus is confirmed on your placement. List the most effective infection prevention and control measures that should be applied to minimise the spread of infection.

Dehydration, such as that experienced in patients following norovirus infection, is very common. More rarely, nurses will encounter patients who have too much water in their body.

Water intoxication (water toxaemia)

Water intoxication can be thought of as the opposite of dehydration and is caused by consuming too much water. It is frequently seen in endurance athletes such as cyclists and marathon runners who may routinely consume large quantities of water at drink-ing stations along the routes of their races. Occasionally it occurs following the use of recreational drugs such as ecstasy (MDMA), which can induce thirst and also upset the normal water balance of the body by reducing urine output. Young babies who are fed on formula milk may also be at risk, particularly in poorer households where the milk powder may be over-diluted to make it last longer.

Consuming large quantities of water dilutes the blood, in effect making it hypotonic and at a lower concentration to the cytosol within cells. The dilution of blood in these patients will also lead to hyponatraemia (low blood sodium). Water will gradually move from the blood into the cells by osmosis, causing the cells to swell. Since all the tis-sues of the body are composed of cells, during water intoxication all the soft tissues will begin to swell and internal organs will enlarge. Early signs of water intoxication will include headache, nausea and vomiting. In more serious cases, the patient may experi-ence confusion, visual disturbances, drowsiness, breathing difficulties, muscle weakness and cramping.

Since the brain is enclosed within the cranium of the skull, there is minimal space available to accommodate cerebral enlargement, and the intracranial pressure will increase restricting blood flow and reduce cerebral perfusion. As a result, the patient will gradually lose consciousness, commonly slipping into a coma and, unless quickly treated, they will suffer permanent brain damage and may die.

Treatment will be determined by the cause and severity of water intoxication. Firstly, the amount of fluid taken on board must be reduced and excess water expelled. This can be achieved by the administration of diuretics to increase urine output. If the condition has been caused by medication, the patient's medication must be reviewed and the drug causing the problem should be discontinued.

The importance of following the manufacturer's instructions when mixing infant formula must be reinforced and where financial hardship is a contributing factor, parents should be advised on appropriate support networks and benefits that might be available. Sodium levels should be corrected by careful administration of intravenous fluids with a relatively high concentration of sodium. Diuretics will also help increase sodium levels as excess fluid is excreted; however, these have to be used with care as some can cause significant loss of potassium, leading to hypokalaemia (low blood potassium).

Other forms of membrane transport

In addition to allowing the passage of single molecules into and out of the cell, the plasma membrane can allow larger groups of molecules and even solid materials/fluids to enter the cell via endocytosis or leave the cell via exocytosis (Figure 1.7).

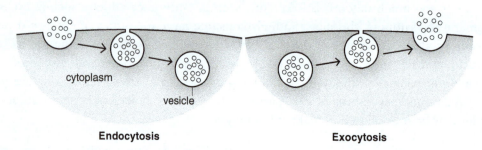

Endocytosis   **Exocytosis**

Figure 1.7   Endocytosis and exocytosis

Phagocytosis

This is the form of endocytosis by which cells can take up solid particulate materials. The term phagocytosis literally means 'cell eating' and is particularly important in the cells of the immune system which are actively engaged in removing pathogenic material such as bacteria, fungal cells and viral particles. The process of phagocytosis utilises the fluid nature of the plasma membrane. When a pathogen such as a bacterium is encountered the plasma membrane flows around it, engulfing it and enclosing it in a membrane-bound vesicle. Once internalised within the cytoplasm, the lysosomes produced by the Golgi fuse with the vesicle and discharge their enzymes into its interior, killing the pathogen and initiating intracellular digestion.

Exocytosis

Following the intracellular digestion of solid particulates such as bacteria, waste materials such as components of bacterial cell walls are released from cells by exocytosis (Figure 1.7). This process of exocytosis is also the mechanism by which cells of endocrine glands release their hormones into the blood and neurons release their neurotransmitters into synapses (Chapters 5 and 6).

Pinocytosis

This form of endocytosis allows cells to take up small droplets of fluid from the extracellular environment. The term pinocytosis literally means 'cell drinking', with most cells capable of taking up droplets of the interstitial fluid which surrounds them.

Histology

Histology is the study of biological tissues. A tissue can be defined as a collection of one or more cell types that work together for a common purpose. In the human body tissues can be thought of as the building blocks of organs. As highlighted in Josie's case study at the beginning of this chapter, tissue samples can be collected via biopsy to screen for disease.

Although the human body is incredibly complex, only four major categories of tissue are present: epithelial tissues, connective tissues (e.g. bone, cartilage, blood, adipose tissue and fat), muscle (skeletal muscle, cardiac muscle and smooth muscle) and nervous tissue (neurons and neuroglial cells).

As we move through this list from epithelial tissue through to nervous tissue, there is a gradual increase in complexity, with epithelial tissues regarded as the simplest human tissues and nervous tissue the most highly organised and complex. In this chapter we will only examine the nature of the epithelial tissues since the other tissue types are explored throughout the book.

The nature of epithelial tissue

Epithelial tissues are found throughout the body and have many diverse roles that are typically associated with absorption, protection and secretion. Epithelial tissues are recognisable since they rest on a thin delicate basement membrane (Figure 1.8).

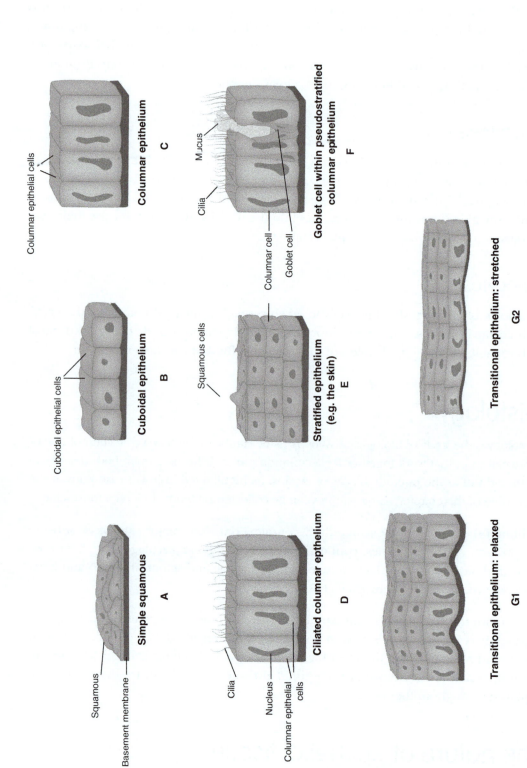

Figure 1.8 Some of the major epithelial tissues

Epithelial tissues can be broadly split into the simple epithelia, which consist of a single layer of cells, and the stratified epithelia, which consist of multiple layers of cells stacked one on top of the other like bricks in a wall.

The simple epithelia

Simple squamous epithelium

The term squamous means resembling the scale of a fish, therefore squamous cells are described as being thin and flat in appearance (Figure 1.8A). This tissue is found in multiple locations within the body including the alveolar walls of the lung, endothelial lining of blood vessels and capillary walls, and lining the major serous membranes and serous layers of organs.

Since the cells of squamous epithelium are so thin and flat, they are perfectly adapted to locations where simple diffusion takes place such as the alveoli of the lungs. Their thinness also imparts elasticity to the alveolar wall, allowing inflation of the lungs when air is inspired.

From a surface (apical) view, squamous epithelial cells have an appearance that resembles 'crazy paving', and for this reason this tissue is also commonly referred to as pavement epithelium. Many of the body's internal membranes, such as the peritoneal membrane which lines the abdominopelvic cavity, the pericardial membranes that surround the heart and the pleural membranes that surround the lungs, have a layer of squamous epithelial cells associated with them. These membranes are referred to as serous membranes since their resident squamous cells secrete a thin watery fluid called serous fluid.

This fluid is very slippery and acts as a natural internal lubricant within the body, reducing friction between the visceral organs during bodily movement. Many of the body's internal organs such as the outer layers of the gut (serosa) and the uterus (perimetrium) also have a thin serous layer composed of squamous cells, which contribute further to the secretion of this internal lubricant. When major body cavities are opened during surgery this serous fluid is clearly visible as a glistening shiny surface coating the internal organs.

Simple cuboidal epithelium

This consists of a single layer of cube-shaped cells (Figure 1.8B) and is found forming the walls of the kidney tubules where it plays a key role in regulating the composition of the urine. Within the brain are specialised cuboidal epithelial cells called ependymal cells which produce cerebrospinal fluid which surrounds the brain and spinal cord.

Simple columnar epithelium

This consists of a single layer of tall, thin, column-shaped cells (Figure 1.8C) found forming the mucosal lining of many areas of the gastrointestinal tract. These relatively thick cells allow gradual absorption of nutrients across the gut into the blood. A specialised ciliated columnar epithelium (Figure 1.8D) is located in the lining of the fallopian tubes; here the cilia beat in coordinated waves, playing a key role in transporting ova from the ovaries to the uterus.

Stratified epithelium

Stratified squamous epithelium

This consists of several layers of thin, flat cells (Figure 1.8E). The epidermis which forms the outer layer of the skin is composed of a stratified squamous epithelium. The initial layer of cells that resides on the basement membrane is continually dividing by mitosis and is the origin of the cells above. As cells move up through the layers, they accumulate the tough, dense protein called keratin. This makes the epidermal layer very strong but also renders the cells near the surface impermeable to oxygen so that they gradually die.

This means that the outer layer of the epidermis is composed of entirely dead skin cells which gradually slough off and flake away from the surface. There are examples of stratified cuboidal epithelium found surrounding developing ovarian follicles and stratified columnar epithelium found lining the male urethra, and these are discussed further in subsequent chapters.

Pseudostratified epithelium

Lining the nasal cavity, trachea and upper portions of the bronchial tree is a specialised ciliated epithelium. This is composed of a combination of tall column-shaped cells and smaller cells squashed between. This gives the false appearance of a tissue that is stratified (multilayered). The term pseudostratified (which literally means falsely layered) is often used to describe this tissue. In reality, all the cells within this tissue are in contact with the basement membrane and so pseudostratified epithelium is actually a specialised simple epithelium (Figure 1.8F).

Transitional epithelium

The bladder is lined by an elastic stratified epithelium with cells that change shape according to the volume of urine currently stored. When the bladder is full, the pressure exerted by the urine compresses this tissue and the cells take on a thin, flat, squamous appearance (Figure 1.8G2). As the bladder empties, the cells become progressively less compressed, gradually adopting a cuboidal and then a columnar appearance (Figure 1.8G1).

Prokaryotic cells

Cells which contain their DNA within a nuclear membrane are referred to as eukaryotic cells. The cells which make up the bodies of animals (including humans), plants and fungi are all eukaryotic. Human erythrocytes (red blood cells) lose their nucleus as they mature; this loss of the nucleus allows more haemoglobin molecules to be packed into the cell, improving the efficiency of oxygen transport. However, since erythrocytes are derived from nucleated cells, they are still eukaryotic in origin.

Unlike eukaryotic cells, bacterial cells do not have their DNA enclosed within a nuclear envelope and are referred to as prokaryotic cells.

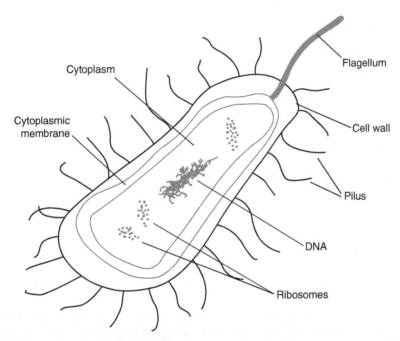

Figure 1.9   Structure of prokaryotic cells

Prokaryotic cells typically have other differences from eukaryotic cells; most are surrounded by a thick, robust cell wall which allows them to survive in fluctuating environmental extremes of temperature, pH and dryness (Figure 1.9). A key feature of bacteria is that they are able to replicate incredibly fast. This allows huge populations to be generated in relatively short periods of time; in the human body this can have disastrous consequences, particularly if bacteria gain access to the blood.

Sepsis is often defined as an overwhelming life-threatening infection. It is more common than myocardial infarction (heart attack) and kills more people in the UK than breast, bowel and prostate cancer combined. Sepsis is more common in the very old and very young whose immune systems are in decline or not fully developed, while patients on immunosuppressive medications such as certain steroids are also at increased risk (Knight and Hore, 2018).

Symptoms of sepsis vary according to the age of the patient. According to the UK Sepsis Trust, the signs of sepsis in an adult include:

1. 'Slurred' speech or confusion
2. Extreme shivering or muscle pain
3. Passing no urine (in a day)
4. Severe breathlessness
5. It feels like you're going to die
6. Skin mottled or discoloured.

In children, sepsis should be suspected if the child:

1. Is breathing very fast
2. Has a 'fit' or convulsion
3. Looks mottled, bluish, or pale
4. Has a rash that does not fade when you press it
5. Is very lethargic or difficult to wake
6. Feels abnormally cold to touch.

A child under five may have sepsis if he or she:

1. Is not feeding
2. Is vomiting repeatedly
3. Has not passed urine for 12 hours.

(UK Sepsis Trust, 2019)

Since sepsis is life-threatening and so common, it is essential that nurses learn to recognise some of the key features of this medical emergency early in their training. To help develop your knowledge, read through Mary's case study.

Case study: Mary – sepsis evidence-based practice

Mary is 72 and has become extremely unwell over the last 24 hours. She has become increasingly breathless and is expectorating green sputum. She was seen by her GP who sent her into her local hospital as an emergency admission. On admission, Mary was fully conscious and alert but slightly confused. Her temperature was 38 °C, her heart rate was 125, her blood pressure 110/58, respiratory rate 26 breaths per minute and oxygen saturation 92 per cent on room air. Mary's vital signs were recorded using the NEWS 2 (National Early Warning Scoring) system (Royal College of Physicians, 2017) and her total score was calculated as 11. Any score of 7 or above should trigger an emergency response by a clinical team with experience in caring for critically ill patients.

Mary was seen by the critical care outreach team and transferred to the High-Dependency Unit where the Sepsis Six Pathway (Sepsis Trust, 2019) was initiated: oxygen was administered, blood cultures were taken, intravenous antibiotics were commenced and a urinary catheter was inserted to measure Mary's urine output accurately. Serial lactates were checked. A raised serum lactate (> 4 mmol/L) is associated with a significantly increased mortality rate. Lactate levels rise during sepsis from both aerobic and anaerobic sources as well as reduced lactate clearance. Mary gradually recovered and was able to return home two weeks after her admission.

Mary's case study highlights that although sepsis is immediately life-threatening, if it is recognised early and treatment initiated quickly, even elderly patients can recover.

Not all bacteria are pathogenic or harmful; indeed, some are essential to human survival and health. Bacteria are found in huge numbers within and on the surface of the human body where, together with other microorganisms, they form the microbial biome. It has been estimated that there are around 23 times more bacterial cells associated with the human body than human cells, and although it has been known for a long time that certain bacteria such as those found in the colon play key roles such as synthesising vitamin K (a key clotting factor), the complex roles of the microbial biome are still poorly understood.

Cells as targets for drugs

Virtually all drugs used by nurses exert their effects at a cellular level. A good example would be synthetic insulin that is used to control the blood sugar levels of patients with diabetes mellitus. Synthetic insulin mimics the naturally produced insulin of the pancreas, stimulating human cells to take up glucose from the blood. Human cells are able to recognise each other using the glycoproteins embedded in their cell membranes; these protein markers can also allow drugs to target specific cell types within the body. To conclude this chapter, we will return to Josie who was recently diagnosed with breast cancer.

Case study: Josie revisited – breast cancer evidence-based practice

Josie was fortunate to detect the lump in her breast while the tumour mass was small and quickly underwent surgery (lumpectomy) to remove the cancerous tissue. Following histological examination it was determined that the malignant cells forming Josie's tumour expressed the human epidermal growth factor receptor 2 (HER2).

(Continued)

(Continued)

Drugs that block this receptor such as Herceptin have recently become available, which provide a new tool for treating breast cancer.

Herceptin can slow the growth of breast tumour cells and when used in early breast cancer can reduce the risk of recurrence. Josie was relieved to be told by her consultant that since her tumour mass was small, chemotherapy would not be required and since beginning her Herceptin treatment six months ago tests have revealed that Josie is currently free of the disease.

Targeted drugs such as Herceptin are revolutionising the treatment of many forms of cancer, with new targeted therapies continually being developed and made available.

Now that you have completed the chapter, attempt the multiple-choice questions in Activity 1.5 to assess your knowledge.

Activity 1.5   Multiple-choice questions

1. DNA is found wrapped around

   a) Histamine
   b) Histone protein
   c) Myosin protein
   d) Keratin protein

2. The region of a cell primarily involved in protein synthesis is

   a) The smooth endoplasmic reticulum
   b) The lysosomes
   c) The plasma membrane
   d) The rough endoplasmic reticulum

3. The diploid number of human chromosomes is

   a) 46
   b) 23
   c) 48
   d) 52

4. Release of energy within the mitochondria in the presence of adequate oxygen is referred to as

   a) Anaerobic respiration

   b) Aerobic respiration

   c) Glycosylation

   d) Gluconeogenesis

5. Which of the following is *not* a function of the Golgi apparatus?

   a) Production of lysosomes

   b) Preparing material for export out of the cells

   c) Refining of crude proteins from the rough endoplasmic reticulum

   d) Production of mitochondria

6. Which of the following commonly results in dehydration?

   a) Vomiting

   b) Poorly controlled diabetes

   c) Not drinking enough fluid

   d) All of the above

7. Cells will show crenation when placed in a

   a) Hypertonic solution

   b) Isotonic solution

   c) Hypotonic solution

   d) All of the above

8. Water intoxication can cause death because

   a) Soft organs will rapidly become dehydrated

   b) Swelling of the brain raises the intracranial pressure, reducing blood flow

   c) Excess water increases movement of water into the blood

   d) Blood pressure will rise rapidly

9. The elastic tissue found lining the bladder is

   a) Simple columnar epithelium

   b) Simple cuboidal epithelium

(Continued)

(Continued)

   c) Pseudostratified epithelium

   d) Transitional epithelium

10. Which of the following tissues forms the walls of each alveolar air sac?

   a) Stratified columnar epithelium

   b) Stratified cuboidal epithelium

   c) Simple squamous epithelium

   d) Simple cuboidal epithelium

Chapter summary

Human cells have three major regions called the nucleus, the cytoplasm and the plasma membrane. The nucleus is the control centre of the cell and is the location of DNA. When cells divide the DNA condenses to form chromosomes, which can be visualised and counted. Human cells (with the exception of sperm and ova) have the diploid number of chromosomes (46). Deviations from this diploid number can result in chromosomal disorders such as Down's syndrome.

The cytoplasm of the cell consists of the rough endoplasmic reticulum which is an area of protein synthesis and the smooth endoplasmic reticulum which is responsible for the synthesis of lipids (fats). The cytoplasm is also the location of organelles including: mitochondria which release energy from molecules such as glucose and the Golgi apparatus which prepares and packages material for export.

The plasma membrane which surrounds the cell is composed predominantly of a phospholipid bilayer in which there are a variety of proteins which function as channels and receptors. The plasma membrane holds the cell together, controls what enters and leaves the cell and plays key roles in signalling and recognition between cells.

Cells are grouped together in organised collections termed tissues; these include epithelial, connective, muscle and nervous tissue which are used to construct the internal and external organs. The human body also hosts a diverse community of microorganisms which are collectively referred to as the microbial biome.

Activities: Brief outline answers

Activity 1.1: Reflection (page 8)

As you wind the elastic up tighter and tighter it will begin to fold and loop over itself and progressively become thicker. This process is termed 'supercoiling' and a similar thing happens to DNA as cells begin to divide.

Activity 1.2: Team working (page 14)

Eventually the whole room will start to smell of the aroma as the material evaporates into the room and begins to diffuse in the air from a region of high concentration (the tissue) to a region of low concentration (the room), until an even distribution occurs.

You may have noticed a similar phenomenon when somebody boards a bus with strong-smelling deodorant and eventually everyone on the bus becomes aware of the smell as the deodorant diffuses through the air.

Activity 1.3: Evidence-based practice and research (page 18)

Most saline drips will state 0.9 per cent NaCl which is isotonic to human cells.

Activity 1.4: Evidence-based practice and research (page 19)

Effective infection prevention and control measures include:

- Hand washing with soap and water following the World Health Organization's 5 Moments.
- Wear gloves and aprons for contact with vomit, faeces or contaminated equipment or environment.
- Source isolation preferably in a single room with en-suite facilities or cohort nursing with designated toilets or commodes.
- Specimens of faeces should be sent for microbiological examination.
- Polymerase chain reaction (PCR) tests which detect the presence of norovirus nucleic acid are the preferred tests.
- Prompt decontamination of spillages and increased frequency of environmental cleaning first with detergent and water followed by a 1000 ppm solution of a chlorine-releasing disinfectant.
- Reduce unnecessary movement of patients.
- Discharge home is allowed but transfer to nursing homes should be delayed until the patient has been asymptomatic for 48 hours. Transfer to other wards must only be allowed according to urgent clinical need and following a risk assessment.
- Contaminated linen should be placed in an alginate bag before being placed in a red linen bag and sent to the laundry.
- Waste must be correctly sorted and the appropriate coloured bag used.
- Non-essential visitors must be excluded, e.g. hair dressers, newspaper trolleys.
- All patients' visitors must be informed of the outbreak and advised to wash their hands thoroughly on leaving the ward. In some cases visiting may be discouraged but in the case of terminally ill patients, children, vulnerable adults and those for whom visiting is an essential part of recovery, visiting should be allowed.
- Any staff who become unwell should stay off sick until they have been asymptomatic for 48 hours.
- All patient areas must be thoroughly cleaned at the end of the outbreak. This should include laundering of curtains, and steam cleaning of soft furnishings should be considered.

Activity 1.5: Multiple-choice questions (pages 28–30)

1) a, 2) d, 3) a, 4) b, 5) d, 6) d, 7) a, 8) b, 9) d, 10) c

Further reading

Boore J et al. (2016) Chapter 2: The human cell, in *Essentials of Anatomy and Physiology for Nursing Practice*. London: SAGE Publications Ltd.

A textbook to develop your knowledge of human anatomy and physiology that is aimed specifically at nurses.

Knight J and Andrade M (2018) Genes and chromosomes 1: Basic principles of genetics. *Nursing Times*, 114(7), 42–5.

A gentle overview of how DNA is organised and the nature of chromosomes.

Tortora G and Derrickson B (2017) Chapter 3: The cellular level of organization, in *Tortora's Principles of Anatomy and Physiology* (15th edition). New York: John Wiley & Sons.

In-depth coverage of human anatomy and physiology.

Useful websites

www.medicalnewstoday.com/articles/320878.php

A simple overview of cell structure and function.

www.kenhub.com/en/library/anatomy/introduction-to-histology

An overview of histology including real tissue sections as viewed under a microscope.

Chapter 2 Homeostasis

Chapter aims

After reading this chapter, you will be able to:

- define homeostasis and describe the key elements of negative feedback;
- explain what is meant by the terms 'set point' and 'normal range';
- explain why nurses need to know the normal physiological ranges of major variables such as body temperature, electrolytes and blood glucose;
- describe how positive feedback differs from negative feedback.

Introduction

Case study: Ian – type II diabetes

Recently Ian has been waking up several times during the night to pass urine; as a result, he has a permanently dry mouth and a raging thirst which he has been able to relieve by drinking from the large bottle of water which he now keeps on his bedside cabinet. These disturbances to his sleep have left Ian permanently exhausted and of late it has been a real struggle to even get out of bed in the morning. While at work Ian has been tired and crotchety and has found it increasingly difficult to concentrate on even the simplest tasks.

During an appointment with his GP a random blood glucose reading of 24.5 mmol/l was recorded and a urine sample revealed the presence of large amounts of glucose. Ian was asked to return the following morning after skipping breakfast to have his fasting blood glucose level recorded, which at 11.2 mmol/l confirmed his GP's suspicion of diabetes mellitus and Ian was promptly referred to his local diabetes clinic. Further tests confirmed that Ian has type II diabetes mellitus which he is currently managing via a combination of diet, exercise and drugs.

Introduction

To ensure optimal health, the cells of the human body need to be maintained within a stable environment with minimal fluctuations in temperature, pH and chemical composition, otherwise pathological states may arise. This chapter will explore the mechanisms by which key internal variables of the body are maintained and balanced. We shall begin by defining homeostasis and exploring the nature of the negative feedback mechanisms that allow variables to be held within their normal ranges. We shall then examine the role of the endocrine and nervous system in maintaining homeostasis and highlight problems that may occur when these mechanisms do not function optimally. Finally, we shall introduce the concept of positive feedback and highlight how positive feedback mechanisms differ from those of negative feedback. Throughout the chapter we shall link the often abstract concepts of homeostasis to common clinical scenarios encountered by nurses.

Homeostasis

Homeostasis can be defined as the ability to maintain a relatively constant internal environment. There are multiple physical and chemical variables within the body that are subject to fluctuation; these include: temperature, pH, blood pressure and all of the dissolved components of plasma such as glucose, sodium, potassium, calcium and bicarbonate.

Negative feedback mechanisms

For each physiological variable there is an optimal value termed the 'set point'.

For example, the set point for blood glucose is around 5 mmol/l. At this optimal concentration cells throughout the body will have a steady supply of glucose, allowing them to undertake efficient cellular metabolism. The body attempts to maintain each variable as close to its set point as possible by a process called negative feedback. During negative feedback deviations from the set point are minimised and resisted to constrain the variable within its 'normal range'.

Requirements for negative feedback

All homeostatic processes that rely on negative feedback must have the following elements.

- A stimulus: this is the trigger that causes the variable to deviate from its set point, e.g. moving to a cold environment will lower the core temperature.
- A sensor: to detect deviations from the set point, e.g. the core and skin thermoreceptors that measure temperature changes.

- A control centre: to decide how to bring the variable back towards its set point, i.e. the thermoregulatory centre of the hypothalamus.
- Effector organs and tissues: to effect the physiological changes necessary to bring the variable back towards its set point, e.g. the sweat glands and blood vessels in the dermis of the skin that help control heat loss and retention.

Homeostatic control of blood glucose

The normal range for blood glucose is roughly between 4 and 6 mmol/l (Figure 2.1). When blood glucose rises, for example after eating a slice of sweet cake, this is detected by the pancreas and the hormone insulin is released. Insulin stimulates cells throughout the body to take up glucose from the blood; gradually blood glucose levels return back towards the set point. Conversely, if carbohydrates are not consumed for a few hours, e.g. you have just gone to bed and fallen asleep, blood sugar will fall and the hormone glucagon is released from the pancreas, stimulating the liver to release glucose increasing concentrations back towards the set point.

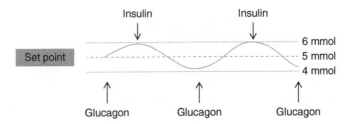

Figure 2.1   Homeostatic control of blood glucose via negative feedback

The regulation of blood glucose described above is a classic example of negative feedback; here two antagonistic hormones are constraining a variable within its normal range by minimising any deviations from the physiological set point.

If a variable remains consistently outside of its normal physiological range then pathological (disease) states usually occur. In the case study at the start of the chapter, Ian's blood glucose was recorded at 24.5 mmol/l, which is greatly outside its normal range of 4–6 mmol/l. As a patient with type II diabetes, over time Ian had become progressively resistant to the effects of his own insulin. Without an effective insulin response to reduce his blood glucose, Ian arrived at his GP surgery with pronounced hyperglycaemia (see next section).

In some patients with type II diabetes insulin injections are also prescribed to help lower their blood glucose. Occasionally, particularly when the patient has not eaten enough carbohydrate, insulin injections can lead to blood glucose dropping below its normal range; this is referred to as hypoglycaemia. Hypoglycaemia is extremely dangerous and can potentially lead to coma and death unless treated quickly. Fortunately, most patients who use insulin learn to become aware of the early warning signs of hypoglycaemia (e.g. feeling shaky and disorientated) and carry something sweet such as a bar of chocolate or some biscuits to quickly boost their blood glucose.

Hyper and hypo prefixes

In clinical practice, the terms hyper (meaning high) and hypo (meaning low) are commonly used as prefixes when a named variable is outside of its normal range. In Ian's case the term hyperglycaemia literally means: hyper (high) glyc (sugar/glucose) aemia (in blood), so hyperglycaemia is the medical term for high blood sugar. Similarly, if a patient injects too much insulin, this results in hypoglycaemia, which means hypo (low) glyc (sugar/glucose) aemia (in blood) or low blood sugar.

Now that you have been introduced to the prefixes hyper and hypo, attempt Activity 2.1 to reinforce your understanding.

Activity 2.1 Evidence-based practice and research

Write down the medical terms for the following pathological states. Hint: you will need to know the chemical symbols for each of the electrolytes below.

High blood calcium and low blood calcium

High blood sodium and low blood sodium

High blood potassium and low blood potassium

There are some possible answers to all activities at the end of the chapter, unless otherwise indicated.

Activity 2.1 reveals the importance of learning medical terminology since all of the pathological states highlighted in the activity will be routinely encountered in clinical practice. We will now develop your understanding of negative feedback by examining how a stable body temperature is maintained.

Regulation of body temperature: thermoregulation

Most of the cellular enzymes that drive the biochemical reactions necessary for life have an optimal temperature which is usually close to that of the core temperature of the body. In health, core temperature is maintained close to 37°C and this can be regarded as the physiological set point.

The normal range for core temperature is extremely narrow at between 36.1°C and 37.2°C (Figure 2.2). To ensure core temperature is maintained close to 37°C, the human body has some very elaborate and highly coordinated physiological responses.

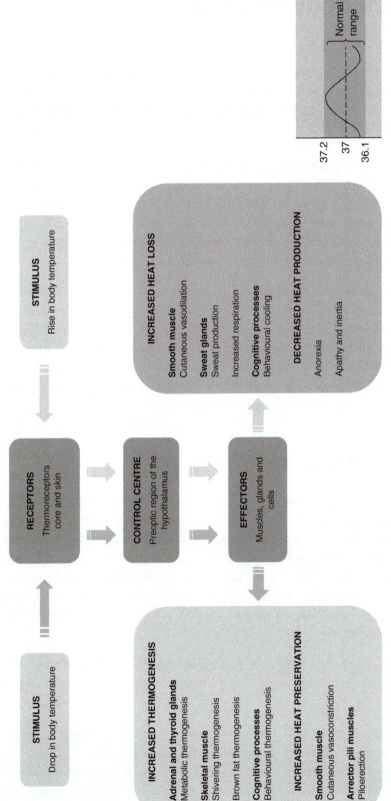

Figure 2.2 Homeostatic control of body temperature

Increased body temperature (hyperthermia)

As core temperature begins to rise (e.g. following a bout of intense exercise) temperature sensors (thermoreceptors) detect this rise and feed information to the hypothalamus. This region of the brain functions as the thermoregulatory control centre initiating the physiological changes that will lower core temperature towards the set point of 37°C. When the core temperature is high, the hypothalamus increases blood flow to the skin by initiating the vasodilation of blood vessels in the dermis. Since the skin has a large surface area of over 1.5–2 square metres, this allows rapid heat loss through conduction, convection and radiation. If the core temperature remains high then eccrine sweat glands in the skin can be activated. These produce a thin watery sweat that will evaporate at the skin's surface to allow rapid cooling; however, if water intake is not maintained then prolonged sweating can lead to dehydration (Chapter 1).

If the core temperature cannot be reduced, this can lead to hyperthermia (remember, hyper means high), and this is commonly seen in heatstroke, for example in endurance athletes. Heatstroke is a life-threatening medical emergency since having a persistently high core temperature reduces the activity of the enzymes essential for cellular metabolism and energy release. It is treated initially by cooling the body by whatever means are available; initially this will involve removing layers of clothing and immersing the body in cool water or using ice packs.

Low body temperature (hypothermia)

Unlike many animals, humans do not have a layer of fur to minimise heat losses. The thin layer of hair that we possess can only trap a small amount of warm air close to the skin, which leaves the human body very vulnerable to heat loss. Without adequate shelter and heat, in cold environments the core temperature can rapidly drop, slowing the rate at which cellular enzymes can function. As the core temperature drops, thermoreceptors relay information to the hypothalamic thermoregulatory control centre, which responds by switching off the production of sweat and reducing blood flow to the skin by initiating vasoconstriction in the dermis.

This minimises heat loss at the skin surface and typically results in the skin taking on a pallid and sometimes bluish appearance (think of how your fingers look when making a snowball).

If this is not sufficient to raise the core temperature towards the set point quickly enough, shivering is initiated where the major skeletal muscle groups contract in spasmodic movements to generate extra heat. If an individual remains in a cold environment for extended periods of time, hormonal adaptations occur such as enhanced release of adrenaline and the thyroid hormones (T3 and T4). This increases the metabolic rate in the longer term (Figure 2.2), generating further internal heat via metabolic thermogenesis. These hormonal adaptations allow the body to adapt to living in a colder environment.

Beneath the dermis of skin is a layer of subcutaneous fat called the hypodermis. This acts as a layer of insulation helping prevent heat loss by holding the heat generated through metabolism within the core of the body. Individuals that are overweight or obese often find it difficult to lose heat because their subcutaneous layers are thicker and this can put them at greater risk of heatstroke, particularly when exercising on hot days. Conversely, older individuals often lose a significant amount of subcutaneous fat as they age and consequently find it harder to retain heat and maintain their core temperature.

Older people also tend to have a lower metabolic rate and a reduced shivering response which places them at increased risk of hypothermia. Hypothermia (remember, hypo means low) is defined as a core temperature of 35°C or lower. At these temperatures cellular enzymatic activity will have slowed significantly and the patient will initially show increased shivering and progressive mental confusion. As hypothermia progresses, the shivering response may be lost, allowing the core temperature to drop further. In severe hypothermia behaviour may become increasingly erratic and illogical. As the core temperature drops below 35°C, the heart rate begins to progressively slow, leading to bradycardia which is defined as a resting heart rate of 60 bpm or less. This leads to reduced tissue and organ perfusion.

Unless treated, severe hypothermia may progressively lead to cardio-respiratory failure and death. However, clinicians have to be extremely careful when pronouncing someone dead as a result of hypothermia since the heart rate and brain activity can be reduced significantly, leading to a torpid state that closely resembles death. Hypothermia is usually treated by moving the patient to a warm environment, ensuring that they are adequately clothed, ideally in multiple layers of dry clothing, and if necessary re-warming the body using heated blankets, water bottles or devices that blow warm air over the body.

Elderly patients are particularly vulnerable to hypothermia in the winter months and this is explored in Grace's case study.

Case study: Grace – hypothermia

Grace is 82 and lives on her own in a small two-bedroom terraced house. Her only regular income is her state pension, which she proudly manages very effectively using little boxes to put aside money each week for food, utility bills and a small amount of pocket money for her four grandchildren.

(Continued)

(Continued)

This winter has been cold with several heavy snowfalls and Grace has been worrying about her heating costs. Instead of using her central heating, since the beginning of January she has been spending most days in her living room using a small fan heater for warmth and taking a hot water bottle to bed. Amy is Grace's youngest daughter and travels from Brighton to visit her mother once a week. During her last visit Amy was horrified to find all of the heating turned off and her mother wandering the house in a very confused state.

From what you have learnt in this chapter it should be clear that Grace is suffering from hypothermia. Nurses are often required to pass on advice to patients and their families, and this is highlighted in Activity 2.2.

Activity 2.2   Evidence-based practice and research

What advice would you give to Grace and her family to reduce the chances of Grace suffering hypothermia again?

Grace's case study illustrates well the negative impact of a variable such as body temperature straying too far from its ideal physiological set point. However, set points are not always fixed and can be shifted when necessary.

Pyrexia: the fever response

Since the core temperature of the body is maintained at around 37°C, many human pathogens have adapted to replicate fastest at this temperature. During infection their numbers can grow exponentially, placing the body at risk of systemic infection and potentially sepsis and septic shock. Fortunately, the human body can respond by increasing body temperature to help slow down pathogenic replication. When leukocytes (white blood cells) begin to fight infection by trapping and killing pathogens, they release a small protein called interleukin-1 (IL-1). IL-1 can initiate a fever response by binding to receptors on the hypothalamus (Dinarello, 2015).

In response to IL-1 the hypothalamus releases a chemical called prostaglandin E_2 (PGE_2) which functions to shift the set point of the hypothalamus up from 37°C to 38–9°C. This increases the temperature of the body and takes it outside the favourable range for bacterial and viral replication, and as a result the rate of infection will slow. A fever response also allows more rapid trapping and killing of pathogens by leukocytes, some of which function more efficiently at these higher temperatures. Unfortunately, the other cells within the body are now outside of their optimal temperature range and their enzymatic activity slows; as a result, during a fever response we suffer malaise, feeling very ill and lacking in energy.

A normal fever response of 38–9°C is generally regarded as being healthy and beneficial to the body since it slows pathogen growth and speeds up killing, but when the fever response goes beyond 39°C, e.g. 40°C and beyond, this can be dangerous since cellular enzymes may be denatured and life-threatening convulsions can occur. Most non-steroidal anti-inflammatory drugs, e.g. aspirin, are very effective at reducing fever and function by blocking the production of PGE_2 in the hypothalamus, thereby preventing the set point being shifted upwards.

To further your understanding of pyrexia, read through Prisha's case study.

Case study: Prisha – tonsillitis

Prisha is a 19-year-old undergraduate student and for the last week has been suffering from a sore throat. Initially she thought she was suffering from a common cold, but on looking at her throat in a mirror she was horrified to see that her tonsils were enlarged and purulent. The campus GP recorded her tympanic temperature at 39.1°C and, on noting her inflamed tonsils, took mouth swabs and palpated her cervical lymph nodes (in the neck), and noted they were swollen and tender. She was immediately diagnosed with tonsillitis, put on a course of antibiotics and advised to rest. A few days later Prisha was informed that the throat swabs had revealed she had streptococcal tonsillitis; her GP was happy that this was responding well to the prescribed antibiotics.

Throughout this chapter we have seen that homeostasis is reliant on negative feedback mechanisms to minimise deviations from the physiological set point to constrain a variable within its normal range. However, in some physiological situations it is desirable for the overall health of the body to temporarily deviate dramatically from a physiological set point.

Positive feedback

The term positive feedback is used to describe situations where deviations from the physiological set point are amplified and made larger. In humans the classic example of positive feedback occurs during childbirth (Figure 2.3). As the time of delivery nears at around 9 months, the muscular wall (myometrium) of the uterus is progressively stretched. This activates stretch receptors in the uterine wall and nerve impulses are generated and relayed to the brain. The posterior pituitary gland releases the hormone oxytocin, which circulates in the blood before binding to receptors on the smooth muscle cells of the myometrium, initiating uterine contraction.

This process is then perpetuated with uterine contraction leading to further oxytocin release, which then itself leads to further uterine contraction. This establishes a positive feedback loop during which the uterine contractions get more and more powerful and closer together until eventually the baby is delivered. Levels of oxytocin remain high in the mother's blood following delivery; this hormone is often referred to as the 'love hormone' since it promotes feelings of love and affection which play a key role in the bonding between mother and newborn baby. Oxytocin also stimulates the 'let-down reflex' which pushes milk into the milk ducts of the breast towards the nipple to allow the baby to feed.

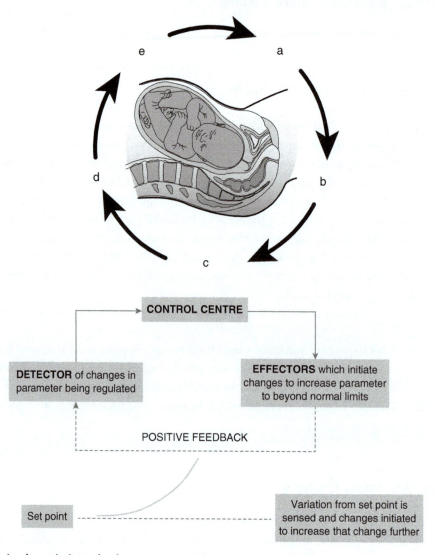

a. Brain stimulates pituitary gland to secrete oxytocin
b. Oxytocin carried in bloodstream to uterus
c. Oxytocin stimulates uterine contractions and pushes baby towards cervix
d. Head of baby pushes against cervix
e. Nerve impulse from cervix transmitted to brain

Figure 2.3 Childbirth (parturition)

Source: OpenStax (2013) Anatomy and Physiology. Rice University. Available at: https://openstax.org/books/anatomy-and-physiology/pages/preface

Now that you have completed the chapter, attempt the multiple-choice questions in Activity 2.3 to assess your knowledge.

Activity 2.3   Multiple-choice questions

1. The set point of a variable is

    a) The value that the variable is always kept at in health
    b) The optimal value for the variable
    c) The point at which the variable is too high to allow normal physiological processes
    d) The point at which the variable is too low to allow normal physiological processes

2. Most homeostatic mechanisms rely on

    a) Negative feedback
    b) Positive feedback
    c) Glycolysis
    d) All of the above

3. Which of the following is essential for negative feedback?

    a) A stimulus
    b) A sensor
    c) A control centre
    d) All of the above

4. Which of the following hormones increases blood glucose?

    a) Insulin
    b) Glucagon
    c) Oxytocin
    d) Thyroxine

5. Low blood glucose is clinically referred to as

    a) Isoglycaemia
    b) Hyperglycaemia

(Continued)

(Continued)

    c) Hypoglycaemia

    d) Endoglycaemia

6. Which of the following would be regarded as a normal body temperature?

    a) 36.9°C

    b) 38.2°C

    c) 34.9°C

    d) 39.1°C

7. Which of the following acts as an endogenous pyrogen?

    a) Interleukin 2 (IL-2)

    b) Interleukin 3 (IL-3)

    c) Interleukin 1 (IL-1)

    d) Interleukin 4 (IL-4)

8. Which of the following drug groups is frequently used to reduce fever?

    a) Opioids

    b) Diuretics

    c) Beta blockers

    d) Non-steroidal anti-inflammatory drugs (NSAIDs)

9. During positive feedback

    a) Variables are kept exactly at their set point

    b) Variables are kept within their normal range

    c) Any deviations from the set point are amplified

    d) Hormones are never involved

10. Which of the following hormones triggers uterine contraction?

    a) Oxytocin

    b) Prolactin

    c) Oestrogen

    d) Progesterone

Chapter summary

Homeostasis is the ability to maintain a relatively stable internal environment that is conducive to the optimal functioning of the body's cells and tissues. Each variable in the human body has an optimal value known as the set point. Homeostasis relies on negative feedback mechanisms to minimise any deviations from the set point and constrain these deviations within a normal range. When variables are consistently outside of their physiological normal range, pathological states can occur, and medical interventions may be necessary to restore the variable to within its normal range. Positive feedback mechanisms can be thought of as the opposite of negative feedback and here any deviations from the set point are amplified and made greater.

Activities: Brief outline answers

Activity 2.1: Evidence-based practice and research (page 36)

High blood calcium is referred to as hypocalcaemia and low blood calcium is referred to as hypocalcaemia.

High blood sodium is referred to as hypernatraemia and low blood sodium is referred to as hyponatraemia.

High blood potassium is referred to as hyperkalaemia and low blood sodium is referred to as hypokalaemia.

Activity 2.2: Evidence-based practice and research (page 40)

The very old and the very young are particularly susceptible to drops in their core body temperature. To avoid hypothermia people need to remain warm indoors in the following ways:

Keep your home at a temperature of at least 18°C

Babies' rooms should be kept between 16 and 20°C

Keep windows and internal doors shut

Wear warm clothes; the more layers the better

Use a room thermometer to monitor temperature

(NHS, 2019a)

Activity 2.3: Multiple-choice questions (pages 43–4)

1) b, 2) a, 3) d, 4) b, 5) c, 6) a, 7) c, 8) d, 9) c, 10) a

Further reading

Boore J et al. (2016) Chapter 1: Homeostasis in person-centred care, in *Essentials of Anatomy and Physiology for Nursing Practice*. London: SAGE Publications Ltd.

A textbook to develop your knowledge of human anatomy and physiology that is aimed specifically at nurses.

Tortora G and Derrickson B (2017) Chapter 2: The chemical level of organization, in *Tortora's Principles of Anatomy and Physiology* (15th edition). New York: John Wiley & Sons.

In-depth coverage of human anatomy and physiology.

Useful websites

www.sciencedirect.com/topics/immunology-and-microbiology/homeostasis

An overview of homeostasis.

Chapter 3 The cardiovascular system

Chapter aims

After reading this chapter, you will be able to:

- describe the key functions of the cardiovascular system;
- identify the major structures of the cardiovascular system;
- explain what is meant by the pulmonary and systemic circulations;
- describe the events of the cardiac cycle;
- provide an overview of the coronary circulation and the nature of coronary artery disease (CAD);
- describe the structure of arteries, veins and capillaries;
- explain how blood pressure is regulated via neural and hormonal mechanisms.

Introduction

Case study: George – myocardial infarction

George was unloading shopping from his car when he suddenly felt a crushing heavy pain in the central part of his chest which spread down the inside of his left arm. By the time he sat down, he was feeling breathless with cold, clammy skin and experiencing a feeling of absolute terror. After ringing for an ambulance George's wife was told to give him an aspirin to chew on and he was rapidly transferred to the local A&E department where, based on ECG evidence, he was immediately diagnosed with a major myocardial infarction (MI). George quickly had stents fitted in to open up his occluded blood vessels and felt almost immediate relief of his pain.

Cardiovascular disease such as that which led to George's heart attack is a major cause of death and disability throughout the world. Nurses will spend a great deal of their time caring for patients with a variety of both heart and blood vessel disease. Many of the routine physiological measurements carried out by nurses such as recording heart rate, blood pressure and blood oxygen saturation provide snapshots of the patient's current cardiovascular status.

This chapter will begin by describing the major functions of the cardiovascular system before examining the structure of the heart and its associated structures. Once you have an understanding of the anatomy of the heart, we will explore how the heart functions as a mechanical pump and examine the control mechanisms that ensure its optimal function. The second section of the chapter will examine the structure of blood vessels and explain how the cardiovascular system maintains cardiac output to ensure that blood pressure and tissue perfusion are adequately maintained. To reinforce the key points, we will explore the nature of some of the cardiovascular diseases that nurses routinely encounter in clinical practice.

Overview of the cardiovascular system

The cardiovascular system (Figure 3.1, Table 3.1) consists of the heart (cardio) and the blood vessels (vascular). It is primarily a pumped system reliant on both the efficient coordinated contractions of the heart and a system of vessels which act as conduits through which the blood is circulated.

Heart structure and function

Position of heart within the thorax

The heart has a relatively central position within the thoracic cavity (Figure 3.1) with the bulk of its structure found behind the sternum (breastbone). On average, an adult human heart weighs around 250–350 g and is around 12–14 cm long and 9–11 cm wide. There is much variation in heart size, with larger people unsurprisingly having larger hearts compared to their smaller counterparts. It is commonly stated that an individual's own heart is roughly the same size as their own clenched fist.

The heart is located in the mediastinum (region between the right and left lung) and is positioned obliquely between the second rib and the fifth intercostal space.

In individuals with a normal body mass index (BMI), the apex heartbeat can usually be detected in the left fifth intercostal space around 8 cm to the left of the central point of the sternum.

The pericardium

The heart is surrounded, protected and anchored in position by a compound membrane called the pericardium which consists of two major layers. The first of these is the fibrous pericardium, which forms an outer protective sheath and is composed of collagenous connective tissue. It anchors the heart in position within the thoracic

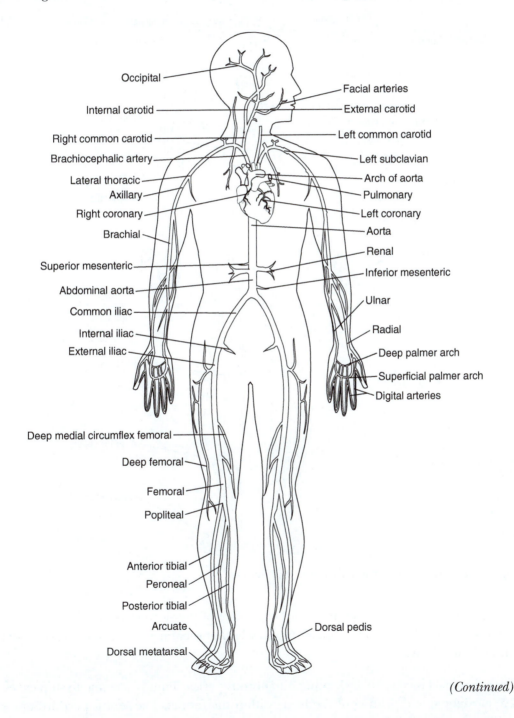

(Continued)

Figure 3.1 (Continued)

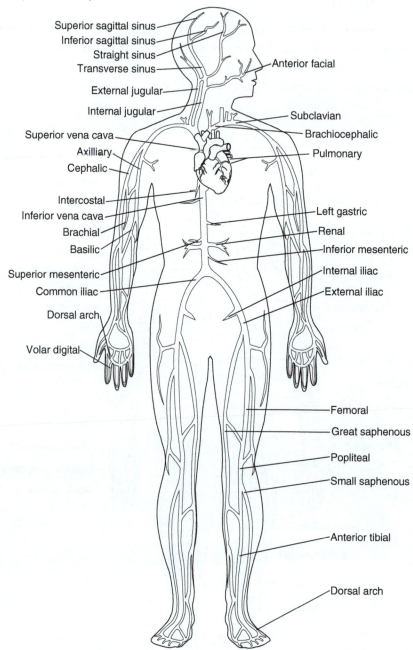

Superior sagittal sinus
Inferior sagittal sinus
Straight sinus
Transverse sinus
Anterior facial
External jugular
Internal jugular
Subclavian
Superior vena cava
Brachiocephalic
Axilliary
Pulmonary
Cephalic
Intercostal
Left gastric
Inferior vena cava
Renal
Brachial
Inferior mesenteric
Basilic
Superior mesenteric
Internal iliac
Common iliac
External iliac
Dorsal arch
Volar digital
Femoral
Great saphenous
Popliteal
Small saphenous
Anterior tibial
Dorsal arch

Figure 3.1   Overview of the cardiovascular system

cavity; anteriorly it is attached to the inner surface of the sternum and inferiorly to the diaphragm, the dome-shaped breathing muscle that separates the thoracic cavity from the abdominal cavity.

Since the heart is continually beating, the fibrous pericardium is essential to stop excessive movement and drifting of the heart within the thorax. The serous pericardium is

Table 3.1 Functions of the cardiovascular system

Transport	In the average adult, around 5 litres (9 pints) of blood is continually circulated throughout the body. Blood functions as a fluid medium facilitating the delivery of oxygen, nutrients and chemical signals termed hormones to all organs and tissues. Simultaneously, waste products such as carbon dioxide and urea are transported from their sites of production to the organs of elimination such as the lungs and kidneys
Maintaining blood pressure (BP)	A normal blood pressure of around 120/80 mmHg is essential to maintain blood flow to all regions of the body. BP must be continually adjusted in response to changes in posture, fluid volume and levels of exercise
Thermoregulation	Circulation of warm blood plays a key role in the dissipation of heat throughout the body. The diversion of blood flow to and from the skin helps to regulate heat loss and maintain an optimal core temperature of around 37°C
Immune function	By circulating white blood cells (leukocytes) to all regions of the body, the cardiovascular system reduces the chance of infection from invading pathogens. Increased blood flow and therefore leukocytes can also be diverted to infected organs and tissues as part of the normal inflammatory response (Chapter 9)

the inner portion of the pericardium and is itself composed of two distinct layers of tissue: the parietal pericardium, a fluid-producing membrane that is attached to the inner portion of the fibrous pericardium, and the visceral pericardium, which is actually the outer layer of the heart and is also known as the epicardium (see below).

The two layers of the serous pericardium secrete a watery fluid termed pericardial fluid which fills the narrow pericardial space between the visceral and parietal pericardium. In health around 10–20 ml of this slippery pericardial fluid surrounds the heart, acting as a lubricant to prevent abrasion and damage to the beating heart and the surrounding tissues. This fluid also functions as an effective shock absorber, cushioning the heart against any knocks and bumps.

Pericarditis, pericardial effusions and cardiac tamponade

Viral and bacterial infections of the pericardium are not uncommon and these can trigger an inflammatory response within the pericardial membranes. This is termed pericarditis and is often accompanied by chest pain and a fever. A major issue with pericarditis is that infection can cause pericardial effusion where there is an increase in fluid volume within the pericardial space. This extra fluid typically consists of inflammatory exudate, pus or blood or a combination of these. Pericardial effusion can quickly develop into a life-threatening emergency as fluid builds up around the heart and begins to compress the ventricles, preventing the heart from functioning as an efficient pump.

This phenomenon is termed cardiac tamponade and is usually treated by inserting a needle into the pericardial sac (needle decompression) to drain off the excess fluid that is crushing the heart. Once decompressed, cardiac function is quickly restored since the ventricles can then fill and pump blood normally. Pericardial effusions that may lead to cardiac tamponade can also be caused by blunt trauma to the chest (e.g. following a car accident when the patient's chest impacts the steering wheel).

Layers of the heart

The heart can be regarded as a simple muscular cone consisting of three distinct layers of tissue (Figure 3.2): the endocardium is the smooth inner layer of the heart that forms the lining of the chambers. The myocardium forms the thick, muscular, middle layer of the heart that makes up the vast bulk of the heart's mass and is composed of specialised cardiac muscle fibres. The final outermost layer of the heart is called the epicardium; confusingly, this is the same layer of tissue that is also commonly referred to as the visceral pericardium. It is important that nurses are familiar with both terms as they are used interchangeably in clinical practice.

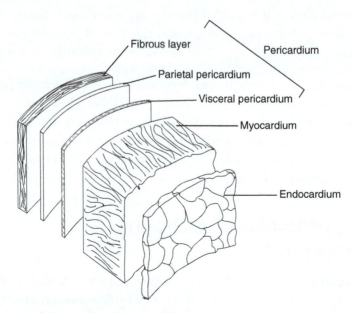

Figure 3.2   Layers of the pericardium and heart

Internal structure of the heart

Internally the heart consists of four distinct chambers (Figure 3.3).

Atria

The atria (sometimes known by the older term auricles) are the two superior (upper) chambers of the heart. These are thin-walled, elastic structures that function primarily as simple collecting chambers. The right atrium collects deoxygenated blood from the two great veins (the superior vena cava and the inferior vena cava). The left atrium receives highly oxygenated blood directly from the lungs via the pulmonary veins. Following collection the atria rapidly deliver blood to their corresponding ventricles. During foetal development the left and right atria are connected to each other via a small opening termed the foramen ovale.

When a baby is born and takes its first breath, changes in blood pressure cause this aperture to close, forming a thin interatrial septum which permanently separates the right- and left-hand sides of the heart. Sometimes this closure does not occur or is incomplete, resulting in a patent foramen ovale (PFO) which is often referred to as a 'hole in the heart'. This is a common congenital birth defect (affecting around 25 per cent of the population) and frequently seen in babies with chromosomal abnormalities such as Down syndrome. Septal defects such as PFO allow abnormal mixing of oxygenated and deoxygenated blood which can lead to reduced blood oxygen saturation and also may increase the risk of stroke in later life. Such congenital defects, if severe, often require surgery to correct.

Ventricles

The ventricles are the two inferior (lower) chambers of the heart; these are much thicker than the atria, containing the bulk of the cardiac muscle mass of the myocardium. The ventricles function as the primary pumping chambers of the heart and are responsible for pumping around 7,200 litres of blood around the body per day. The left and right ventricles are separated by a thick muscular interventricular septum which effectively separates the heart into two distinct pumping mechanisms. Internally within the heart there are four valves which ensure that blood flows in the correct direction.

The two upper valves are semi-lunar valves called the pulmonary and aortic valves which close to prevent blood flowing back into the heart following contraction of the ventricles. The lower two valves are termed atrioventricular (AV) valves since they separate the atria from the ventricles. The AV valve on the right side consists of three flaps (cusps) of tissue and is therefore called the tricuspid, while the AV valve on the left consists of two cusps and is termed the bicuspid or mitral valve. The role of the AV valves is to close and prevent blood flowing back into the atria during ventricular contraction.

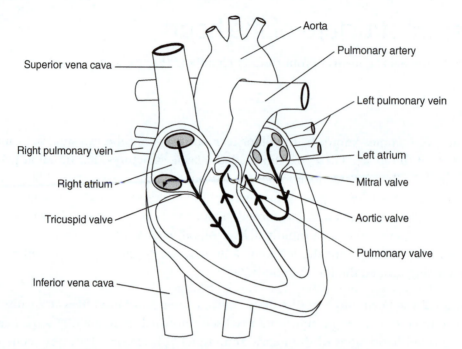

Figure 3.3   Internal structure of the heart showing direction of blood flow

Pulmonary and systemic circuits of blood

The heart can conveniently be thought of as two separate pumps which circulate blood in series (Figure 3.4). The right-hand side of the heart pumps deoxygenated blood to the lungs via the pulmonary circuit and the left-hand side of the heart pumps oxygenated blood from the lungs to all other organ systems via the systemic circuit. The pulmonary arteries and pulmonary veins are unusual blood vessels; unlike most arteries (which usually carry oxygenated blood) the pulmonary arteries carry deoxygenated blood to the lungs, and unlike most veins (which usually carry deoxygenated blood) the pulmonary veins carry oxygenated blood from the lungs.

Nurses are expected to know the basic circulation of blood through the heart including the names of the major blood vessels, chambers of the heart and heart valves through which the blood will pass. Activity 3.1 will help you to learn the names and the correct sequence of blood flow.

Now that you understand the circulation of blood through the pulmonary and systemic circuits, we will explore the nature of the heartbeat.

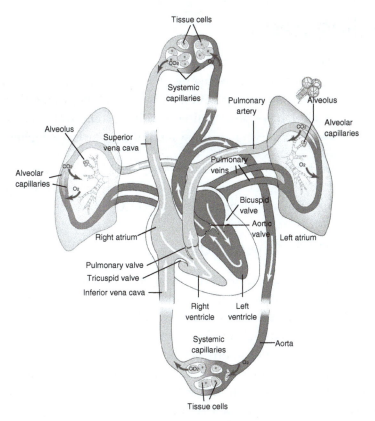

Figure 3.4 Circulation of blood and major blood vessels of the pulmonary and systemic circuits

Activity 3.1 Research and revision

Beginning at the vena cavae and ending at the aortic arch, draw a flow diagram using arrows to illustrate the passage of blood as it passes sequentially through the pulmonary and systemic circuits. The first three steps are:

Vena Cavae → Right Atrium → Tricuspid Valve → ....→ Aortic Arch

Use the following terms to complete your flow diagram:

Left Atrium, Lungs, Bicuspid Valve, Pulmonary Valve, Right Ventricle, Aortic Valve, Pulmonary Veins, Left Ventricle, Pulmonary Artery.

You may find it useful to design your own mnemonic to use as a memory aid.

There are some possible answers to all activities at the end of the chapter, unless otherwise indicated.

The beating heart

Following vigorous exercise or when we are resting and quiet, most people become aware of the sensations and sounds of their beating heart. In young healthy adults, typical resting heart rates range from 60 to 80 beats per minute. In general the resting heart rate relates to the individual's current level of physical fitness; indeed, some athletes may have resting heart rates in the 40s while those who are physically unfit tend to have higher rates.

There are many ways of measuring a patient's heart rate including: taking their pulse, listening to the heart using a stethoscope or other device such as a Doppler probe or viewing the visual display on an electrocardiogram (ECG) machine.

Bradycardia and tachycardia

When recording a patient's resting heart rate sometimes it may be either slower or faster than expected. The term bradycardia is used to describe a resting heart rate of 60 bpm or lower. In most cases bradycardia is not indicative of disease; indeed, the most common cause of a slow heart rate is a high level of physical fitness. Bradycardia is also associated with the use of certain medications, particularly beta blockers (β blockers) which are frequently used to treat high blood pressure by slowing the heart. However, there are some medically significant causes of bradycardia such as hypothermia (see Chapter 2) or damage to the electrical conductive tissues of the heart.

Tachycardia is the opposite of bradycardia and is defined as a resting heart rate of 100 bpm or above. Tachycardia can have many causes ranging from increased release of adrenaline when a person is frightened, to more serious causes such as a major infection or severe haemorrhage.

It is essential to recognise that the terms bradycardia and tachycardia are only applied to a patient's resting heart rate; so a heart rate above 100 bpm during exercise would not be referred to as tachycardia.

Systole and diastole

Contraction of the heart's chambers is referred to as systole while relaxation is referred to as diastole. For the heart to function as an efficient pump, it needs to contract and relax in a precisely timed sequence. This sequence ensures the upper chambers contract first (atrial systole), allowing the ventricles to fill, which then contract (ventricular systole) to eject blood from the heart.

The cardiac cycle

Each heartbeat can be divided into series of five distinct phases termed the cardiac cycle (Figure 3.5). Each phase is perfectly timed and coordinated by the cardiac conductive

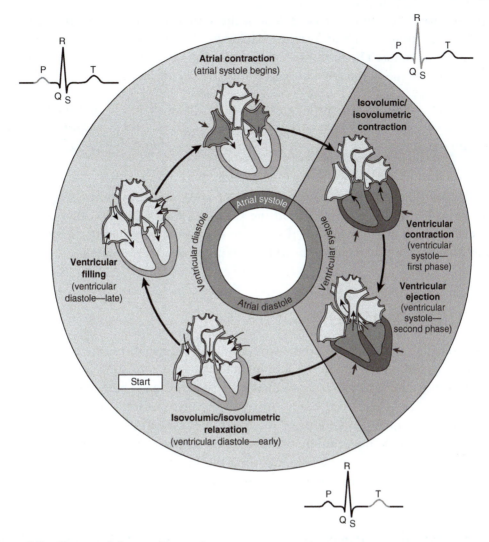

Figure 3.5   Phases of the cardiac cycle

Source: OpenStax (2013) *Anatomy and Physiology*. Rice University. Available at: https://opentextbc.ca/anatomyandphysiology/chapter/19-3-cardiac-cycle

system to ensure that the chambers of the heart contract and relax at the correct time, allowing the heart to function as an efficient pump.

The first phase is called the passive ventricular filling stage, where for a short time both the atria and the ventricles of the heart are in diastole and the atrioventricular valves (bicuspid and tricuspid) are open. This allows approximately 70 per cent of atrial blood volume to flow passively from the atria into the dilated ventricles under the influence of gravity and the elastic recoil of the atria.

This is followed by phase two, atrial systole, where the atria contract, forcing the remaining 30 per cent of atrial blood volume into the dilated ventricles.

In phase three, isovolumetric contraction, the ventricles are rapidly undergoing systole, forcing closure of the atrioventricular valves. This phase is very fast, occurring in around 0.05 seconds. The term isovolumetric means at constant volume, reflecting the fact that the volume of the left and right ventricle is identical.

Phase four is known as ventricular ejection; as the pressure in the ventricles increases, the aortic and pulmonary valves are forced open and blood is ejected into the pulmonary and systemic circuits.

The final fifth phase is isovolumetric relaxation; here the ventricles undergo diastole and blood begins to flow back against the aortic and pulmonary valves, snapping them shut. Pressure continues to fall within the ventricles until it is below that of the atria. The elastic recoil of the atria and effects of gravity push blood onto the atrioventricular valves which open, returning the heart back to phase one, passive filling.

Cardiac muscle

Unlike skeletal muscle which consists of parallel running fibres, the cardiac muscle, which forms the myocardium, has a branched structure consisting of individual cells joined together by tight junctions termed intercalated discs. These allow efficient and rapid movement of electrical signals through the myocardium, allowing the component fibres to contract in synchrony to ensure the myocardium contracts as a single unit. Cardiac muscle has a unique feature called intrinsic rhythm which is an inbuilt ability to contract at a regular rate, allowing the heart to beat at a relatively regular rhythm even if its natural pacemaker is damaged.

The cardiac conductive system of the heart

As we have seen above, each heartbeat involves precise and accurately timed contraction and relaxation of the heart's chambers during the cardiac cycle. The five phases of the cardiac cycle are coordinated and timed to split-second accuracy via the cardiac conductive system. This consists of a series of specialised interconnected cardiac muscle fibres which originate in the atria before permeating deep into the ventricles (Figure 3.6a). You may find it useful to think of this system as behaving in a similar way to the cells of the nervous system in that it conducts electrical signals. As these electrical impulses travel through the heart, a coordinated wave of muscular contraction is initiated within the myocardium which corresponds to a single heartbeat. Since the heart is continually beating, this electrical activity within the conductive tissues is continuous and is readily recordable on an ECG.

The cardiac conductive system consists of several distinct regions, as follows: the sinoatrial node (SAN), commonly referred to as the heart's natural pacemaker because it sets the basic rhythm of the heart. Within the SAN, pacemaker cells spontaneously generate regular electrical impulses called action potentials which then travel rapidly over the atria, initiating atrial systole; the atrioventricular node (AVN), a key region of the conductive system located in the lower portion of the right atrium. Action potentials that have spread over the atria rapidly converge on the AVN and are delayed here for around a tenth of a second, allowing time for blood to pass from the atria into the ventricles. Should the SAN be damaged (e.g. following infarction), the AV node is able to take over the role of pacemaker. The AVN is connected to atrioventricular bundle (AVB), frequently referred to as the bundle of His; this consists of a relatively thick bunch of fibres that extends the length of the interventricular septum before splitting into the right and left bundle branches.

Following the delay at the AVN, the AVB and bundle branches rapidly conduct action potentials into the ventricles to initiate ventricular depolarisation and contraction (systole). The right and left bundle branches split into fine extensions called Purkinje fibres which permeate deeply into the myocardium of the left and right ventricles. These allow rapid propagation of action potentials through the ventricles, ensuring that all the muscle fibres of the ventricles contract in synchrony to enable the most efficient ejection of blood from the heart by ensuring that the pumping chambers contract as a single unit (termed a syncytium).

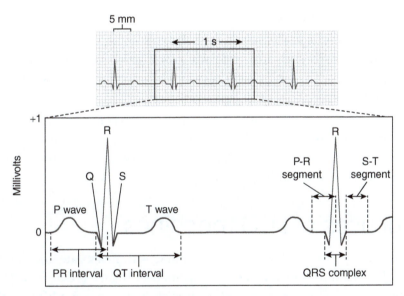

Figure 3.6a and b   The electrical conductive tissues and ECG waves

Source: OpenStax (2013) *Anatomy and Physiology*. Rice University. Available at: https://openstax.org/books/anatomy-and-physiology/pages/1-introduction

The ECG (electrocardiogram)

The ECG is an important diagnostic tool. ECG machines monitor the conduction of action potentials through the heart's electrical conductive tissues and the cardiac muscle that forms the myocardium.

Electrical waves and time intervals viewable on an ECG

Ideally when learning the components of an ECG, it is suggested that you should continually refer to the cardiac conductive system, and for this reason the two are presented together (Figure 3.6a and b). The electrical activity shown in Figure 3.6b corresponds to a single heartbeat and consists of:

The P wave: This small wave corresponds to the action potentials generated by the heart's natural pacemaker, the sinoatrial node (SAN), and their passage across the atria. Therefore, nurses can regard this small initial peak (P) as corresponding exactly to the time when the patient's atria are undergoing atrial systole. It may be a useful memory aid to think of the P wave as corresponding to activity generated by the pacemaker (p for pacemaker).

The P-R interval: This short time period corresponds to atrial contraction and the short delay in action potentials that occurs at the AV node to allow ventricular filling.

The QRS complex: Since the ventricles are so thick and muscular when action potentials spread through these lower chambers, a much larger electrical signal is generated. This is recorded on an ECG as a large spike termed the QRS complex. It is useful to regard this portion of the ECG as corresponding to the time when the ventricles are undergoing ventricular systole.

The T wave: This final major electrical peak corresponds to the ventricles returning to their resting state (ventricular repolarisation). Nurses can regard the T wave as corresponding to the time when the ventricles are relaxing as they undergo ventricular diastole.

The S-T segment: The period of electrical activity between ventricular depolarisation and repolarisation. Characteristic changes to this segment are frequently seen in patients with CAD, particularly when the patient has their ECG recorded when on a treadmill (stress ECG).

Clinical uses of ECG machines

Nurses routinely monitor ECGs, looking for changes in heart rate and rhythm. Most modern machines will provide an alert if a rhythm disturbance is detected. The P wave, QRS complex and T wave are repeated, with each heart beat resulting in the standard sinus rhythm that nurses observe on an ECG machine. The distance and timing between QRS complexes on an ECG trace provide an accurate measure of the patient's current heart rate. Most ECG machines calculate this automatically to display a real-time reading of the heart rate.

Recording of an ECG may be deemed necessary in many circumstances including:

- irregular heart beat (palpitations);
- chest pain (angina pectoris);
- suspected myocardial infarction (heart attack);

- suspected electrolyte disturbances/imbalances;
- loss of consciousness (syncope);
- bradycardia (slow heart rate) or tachycardia (rapid heart rate);
- to investigate the condition of the myocardium, in conditions such as heart failure, cardiomyopathy or long-standing hypertension.

Cardiac arrhythmias

The term cardiac arrhythmia is used to describe any changes to the transmission of action potentials through the cardiac conductive system that leads to an abnormal heart rhythm or heart rate. Many arrhythmias such as simple ectopic beats are benign with no major physiological effects, while others may result in a heart that pumps blood less effectively, leading to a reduction in cardiac output. In the most severe arrhythmias cardiac output may cease completely, leading to sudden cardiac death.

Changes to the cardiac conductive system

By the age of 50 around 50–75 per cent of the pacemaker cells of the heart's natural pacemaker SAN have been lost, while the cardiac muscle fibres of the atrioventricular bundle (bundle of His) undergo varying degrees of fibrosis. These changes may reduce the efficiency of cardiac conduction and contribute to the increased risk of ectopic beats (palpitations) seen in older people.

Ectopic beats

Two major types are recognised and are classified according to which chambers are affected. Premature atrial contractions (PACs) occur when there is an early contraction of the atria and can usually be recognised on an ECG as an extra P wave. PACs are minor events and often not even perceived by the patient. Premature ventricular contractions (PVCs) occur as a result of early contraction of the ventricles; these are usually more noticeable to the patient. Often the patient will complain that it feels as if their heart has paused (or lurched) in their chest followed by a more powerful subsequent recovery beat.

Frequently PVCs may be experienced in clusters or in predictable patterns before disappearing and returning hours, days or even months or years later. Since PVCs occur as a result of abnormal conduction in the ventricles, they are more easily recognisable as irregular spikes on an ECG that interrupt the normal sinus rhythm. Most PVCs, while quite scary for the patient, are benign and often related to stress, dehydration or use of stimulants such as caffeine or nicotine. They are also very common in women going through the menopause. When PVCs occur sequentially one after the other, they may develop into more serious arrhythmias such as ventricular tachycardia.

61

Atrial fibrillation (AF)

This common arrhythmia is characterised by the rapid and uncoordinated contraction of the atria (fibrillation) which can reduce ventricular filling. Since the atria are only responsible for the last 33 per cent of ventricular filling, symptoms of AF such as weakness, dizziness or breathlessness may only be experienced during exercise or periods of excitement when cardiac output increases. Some individuals may never experience symptoms even with long-standing AF and are only diagnosed following a routine check-up. During periods of sustained AF the uncoordinated irregular contractions cause turbulent blood flow, allowing blood to collect in the atrial recesses, particularly in the left atrial appendage. This static blood can remain for long periods and begin to coagulate, resulting in a progressively enlarging clot (thrombus).

At any time, these thrombi can embolise and travel up into the cerebral circulation, resulting in stroke. If only small clots are dislodged then transient ischaemic attacks (TIAs) may occur, but if clots forming in the left atrial appendage are large and embolise, major cerebral vessels may be occluded, leading to severe CVAs that may be fatal. It has been estimated that the risk of thromboembolic stroke increases around fivefold in patients with persistent AF (Wolf et al., 1991), and so to minimise risk these patients are usually placed on long-term anticoagulation therapies such as warfarin or apixaban.

AF is commonly seen in patients with coronary artery disease or in those that have previously suffered MI; however, age is recognised as the major risk factor for developing AF (Steenman and Lande, 2017). AF is readily diagnosed by reference to a patient's ECG where the presence of multiple P waves and an irregular heart rate are commonly observed. Since AF is so frequently encountered by nurses, to further your understanding of this important arrhythmia read through Gerald's case study before attempting Activity 3.2.

Case study: Gerald – atrial fibrillation

Gerald is a 62-year-old man who recently visited his GP complaining of feeling constantly tired and washed out and experiencing breathlessness when climbing his stairs and doing his gardening. His GP noted that his pulse rate was high at 107 bpm and was also very irregular, and he was referred to a local cardiac clinic where he was diagnosed with persistent atrial fibrillation. Following unsuccessful cardioversion (where a controlled electrical shock is given to restore sinus rhythm), Gerald was prescribed apixaban and a beta blocker (sotalol) to manage his condition. Gerald has been taking his medication sporadically. Two days ago Gerald was admitted to hospital after suffering a minor stroke and on questioning it was discovered that he had stopped taking his apixaban, which almost certainly increased the coagulability of his blood, leading to his stroke.

From the case study above it is apparent that Gerald is still unclear about the risks associated with his condition. A key role of nurses is to help educate patients and explain the purpose of their medications. Activity 3.2 highlights this role.

Activity 3.2   Communication

Describe how you would explain the nature of his condition to Gerald and highlight why it is important that he should take *all* of his prescribed medications.

This activity highlights the importance of communication between nurse and patient in encouraging compliance with treatment regimes. While AF is a common chronic but manageable arrhythmia, other rhythm disturbances are emergencies requiring immediate medical intervention.

Ventricular fibrillation (VF)

Ventricular fibrillation is a serious life-threatening arrhythmia that commonly occurs following major MIs, chronic heart disease and occasionally following an electrical shock. During VF the ventricles are not contracting in an organised manner and the heart can no longer function as an effective pump. Unless the heart can be restored to its original sinus rhythm via the use of a defibrillator, the patient will die. VF is usually very clear on an ECG since no QRS complexes or sinus rhythm are visible.

In the first part of this chapter we examined how the heart functions as an efficient pump to ensure continuous circulation of blood. We now need to explore in greater detail the role played by blood vessels in distributing blood and maintaining blood pressure.

Blood vessels: the vasculature

Amazingly, the human body has between 60,000 and 100,000 miles of blood vessels which function as conduits through which our 5 litres of blood is continuously circulated. There are three major types of blood vessel: arteries, veins and capillaries.

Arteries and veins are the largest blood vessels and both consist of three distinct layers (tunics) of tissue, outlined in Figure 3.7.

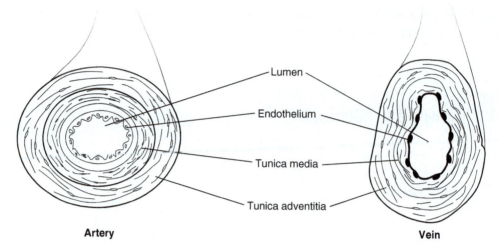

Figure 3.7 The internal structure of an artery and vein

The tunica externa: This is the protective outer layer of the vessel composed predominantly of collagen-rich connective tissue. It is usually continuous with the surrounding tissues, serving to anchor the blood vessel in position within the body and prevent vessel movement following ejection of blood from the heart or during the physical movement of the body.

The tunica media: Composed of involuntary smooth muscle, this middle layer can contract (vasoconstriction) or dilate (vasodilation) to change the diameter of the blood vessel and alter the rate of blood flow. The tunica media is much thicker in arteries than in veins since arteries are usually carrying blood under high pressure and their walls require extra reinforcement. The smooth muscle layers are innervated by sympathetic nerve fibres which are under the influence of the vasomotor centre within the medulla oblongata of the brain. This is the region of the brain that regulates vascular tone and therefore blood pressure by controlling the processes of vasoconstriction and vasodilation.

The tunica intima: This is the thinnest and innermost layer of the blood vessel. It is composed of a single layer of incredibly smooth squamous epithelial cells (the endothelium) and is separated from the smooth muscle cells of the tunica media by a thin layer of collagen-rich tissue termed the lamina. In arteries the smooth, silky nature of this innermost layer affords minimal resistance, ensuring that blood flows rapidly in concentric layers (laminar blood flow).

Arteries

Arteries are muscular, pulsatile, elastic blood vessels that circulate blood under high pressure with most carrying oxygenated blood away from the heart. The aorta is the major systemic artery and has a greater stretch than other arteries because its walls have a higher elastin content. It carries blood directly away from the left ventricle of the heart into the systemic circuit. On exiting the left ventricle, the aorta curves over the superior portion of the heart (aortic arch), delivering blood into its descending portion which branches and supplies blood to the major abdominal and pelvic organs. The major arteries of the body are typically named according to the organ or region that they supply, e.g. the hepatic artery supplies blood to the liver, the splenic artery to the **spleen** and the renal arteries to the kidneys. The large arteries continually subdivide into smaller and smaller vessels before eventually terminating in arterioles which are the smallest arteries of the body.

Capillaries

Arterioles supply high-pressure blood directly into complex vascular structures termed capillary beds (Figure 3.8). These function as distribution vessels ensuring that all cells within a tissue or organ are adequately perfused with oxygenated blood. It is useful to visualise capillaries as completing the circuit of blood flow by forming bridges between the arteries and veins of the body. Pre-capillary sphincters are tiny rings of smooth muscle which act as valves to regulate the flow of blood into each capillary bed; these are under the control of the autonomic nervous system and a variety of locally acting chemical signals and hormones.

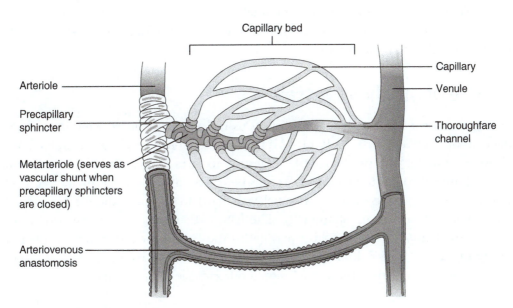

Figure 3.8   Capillary bed structure

Source: OpenStax (2013) *Anatomy and Physiology*. Rice University. Available at: https://openstax.org/books/anatomy-and-physiology/pages/1-introduction

Haemodynamics of the capillary bed: filtration and the formation of interstitial (tissue) fluid

When the pre-capillary sphincters open, blood flows into the capillary beds under high pressure (around 35 mmHg) directly from the arterioles. Each individual capillary is composed of a tube of squamous epithelial cells.

Capillaries are just wide enough to allow erythrocytes to squeeze through and travel along their length. Erythrocytes themselves are deformable because of their biconcave structure (Chapter 9); this allows the membranes of each erythrocyte to be in close proximity to the capillary wall, increasing the efficiency of oxygen diffusion into the tissues.

The adjacent cells in a capillary have regular tiny slits/gaps in their junctions which function as crude mechanical filters. When blood is forced into these porous vessels, fluid containing low-molecular-weight molecules such as oxygen, salts (sodium, potassium calcium, chloride), amino acids and sugars such as glucose is driven out through the vessel wall by a process called filtration. This fluid is termed interstitial or tissue fluid and is continually being produced to act as a medium to deliver useful molecules to the local cells. Most cells are continually bathed in a thin layer of this interstitial fluid, which also forms a medium into which waste materials such as carbon dioxide and urea can be discharged.

During the process of filtration larger molecules such as plasma proteins are too big to fit through the porous capillary walls and are therefore retained in the capillary blood. This retention increases the osmotic potential of the blood towards the venous end of the capillary bed, which serves to pull tissue fluid, now rich in dissolved waste products, back in through the capillary walls.

The role of lymphatic vessels

Resting within the interstitial spaces of most tissues are blind-ended lymphatic vessels which absorb excess interstitial fluid. This fluid is discharged into larger lymphatic vessels where it mixes with products of fat digestion to form a milky fluid termed lymph. Lymph travels through the lymphatic vessels before eventually being discharged back into the blood (at the right and left subclavian vein) to maintain the total blood volume (explored further in Chapter 9). The lymphatic system can be regarded as a second circulatory system that runs parallel to the cardiovascular system. It is often referred to as the body's drainage system since it plays a key role in preventing over-accumulation of interstitial fluid which would otherwise lead to oedema.

Veins

Blood exiting the venous end of the capillary bed does so under very low pressure, entering the venules which are the smallest veins of the body. Venules from multiple capillary beds join up to form larger and larger veins. Most large- and medium-sized veins are equipped with semi-lunar valves to help prevent the backflow of blood under the influence of gravity. Since the pressure in veins is so low, physical movement of the body is essential to keep blood moving and avoid venous stasis, which can increase the risk of thrombosis. During bodily movement, contraction of the major muscle groups, such as those in the legs, will squeeze the thin-walled veins, ensuring blood is kept mobile, while the valves ensure the blood flows in the correct direction towards the heart.

This mechanism is termed the skeletal muscle pump and is particularly important for ensuring venous return from the lower regions of body. All veins ultimately drain into the superior and inferior vena cavae which deliver deoxygenated blood directly to the right atrium of the heart. Since veins are thin-walled vessels, they show a high degree of compliance (ability to distend) and many of the larger veins of the body act as capacitance vessels with around 60 per cent of the total blood volume found within the venous system.

Immobility and hospital bed rest

In immobile patients, e.g. those with severe disabilities or those confined to hospital beds, the skeletal muscle pump may no longer remain active, resulting in accumulation of blood in the legs and an increased risk of static blood (venous stasis) and thrombus (clot) formation. Risk of thrombosis in hospital patients confined to bed may be reduced by encouraging as much physical movement as the patient can safely undertake or via nurse-led bed exercises or regular visits from the physiotherapist. If frailty makes exercise difficult or impossible then the use of support stockings to compress the veins of the legs can also be effective in reducing the risk of thrombosis. Some patients undergoing surgery may be given subcutaneous low-molecular-weight heparin, for example enoxaparin and dalteparin, post-operatively to reduce the risk of clot formation (NICE, 2019a).

Peripheral oedema

Oedema occurs as a result of over-accumulation of fluid within the interstitial spaces, resulting in tissue swelling which can be uncomfortable and sometimes painful. Peripheral oedema is most frequently seen affecting the legs and particularly the ankles and feet, often making it very difficult for the patient to wear their usual footwear. When severe, peripheral oedema can lead to leakage of fluid through the skin (weeping oedema) or this fluid may collect in blisters which can burst, breaching skin integrity and increasing the risk of infection.

The coronary circulation

Since the heart is continually active, the cardiac muscle fibres of the myocardium require a continual supply of highly oxygenated blood, and this is supplied via the coronary arteries (Figure 3.9). These are relatively small blood vessels originating directly from the aorta and located on the outer surface of the heart. The term coronary refers to the collective appearance of these vessels as resembling a crown that encircles the heart (corona is Latin for crown). The smaller coronary arteries are interconnected by tiny bridging channels termed anastomoses. Should a blockage (e.g. a clot or detached piece of fatty plaque) occur, blood can be diverted into these anastomotic (collateral) channels which can expand and widen, ensuring that the myocardium in proximity to the blockage remains perfused. The anastomotic nature of the coronary circulation allows small blockages to be effectively bypassed, increasing the chances of survival following an MI.

Although the coronary arteries only receive around 4 per cent of the total blood flow, the continually active myocardium is responsible for approximately 11 per cent of the body's total oxygen consumption. This heavy demand for oxygen renders the myo-cardium susceptible to many factors which can compromise blood flow, particularly narrowing of the coronary vessels due to atherosclerotic occlusion.

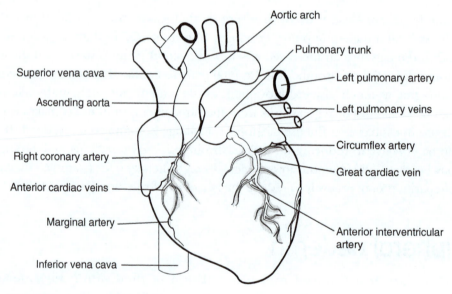

Figure 3.9 The coronary arteries

Coronary artery disease (CAD)

Coronary artery disease (CAD) is the leading cause of heart disease in the UK and worldwide (Bailey and Hall, 2006). The most common form of CAD is caused by ath-erosclerotic occlusion which is characterised by a slow build-up of fatty plaque which progressively hardens and occludes the vessels. The process of atherosclerotic occlu-sion usually follows damage to the delicate endothelial layer that is in contact with the blood. Today many factors are known to cause endothelial damage and therefore to precipitate and accelerate atherosclerosis, including smoking, high blood pressure and high blood glucose, e.g. in patients with diabetes mellitus.

During this process the diameter of the coronary arteries is significantly reduced by a gradual build-up of fatty plaque. Atherosclerotic plaque is dense and has a consistency similar to candle wax which causes a hardening to the vessel wall and reduction in the flexibility of the artery. CAD by itself is the greatest single cause of death in the UK; the figures from 2012 indicate 16 per cent of male deaths and 10 per cent of female deaths were from CAD (predominantly as a result of MI) and this equates to around 74,000 deaths (British Heart Foundation, 2014). CAD is usually diagnosed using a stress ECG (S-T depression) and subsequent angiography which allows the diameter of the coronary arteries to be visualised.

CAD and angina pectoris

As coronary vessel occlusion progresses in CAD patients, less oxygenated blood is delivered to the myocardium and the cardiac muscle cells are forced into anaerobic respiration with lactic acid accumulation. This build-up of lactic acid produces a heavy sensation that is often experienced as central chest pain behind the breastbone. This painful sensation that is associated with CAD is referred to as angina pectoris and commonly spreads from the chest, down the left arm and frequently up the left side of the neck into the left side of the jaw.

Angina can be subdivided into stable angina, where the pain is brought on following physical exertion such as walking up a hill, and unstable angina, where the pain is often unpredictable, frequently occurring without physical exertion at apparently random times during the day and night. Unstable angina is a serious clinical finding since it is often seen in patients prior to suffering an MI.

CAD and myocardial infarction (MI)

A major danger with progressive CAD is that narrowed coronary arteries can easily become completely blocked by a thrombus (clot) or a dislodged piece of fatty plaque. Frequently an area of plaque will rupture, activating the clotting cascade, leading to rapid thrombosis and total vessel occlusion that is indicative of an MI (heart attack).

During infarction the cardiac muscle cells of the myocardium are deprived of oxygen and begin to die. Most MIs result in a characteristic, concentric pattern of tissue damage made up of the area of necrosis (dead tissue), the area of injury (living but damaged tissue) and the ischaemic zone (healthy living tissue but with reduced oxygen supply).

All three concentric areas surrounding the occlusion will collectively reduce the heart's ability to function as an effective pump.

Although MI can come on suddenly and without warning, often a variety of symptoms are initially present. These can include chest pain, shortness of breath (dyspnoea), increased sweating (hyperhidrosis), feeling of impending doom (severe anxiety), confusion or lethargy (NHS, 2018); you may remember all of these were present in George's case study at the beginning of this chapter. However, not everyone will experience MI in the same way; older women often present atypically with research indicating that less than half of women over the age of 75 experienced chest pain during MI (Milner et al., 2004).

To develop your knowledge of heart disease, read through Gloria's case study before attempting Activity 3.3.

Case study: Gloria – peripheral oedema

Gloria is a chatty 86-year-old woman living on her own in sheltered accommodation. For the last 20 years she has suffered chest pain on exertion and five years ago she suffered a major MI followed by two less serious infarctions. Gloria has had stents fitted but based on her health was judged as not fit enough for bypass surgery. During your visit Gloria has been complaining of swollen feet and ankles which, while not painful, are preventing her from wearing even her slippers.

Nurses are required to carefully assess the health status of their patients and draw accurate conclusions based on medical history and current observation.

Activity 3.3   Critical thinking

Based solely on the information that has been provided in the case study, what conclusions can you draw about Gloria's clinical history and the possible cause of her ankle and foot swelling?

We have now examined the structure and function of the heart and blood vessels which work together to enable adequate circulation for healthy tissue perfusion. To ensure that blood is delivered to all regions of the body, an adequate blood pressure must be maintained and regulated.

Blood pressure

Nurses routinely measure blood pressure (BP) using a device termed a sphygmomanometer (sphyg). Because of the past history of using mercury column sphygs (rarely used today because of the toxicity of mercury), BP readings recorded using digital, mercury-free devices are still expressed in mmHg.

A typical reading in a young, healthy adult would be around 120/80 mmHg.

The two figures obtained each time a blood pressure measurement is taken represent:

The systolic BP: This is the upper figure which corresponds to the time during the cardiac cycle when the ventricles are undergoing systole (contraction) and blood is being ejected.

The diastolic BP: This is the lower figure and corresponds to the time during the cardiac cycle when the ventricles of the heart are undergoing diastole (relaxation) and no blood is being ejected.

Currently NICE (National Institute for Health and Care Excellence) recognises BP readings of 140/90 mmHg or higher as being indicative of hypertension (high blood pressure). It is estimated that hypertension affects at least a quarter of all adults in the UK and over half of all adults in the UK over the age of 60. Hypertension is a major preventable cause of mortality in the UK, increasing the risk of MI, stroke (CVA), heart failure, chronic kidney disease and cognitive decline (NICE, 2018).

A normal BP is essential to maintain tissue perfusion (blood supply) throughout the body from the top of the scalp to the tips of the toes. BP can be affected by many parameters, but a normal BP depends on having a healthy heart to ensure adequate cardiac output (CO) and healthy blood vessels to ensure adequate blood flow. The blood vessels provide a collective resistance to blood flow with the total resistance offered by all the blood vessels in the body known as the peripheral resistance (PR).

In simple terms BP can be thought of as a product of multiplying the CO and the PR:

$$BP = CO \times PR$$

As we will explore below, BP can be altered by changing the heart rate to change CO or by altering the diameter of blood vessels to change the PR.

Control of BP

The human body has a variety of elaborate homeostatic mechanisms to ensure that BP is maintained within its normal range. BP control can be broadly split into neural mechanisms, which allow BP to be altered rapidly within seconds, and hormonal mechanisms, which play a key role in the medium- to long-term control of BP.

Neural control of BP

Two specialised regions are located within the medulla oblongata (inferior portion of the brain stem) which can rapidly either raise or lower the BP to match the body's current needs. The cardioregulatory centre or cardiac centre regulates the heart rate and hence the cardiac output (CO). The vasomotor centre regulates vascular tone by controlling the diameter of blood vessels (vasodilation or vasoconstriction).

By regulating vascular tone, the vasomotor centre is able to increase or decrease the peripheral resistance (PR).

Both the cardiac and vasomotor centres require a continuous 'real-time' measurement of the current BP. This is achieved using specialised stretch receptors called baroreceptors which are located in the walls of the aortic arch and carotid sinuses (bulbous regions of the carotid arteries in the neck). Measuring the degree of stretch gives a good measure of current BP, with more stretch equating to a higher BP and less stretch indicative of a lower BP. In humans the aortic arch baroreceptors relay information to the cardioregulatory and vasomotor centres via the vagus nerve and the carotid sinus baroreceptors via the glossopharyngeal nerve (Figure 3.10).

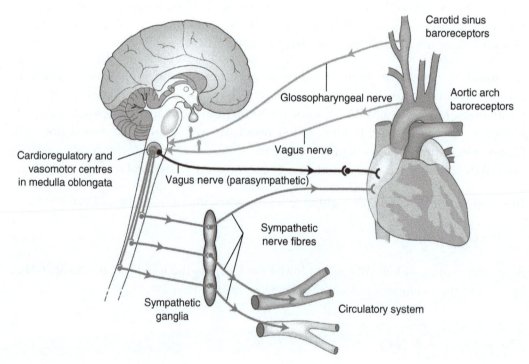

Figure 3.10 Baroreceptor response

The baroreceptor responses

Neural control of blood pressure is particularly important for changes in posture or when engaging in strenuous physical activities. The baroreceptor responses highlighted below are classic examples of homeostatic negative feedback (Chapter 2) where deviations from normal systolic and diastolic BP are resisted and BP is normalised.

Many things can cause a drop in BP but a common cause is suddenly standing up (Figure 3.11).

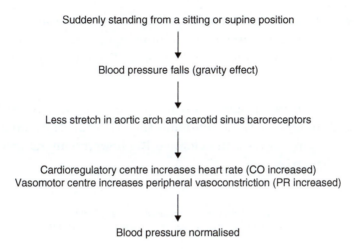

Suddenly standing from a sitting or supine position

↓

Blood pressure falls (gravity effect)

↓

Less stretch in aortic arch and carotid sinus baroreceptors

↓

Cardioregulatory centre increases heart rate (CO increased)
Vasomotor centre increases peripheral vasoconstriction (PR increased)

↓

Blood pressure normalised

Figure 3.11   Neural responses to decreased BP

In the situation in Figure 3.11, gravity will pull arterial blood downwards (arteries have no valves), leading to a significant drop in BP. If BP is not restored rapidly, there is a risk of reducing cerebral blood flow, potentially leading to dizziness and fainting (syncope). This phenomenon is termed postural hypotension or orthostatic intolerance and becomes more common with age. An understanding of postural hypotension is essential for nurses, so to develop your understanding further read through Janet's case study before attempting Activity 3.4.

Case study: Janet – postural hypotension

Janet is a 71-year-old woman who has recently returned home following a long 10-day stay in hospital recovering from a severe bout of pneumonia. Janet has hypertension which has for many years been treated successfully using a combined beta blocker and diuretic. When Janet stood up to make herself a cup of tea she promptly fainted, hitting her head on a coffee table as she fell. Fortunately, her partner was with her and able to drive her quickly to A&E for stitches and a full assessment.

As a nurse, you should be able to link your knowledge of human anatomy and physiology to patient histories.

Activity 3.4   Evidence-based practice and research

From what you have learnt in this chapter, describe what is likely to have caused Janet's faint. Could this be related to her recent hospital stay or blood pressure medication?

You should now have a good understanding of the nature of postural hypotension and the risk of falls associated with this condition. Although postural hypotension becomes more common in older people, high blood pressure affects a much greater proportion of the population.

Increased BP may occur as a result of disease (e.g. atherosclerosis), stress or simply through increased sodium (salt) consumption (Figure 3.12). Hormonal mechanisms tend to be more effective in reducing elevated BP; however, neural mechanisms also play a more immediate role.

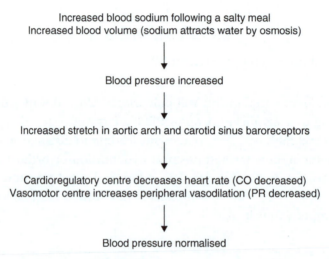

Figure 3.12   Neural responses to increased BP

In addition to the rapid neural adjustments to BP that are required as a result of postural changes, it is essential that BP is controlled and maintained over the longer term. It is here that hormonal mechanisms play the dominant role.

Hormonal control of blood pressure

Hormones are chemical signals which are transported to their sites of action in the blood (Chapter 5). A multitude of hormones are involved in regulating blood pressure and there is much synergy (working together) between these and also much interplay between the hormonal mechanisms and neural mechanisms described above.

Antidiuretic hormone (ADH)

Also known as vasopressin, ADH is a neuropeptide hormone (small protein produced by nerve cells) that is synthesised in the hypothalamus. Once produced, ADH is transported along the axons of hypothalamic neurones to be stored in the posterior pituitary gland. There are several potential triggers that stimulate the release of ADH, including a decrease in BP as detected by the aortic arch and carotid sinus baroreceptors, an increase in blood concentration as detected by hypothalamic osmoreceptors (receptors that measure the osmotic potential of the blood) and the presence of angiotensin-II from the rennin angiotensin aldosterone mechanism (see section on RAAS below).

Physiological actions of ADH

The term antidiuretic hormone is applied to this hormone since its major effect is to reduce urine output by the kidneys, leading to the production of dark, concentrated urine (Chapter 11). When BP is low this is an ideal strategy, since by reducing urine production more water remains in the blood, boosting plasma volume and increasing BP. ADH further increases BP by stimulating arterial vasoconstriction.

Conversely, when the aortic arch and carotid sinus baroreceptors detect an increase in BP the release of ADH from the posterior pituitary is reduced or stopped. This leads to the production of a large volume of dilute urine, effectively allowing the body to 'dump' blood volume in the form of dilute urine to reduce BP. Simultaneously, reduced levels of ADH will reduce arterial vasoconstriction to further reduce BP.

Atrial natriuretic peptide (ANP)

This hormone is produced by the atria of the heart in response to increased blood volume. If blood volume increases, the atria are subjected to increased stretch, with the atrial myocytes (muscle cells) releasing ANP at concentrations proportional to the degree of stretch. ANP is a powerful natural diuretic peptide and stimulates the kidneys to produce a large amount of dilute urine to normalise the total blood volume. ANP and ADH can be seen to be antagonistic to each other in terms of regulating blood volume and blood pressure. The physiology of these hormones and their effects on the kidney are discussed in greater detail in Chapter 11.

Adrenaline (epinephrine)

Adrenaline is produced by the central portion of the adrenal glands (adrenal medulla) and is the body's major fight-or-flight hormone. Adrenaline is released during periods of excitement or fear and functions primarily to prepare the body for immediate action. Adrenaline is a catecholamine hormone which, when released into the blood, has powerful physiological effects, many of which are mediated through activation of the sympathetic nervous system (Chapter 5). Here we focus on its influence on BP.

Cardiovascular effects of adrenaline

Adrenaline increases the heart rate and cardiac output by binding to beta (β) adrenergic receptors at the pacemaker (SAN). The drugs termed β blockers block adrenaline and noradrenaline from binding, thereby slowing the heart rate and reducing cardiac output and BP. Until recently β blockers such as atenolol were frequently prescribed to treat hypertension, but their use in treating this condition has now been largely superseded by ACE inhibitors (see below).

Adrenaline promotes vasoconstriction of blood vessels in the skin and gut: during periods of adrenaline release, the skin may take on an ashen appearance and many people complain of a feeling of butterflies in the stomach, which is thought to correspond to vasoconstriction in the gut. Simultaneously, adrenaline promotes vasodilation of blood vessels in the lungs and muscles, ensuring that blood is diverted to the key areas required for a fight-or-flight response.

The net result of increased cardiac output and changes in vascular tone mediated through adrenaline is a sudden increase in BP.

The renin angiotensin aldosterone system (RAAS)

The RAAS is the most important hormonal mechanism for maintaining blood pressure over the long term. It is a cascade mechanism that involves several major organs working together. At the centre of this cascade is the inert plasma protein angiotensinogen, which is continually produced by the liver and found as a normal component of the blood (Figure 3.13).

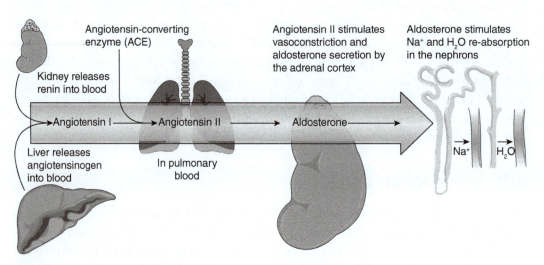

Figure 3.13   Overview of the RAAS

Source: OpenStax (2013) *Anatomy and Physiology*. Rice University. Available at: https://openstax.org/books/anatomy-and-physiology/pages/1-introduction

Biochemical steps in the RAAS

The RAAS is triggered whenever there is a drop in blood pressure and follows a set series of events, which are highlighted below.

When BP falls, the kidneys release an enzyme termed renin (Chapter 11).

- Renin rapidly converts angiotensinogen into the protein angiotensin-I.
- Angiotensin-1 is inert and has no biological activity; it circulates freely in the blood until it reaches the lungs.
- Within the lung tissue are located the angiotensin-converting enzymes (ACEs). These convert the inert angiotensin-I into its biologically active form angiotensin-II.
- Angiotensin-II binds to receptors on smooth muscle cells in the tunica media (muscle layer) of arteries to initiate vasoconstriction. The process of vasoconstriction increases peripheral resistance (PR), helping to restore BP (remember, this mechanism was triggered by a drop in BP).
- Angiotensin-II stimulates the release of aldosterone from the adrenal cortex.
- Aldosterone promotes sodium retention by the kidneys, increasing plasma sodium levels. Sodium attracts water from the tissues into the blood (water follows sodium) by osmosis, increasing blood volume and pressure.
- Angiotensin-II stimulates the release of antidiuretic hormone (ADH) from the posterior pituitary gland. As described previously, ADH increases blood volume by reducing urine output while simultaneously inducing vasoconstriction.
- The end result of the RAAS is that blood pressure is restored and maintained.

Now you have completed this chapter, attempt the multiple-choice questions in Activity 3.5 to assess your knowledge.

Activity 3.5   Multiple-choice questions

1. Which of the following layers of the heart is composed predominantly of branched cardiac muscle fibres?

   a) The endocardium
   b) The epicardium
   c) The myocardium
   d) The visceral pericardium

2. The bicuspid (mitral valve) is located

   a) Between the left atrium and left ventricle
   b) Between the right atrium and right ventricle
   c) At the origin of the pulmonary arteries
   d) At the origin of the aorta

   (Continued)

(Continued)

3. During which phase of the cardiac cycle does 70 per cent of the atrial blood volume pass into the ventricles?

    a) Isovolumetric contraction

    b) Passive ventricular filling

    c) Ejection

    d) Atrial systole

4. Which of the following resting heart rates would be referred to as tachycardia?

    a) 90 bpm

    b) 45 bpm

    c) 112 bpm

    d) 75 bpm

5. Which of the following areas of the cardiac conductive system acts as the heart's natural pacemaker?

    a) The atrioventricular bundle (bundle of His)

    b) The Purkinje fibres

    c) The atrioventricular node (AVN)

    d) The sinoatrial node (SAN)

6. Angina pectoris is usually associated with occlusion of

    a) The aorta

    b) The coronary arteries

    c) The carotid arteries

    d) The pulmonary arteries

7. Which of the following blood vessels do not carry oxygenated blood?

    a) The pulmonary veins

    b) The coronary arteries

    c) The aorta

    d) The pulmonary arteries

8. The major baroreceptors that continually measure arterial blood pressure are located in

   a) The vena cavae
   b) The pulmonary arteries
   c) The jugular veins
   d) The aortic arch and carotid sinuses

9. Antidiuretic hormone (ADH), which is also known as vasopressin, is released when

   a) Blood pressure decreases
   b) The blood is diluted by drinking too much water
   c) The kidneys need to eliminate calcium (Ca)
   d) Blood pressure increases

10. Which of the following statements relating to the renin angiotensin aldosterone system (RAAS) is true?

   a) The system is activated when blood pressure is high
   b) Angiotensinogen is produced by the kidney
   c) Angiotensin-II is a powerful vasoconstrictor
   d) Renin is produced by the liver

Chapter summary

The cardiovascular system, consisting of the heart and blood vessels, functions as the major transport system. Blood acts as the transport medium and is continually circulated throughout the body in the blood vessels. Arteries are muscular, thick-walled vessels that usually carry oxygenated blood under high pressure away from the heart, while veins are thin-walled blood vessels equipped with valves that usually carry deoxygenated blood under low pressure towards the heart.

Capillaries are the smallest blood vessels and found in complex networks termed capillary beds which permeate the tissues of the body and function to distribute blood. The right-hand side of the heart pumps deoxygenated blood to the lungs via the pulmonary circuit, while the left-hand side pumps oxygenated blood to all other

(Continued)

(Continued)

areas (organ systems) via the systemic circuit. The heart is anchored in a relatively central position within the thorax (retrosternal) and protected by a compound membrane termed the pericardium. To function as an efficient pump, the chambers of the heart contract and relax in a five-phase sequence termed the cardiac cycle.

The events of the cardiac cycle are precisely timed and coordinated by the cardiac conductive system. The electrical activity of this system can be recorded on an electrocardiogram. Blood pressure (BP) is a product of cardiac output (CO) and the peripheral resistance (PR) afforded by the blood vessels (BP = CO × PR). Ideally, blood pressure is maintained at around 120/80 mmHg by a combination of neural and hormonal mechanisms.

Activities: Brief outline answers

Activity 3.1: Research and revision (page 55)

Sequence of blood flow through major blood vessels of the heart:

Vena Cavae → Right Atrium → Tricuspid Valve → Right Ventricle → Pulmonary Artery → Pulmonary Valve → Lungs → Pulmonary Veins → Left Atrium → Bicuspid Valve → Left Ventricle → Aortic Valve → Aortic Arch

You may find it useful to make up a mnemonic or other memory aid to help remember this sequence.

Activity 3.2: Communication (page 63)

Atrial fibrillation (AF) is an arrhythmia that becomes increasingly common with advancing age. During AF the atria will be contracting rapidly and in an uncoordinated manner, which can result in poor ventricular filling. AF is often asymptomatic when at rest since 70 per cent of ventricular filling occurs passively; however, Gerald has been experiencing symptoms of breathlessness during exercise (when gardening and walking upstairs). It is during exercise that the full filling of the ventricles becomes increasingly important.

With AF the final 30 per cent of ventricular filling may not occur and as a result the cardiac output (CO) may fall, leading to the breathlessness Gerald is experiencing. AF can cause turbulent blood flow in the atria, increasing the risk of thrombosis. It is almost certainly a mobile clot (embolus) that has caused the stroke which Gerald has just suffered. Although Gerald has not recently been compliant in taking his medication, as a nurse it is vital to reinforce how essential apixiban is to managing his AF since it is this medication that will reduce the chances of clots forming and further strokes occurring.

Activity 3.3: Critical thinking (page 70)

Based on Gloria's prior history, it is clear that she has long-standing coronary artery disease. This would explain why she has experienced chest pain during exertion which is indicative of angina. Her past history of infarction indicates that portions of her heart muscle (myocardium) have been damaged. This new issue of swollen ankles and feet is worrying since peripheral oedema is a clinical feature of right-handed heart failure.

It may be that despite having stents fitted, Gloria has suffered further infarctions or the damage caused by the previous infarctions is gradually reducing the ability of the right-hand side of the heart to collect venous blood and pump it through the lungs. These new symptoms will need careful assessment to determine if any further interventions or new medications are needed to manage Gloria's heart problems.

Activity 3.4: Evidence-based practice and research (page 73)

Janet has experienced postural hypotension which has caused her fainting episode. On standing, blood pressure (BP) will fall as gravity pulls blood downwards. This drop is usually quickly detected by the baroreceptors and the heart rate is increased, and blood vessels undergo vasoconstriction to maintain BP. This baroreceptor response tends to become less efficient (blunted) with age. Janet takes a combined beta blocker and diuretic pill to treat her hypotension and this could significantly increase the risk of postural hypotension.

The beta blocker component slows Janet's heart rate reducing her cardiac output while the diuretic will increase urine production, lowering Janet's blood volume. Janet will require further assessment to determine if there are any other underlying causes for her postural hypotension. Based on this episode, Janet should be advised to rise slowly to allow her BP to normalise and she may have to be switched to a different type of antihypertensive medication.

Activity 3.5: Multiple-choice questions (pages 77–9)

1) c, 2) a, 3) b, 4) c, 5) d, 6) b, 7) d, 8) d, 9) a, 10) c

Further reading

Boore J et al. (2016) Chapter 12: The cardiovascular and lymphatic systems, in *Essentials of Anatomy and Physiology for Nursing Practice.* London: SAGE Publications Ltd.

A textbook to develop your knowledge of human anatomy and physiology that is aimed specifically at nurses.

Tortora G and Derrickson B (2017) *Tortora's Principles of Anatomy and Physiology* (15th edition). New York: John Wiley & Sons.

In-depth coverage of human anatomy and physiology.

Useful websites

www.nhs.uk/conditions/arrhythmia

A simple overview of arrhythmias.

www.cvphysiology.com/Heart%20Disease/HD002

A summary explaining in simple terms the phases of the cardiac cycle.

www.nhs.uk/conditions/high-blood-pressure-hypertension

An overview of hypertension and its causes.

www.nice.org.uk/guidance/ng136

Overview of current criteria for diagnosing and managing hypertension.

Chapter 4 The respiratory system

Nikki Williams

Chapter aims

After reading this chapter, you will be able to:

- describe the key functions of the respiratory system;
- identify the major anatomical structures of the respiratory system;
- highlight the regions of the conducting and respiratory zones;
- describe the processes of ventilation and gaseous exchange;
- explain how oxygen and carbon dioxide are transported in the blood;
- describe the mechanisms of respiratory control and the role played by the respiratory system in acid base balance.

Case study: Jake – asthma

Jake is 13 years old and has had asthma for several years. His asthma is generally well controlled, but it is made worse if he suffers from a respiratory tract infection or is exposed to a substance to which he is allergic. One afternoon, Jake and his classmates were on a cross-country run when after a few minutes Jake complained of a tight chest and started to cough profusely. Unfortunately, Jake had left his salbutamol (bronchodilator) inhaler in his bag in the changing room. Jake's close friend Isaac stayed with him and reassured him, while another friend ran to tell their PE teacher who found Jake's school bag. Within a few minutes, the teacher was able to give Jake his inhaler. After four puffs of salbutamol, Jake was feeling well enough to walk slowly back to school.

Introduction

Chronic respiratory diseases, such as the asthma affecting Jake, are routinely encountered and managed by nurses. Since the respiratory tract is in constant contact with the external environment, it is vulnerable to infection from pathogens and physical damage from toxic irritants. A significant problem in the UK and throughout the world is smoking, which progressively damages the airway and lung tissue, increasing the risk of chronic obstructive pulmonary disease (COPD) and other lung diseases, including cancer. This chapter will focus on the primary role of the respiratory tract in facilitating gaseous exchange.

We will begin by examining the structure and function of the upper and lower respiratory tract and the nature of the conduction and respiratory zones. Since nurses need a thorough understanding of the mechanics of breathing, we will explore the physical principles of inhalation and exhalation and identify the principal lung volumes and capacities. The process of gaseous exchange across the alveolar wall will be described together with the mechanisms of oxygen and carbon dioxide transport in the blood.

We will conclude the chapter by examining how breathing is controlled and how the breathing rate may influence the pH of the blood, contributing to acid base balance. Throughout the chapter we will reinforce key points with exercises and case studies highlighting common pathologies routinely encountered by nurses in clinical practice.

Functions of the respiratory system

The respiratory tract has multiple diverse functions, summarised in Table 4.1.

Table 4.1   Functions of the respiratory system

Function	Key features
Gaseous exchange	Movement of oxygen and carbon dioxide across the air sacs (alveoli) of the lungs. This is often described as the primary function of the respiratory tract
Olfaction (sense of smell)	Since odours are inhaled into the nose along with air, the respiratory tract is intimately associated with olfaction
Vocalisation	Production of sounds via the vocal cords. Vocalisation is the dominant method of communication, and this process is frequently compromised during upper respiratory tract infections
Immunity	The respiratory tract plays a vital role in the clearance of particulate materials including pathogens
Acid base balance	Control of breathing allows the pH of our blood to be regulated. The respiratory system works in conjunction with the kidneys to constrain arterial blood pH within narrow physiological limits
Blood pressure control	The lungs contain angiotensin-converting enzymes (ACEs), which play a key role in regulating blood pressure (Chapter 3)

Overview of the respiratory system

The respiratory system facilitates gas exchange by bringing air from the environment into contact with blood flowing through the pulmonary circulation (Chapter 3). The major structures of the respiratory tract include the nose, pharynx, larynx, trachea, bronchi, bronchioles, alveolar ducts, alveoli and lungs and are highlighted in Figure 4.1.

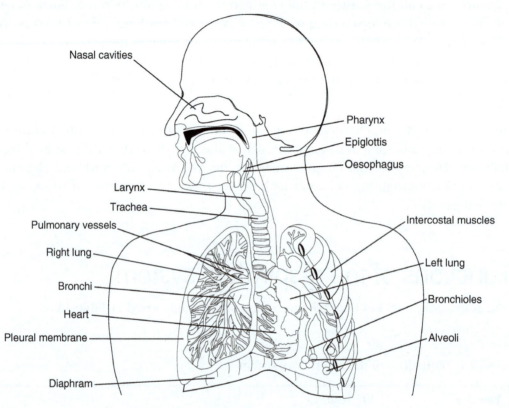

Figure 4.1 Overview of the respiratory tract

The respiratory tract is divided into upper (Figure 4.2) and lower regions.

The upper respiratory tract

The nose and nasal cavity

The nose functions as the primary inlet for air during inspiration. The upper, rigid section of the external nose is formed by the nasal bones and the frontal process of the maxilla (upper jaw bone); the lower and more flexible section is composed of hyaline cartilage. Air enters the nose through the nostrils (external nares) and passes into the nasal cavity which is divided into left and right portions by the nasal septum.

Within the nostrils, coarse hairs called vibrissae provide the first line of defence against larger airborne particles, e.g. soot, sawdust and small insects. The primary function of the nose and nasal cavity is to condition the inspired air by adding moisture (humidification) and progressively warming it so that it is closer to the inner (core) body temperature. The turbinates or conchae are bony structures which form shelf-like projections into the nasal cavities on both sides. As air enters the nose, it diverges into the left and right nasal cavities. On reaching the turbinates, airflow becomes turbulent (swirling movement), slowing its progress and allowing air to remain in contact with the warm respiratory epithelium for longer. The nasal cavities are lined by a pseudostratified epithelium, with microscopic hair-like structures called cilia projecting from the surface.

Mucus, produced by goblet cells, is secreted onto the epithelial surface to form a protective barrier, trapping pathogens and other particulate materials. The cilia move in a coordinated sweeping motion, shifting the mucus, and any trapped particulates, to the pharynx (throat) to be swallowed or expectorated. As well as acting as a physical barrier, mucus contains immune cells, secretory antibodies and an antimicrobial enzyme called lysozyme, which rapidly breaks down bacterial cell walls. A huge network of capillaries sits just below the nasal epithelium, facilitating rapid warming of air which reaches a temperature of approximately 34°C by the time it exits the nasal cavity at the nasopharynx.

The paranasal sinuses

The paranasal sinuses are air-filled cavities in the sphenoid, ethmoid, frontal and maxilla bones of the skull. These function primarily to reduce the weight of the skull and contribute to the conditioning of the inspired air. The sinuses also act as resonance chambers amplifying vocal sounds and giving each voice its own distinctive timbre; this role becomes very apparent when we suffer a head cold with sinus congestion which frequently imparts a tinny quality to the voice.

Infection and allergic responses cause the release of inflammatory mediators such as histamine, which initiates vasodilation of the capillaries underlying the epithelium of the nasal cavity. This can result in swelling and obstruction of the narrow openings to the paranasal sinuses, causing localised pain. In some cases, the sinuses may become chronically infected, leading to a painful condition called sinusitis. Histamine can also increase mucus production in the nasal cavity, leading to a streaming nose which is a common feature of many upper respiratory tract infections and allergies.

The pharynx

The pharynx is a muscular tube running from the nasal cavity to the larynx (voice box) and is often simply referred to as the throat. It consists of three sequential sections: nasopharynx, oropharynx and laryngopharynx.

The nasopharynx is the superior portion of the pharynx, which begins at the nasal cavity. It continues the process of conditioning the inspired air and, like the nasal cavity, contains a ciliated epithelium which continues the trapping and removal of particulates. The tonsils form a ring of lymphoid tissue around the pharynx; these contain populations of immune cells called macrophages which monitor the airway and trap potential pathogens such as bacteria.

There are four groups of tonsils: the pharyngeal tonsils, or adenoids, are situated superiorly and posteriorly in the nasopharynx; the tubal tonsils sit close to the openings of the Eustachian tubes which connect to the middle ear (Chapter 6); the lingual tonsils are embedded in the root of the tongue; and the palatine tonsils are located on either side of the oropharynx. It is the almond-shaped palatine tonsils that frequently become infected and often purulent during tonsillitis.

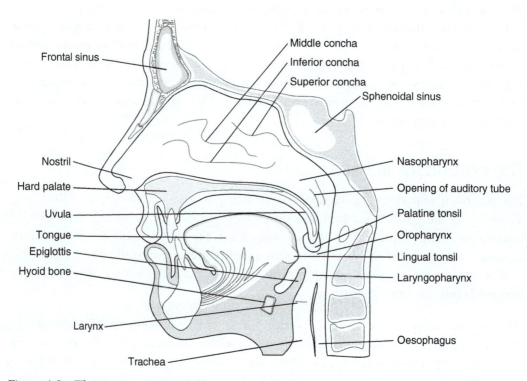

Figure 4.2   The components of the upper respiratory tract

The middle portion of the pharynx, which lies posterior to the oral cavity, is called the oropharynx. This section is part of both the respiratory and digestive systems and is lined by a thicker, non-ciliated, stratified squamous epithelium to resist the abrasive effects of swallowing food and liquids.

The final section of pharynx is called the laryngopharynx because it is continuous with the larynx. As with the oropharynx, it is part of both the respiratory and digestive tracts and is lined by the same type of robust stratified squamous epithelium.

Since these final two sections of the pharynx form a common passageway for air, food and water, there is a danger of the airway becoming occluded should food become stuck when swallowing (deglutition). Difficulty with swallowing is termed dysphagia and this becomes more common with age, increasing the risk of choking and the aspiration of food into the airway.

Obesity is an increasing problem in the UK and is associated with upper airway dysfunction. To further your understanding of this issue, read through the following case study.

Case study: Jack – obstructive sleep apnoea

Jack is a 58-year-old man with type II diabetes who is clinically obese, weighing 115 kg and having a BMI of 33.2. He has a sedentary occupation and takes little exercise. Jack was previously a heavy smoker but gave up cigarettes following a bout of pneumonia. For some months, Jack has complained of tiredness even though he sleeps 7–8 hours a night, and he attributed this to increasing age. Jack's wife has always teased Jack about his snoring, but over the past year it has become worse, and she worries that Jack seems to gasp and stop breathing numerous times throughout the night.

Eventually, Jack was persuaded to visit his GP, who referred him to the local hospital for sleep tests where obstructive sleep apnoea was diagnosed. Jack was provided with a Non-Invasive Positive Pressure Ventilation device (NIPPV) which pushes air under positive pressure into the airways via a close-fitting face mask, which prevents occlusion of the airways and allows Jack to sleep without airway obstruction and snoring.

In addition to getting relief from the use of positive pressure devices, patients such as Jack should be encouraged to lose weight which may eventually allow the use of such devices to be discontinued.

The larynx (voice box)

The larynx or voice box (Figure 4.3) is formed from nine pieces of fused cartilage and is connected superiorly to the laryngopharynx and inferiorly to the trachea or wind pipe. The largest of the laryngeal cartilages is the shield-shaped thyroid cartilage which is so-named because of its close proximity to the thyroid gland. The thyroid cartilage is also known as Adam's apple since in males it usually undergoes rapid expansion during puberty and becomes more prominent.

This expansion corresponds to a general enlargement of the larynx, which usually results in the 'breaking' and deepening of the voice characteristic of adolescent males. Probably the most well known of the laryngeal cartilages is the epiglottis; a piece of flexible elastic cartilage which functions like a 'trap door' to close over the airway during swallowing to prevent aspiration of food and fluids into the lungs (Chapter 10).

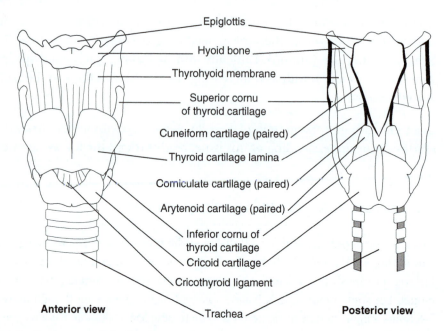

Figure 4.3 Structure of the larynx

The cricoid cartilage lies inferior to and is separated from the thyroid cartilage by the cricothyroid membrane. If the airway is occluded and the patient cannot breathe, an incision can be made in the cricothyroid membrane and a tube inserted to allow artificial ventilation to be established; this procedure is an example of intubation. Inside the larynx are the vocal cords; these are tiny ligaments that vibrate when air is passed over them to generate sound. The tension of the vocal cords can be varied by muscles to alter the pitch of sound produced; this effect is similar to what happens when tightening and loosening a guitar string.

Case study: Phillip – dysphagia

Phillip is 78 and was admitted to your ward following a stroke. While he could be roused, Phillip was experiencing a reduced level of consciousness. In line with current guidance from the National Institute for Health and Care Excellence (NICE, 2019b), the ward manager undertook a rudimentary swallowing assessment by giving Phillip a teaspoon of water to drink. Unfortunately, Phillip couldn't swallow the water, and it trickled out of the side of his mouth. Therefore, he was referred to a speech and language therapist (SALT) for a specialist assessment the next morning. Phillip was kept nil by mouth until he was assessed by the SALT.

Difficulty in swallowing (dysphagia) is common following a stroke if the glossopharyngeal nerve (cranial nerve 9) which coordinates swallowing is damaged.

Failure to recognise and adequately manage dysphagia can result in aspiration pneumonia, which can potentially lead to death.

Depending on the extent of Phillip's dysphagia, a range of measures will be considered including thickened oral fluids and nasogastric or gastrostomy feeding. Hopefully, as Phillip begins to recover from his stroke, his swallowing will improve. His recovery can be supported by the SALT.

A common mistake is to confuse the pharynx with the larynx; this confusion largely arises because these two words sound similar and are spelt in a similar manner. Remember, the term pharynx is generally used interchangeably with throat, while the larynx is the voice box.

Now that we have explored the key components of the upper respiratory tract, we need to examine the nature of the lower respiratory tract and its role in conducting air to the alveolar air sacs and in gaseous exchange.

The lower respiratory tract

The tracheobronchial tree

The airway below the vocal cords marks the beginning of the lower respiratory tract; the trachea progressively subdivides into smaller and smaller airways (Figure 4.4). The tracheobronchial tree usually consists of 23 subdivisions (generations) of the airway before the conditioned air reaches the alveolar air sacs.

The trachea

The trachea is approximately 10 to 12 cm in length and 2.5 cm in diameter. It extends from the lower border of the larynx to the carina, which marks the point where it bifurcates (splits) into the right and left primary bronchi which extend towards their respective lungs. The trachea is held open by a series of stacked C-shaped rings of cartilage which serve to reinforce and prevent the airway collapsing during inspiration and expiration. The oesophagus runs parallel to the trachea, slotting longitudinally into the long posterior groove created by the stacked C-shaped cartilaginous rings.

As in the nasal cavity and nasopharynx, the trachea is lined by a ciliated pseudostratified epithelium which sweeps contaminated mucus and particulates away from the lungs towards the pharynx to be swallowed. This mechanism is known as the mucociliary escalator because it functions in a similar manner to a mechanical stairway, continually clearing and cleaning the airway, reducing the risk of irritation and infection.

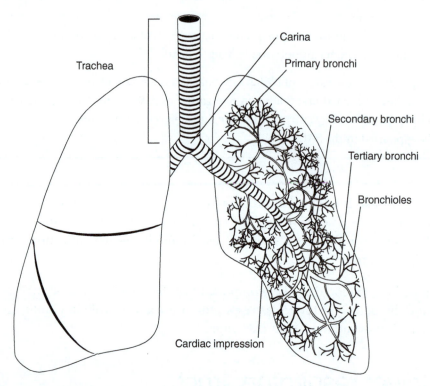

Figure 4.4   Branching structure of the respiratory tract

The carina

Located within the carina are densely arranged sensory receptors which continually monitor the airway for debris. These receptors respond to mechanical stimulation and are ideally positioned since inhaled particles will have to pass through the carina before travelling into the primary bronchi and the lungs. Once activated, these receptors initiate a vigorous coughing reflex where explosive expiration of air will usually clear irritating particulates. Unfortunately, as we grow older, the receptors of the airway become less sensitive to irritation, and this together with age-associated losses in muscle mass and strength means that the coughing reflex is less effective. This contributes to an increased risk of respiratory tract infections in older people.

The primary bronchi

The right primary bronchus is angled at approximately 20 to 30 degrees to the trachea, while the left primary bronchus is angled at between 45 and 55 degrees. This means that foreign objects entering the trachea are more likely to end up in the right bronchus and right lung than the left. As in the trachea, the primary bronchi are reinforced and held open by cartilaginous rings, but rather than being C-shaped, these are complete rings. As the bronchi subdivide, becoming smaller bronchi and bronchioles, the cartilage rings are exchanged for irregular cartilaginous plates. The right lung consists of three lobes and the left lung two (Figure 4.4).

The primary bronchi divide to form the lobar bronchi with each supplying a lobe of the lungs. The subdividing branching structure of the bronchial tree continues into each lung lobe, with each successive division (generation) of airway smaller than the one before.

Bronchioles

Bronchioles arise from the fourth generation of branching; these are small airways with a diameter of less than 1 mm and characteristically lack cartilaginous reinforcement. Structural support for the bronchioles is provided by the lung parenchyma. This is composed predominantly of the alveolar air sacs and elastic connective tissue, which attach to the external surface of these tiny airways, tethering the bronchioles (like guy ropes supporting a tent). This support is necessary to prevent airway collapse, particularly during forced inhalation and expiration.

The bronchioles themselves subdivide into smaller and smaller airways with the terminal bronchioles having a diameter of 0.5 mm or less. Smooth muscle fibres are present in the bronchiolar walls; contraction of this smooth muscle layer leads to bronchoconstriction and a narrowing of the airway. This smooth muscle is physiologically very useful since coordinated bronchoconstriction and bronchodilation can regulate airflow within the lungs. However, uncoordinated bronchoconstriction or bronchospasm can lead to air becoming trapped in the lung, which is one of the key clinical features of asthma.

The conduction zone

The airway extending from the nose all the way through the bronchial tree to the terminal bronchioles is known as the conduction zone because its role is to conduct air to the regions of the lung where gaseous exchange takes place. Jake's asthma case study at the beginning of this chapter perfectly illustrates the importance of a clear, unobstructed conduction zone and highlights why asthma must be carefully managed to ensure an adequate supply of conditioned air to the alveolar air sacs.

The respiratory zone

Each terminal bronchiole branches into several respiratory bronchioles and alveolar ducts which finally terminate in the alveolar air sacs. Collectively, these areas have a berry-like appearance (Figure 4.5) and are referred to as acini (Latin for berries). Acini are the functional units of the lungs where gas exchange takes place. In a healthy young adult, more than 30,000 of these acini are present in each lung, with each acinus having approximately 10,000 alveoli. Around 3 litres (3000 ml) of air is held within the lung acini of a typical adult male. This contrasts with the relatively small volume of air in the conducting airways, which totals only around 150 ml; this volume is known as the anatomical dead space since the air here does not reach the alveoli to participate in gas exchange.

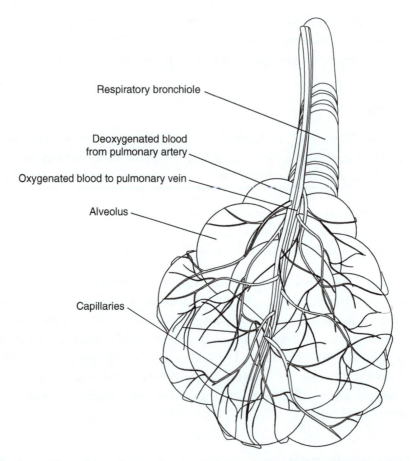

Respiratory bronchiole

Deoxygenated blood
from pulmonary artery

Oxygenated blood to pulmonary vein

Alveolus

Capillaries

Figure 4.5   A small portion of a respiratory acinus, showing alveoli and associated blood capillaries

Alveoli

The alveoli (alveolus = singular) are thin-walled, sac-like structures composed of two major cell types. Type I cells are thin, flat, squamous epithelial cells which make up around 95 per cent of the alveolar wall. These cells are elastic in nature, allowing each alveolus to inflate (like a balloon) during inspiration. The alveolar wall is incredibly delicate with a width as thin as 0.2 μm, which is roughly the same thickness as the wall of a soap bubble. The remaining 5 per cent of the alveolar wall is made up of type II alveolar cells which secrete a material called pulmonary surfactant, which reduces the surface tension of the alveoli to allow easier inflation. Without this surfactant alveolar wall, lung inflation would be extremely difficult, if not impossible.

The importance of pulmonary surfactant in this respect is revealed in premature babies born before 28 weeks' gestation where there is insufficient surfactant present. These babies cannot inflate their lungs adequately, resulting in respiratory distress syndrome; fortunately, synthetic surfactants are available to treat babies born before 28 weeks (Reuter et al., 2014). Inside each alveolus, mobile immune macrophages patrol, ingesting and destroying any particulates and pathogens that have not been cleared by the mucociliary escalator. Because of this role these macrophages are also frequently known as 'dust cells'.

The lungs and pleural membranes

The lungs are elastic organs that reside in the thoracic cavity surrounded and protected by two pleural membranes (Figure 4.6). The left lung is slightly smaller than the right lung because the apex of the heart extends into the left side of the thorax. The left lung is also slightly lower than the right lung, as the position of the heart pushes the left half of the diaphragm downwards, while the liver pushes the right half of the diaphragm upwards.

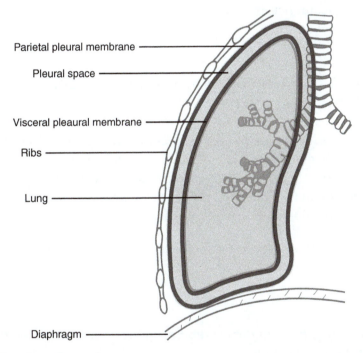

Parietal pleural membrane

Pleural space

Visceral pleaural membrane

Ribs

Lung

Diaphragm

Figure 4.6 The pleural membranes

Source: Cancer Research UK (2016)

The primary role of the pleural membranes is to hold the lung tissue up flush against the inner surface of the ribcage to facilitate the processes of inspiration and expiration (see below). There are two pleural membranes: the visceral pleural membrane is attached to the outer surface of the lungs, while the parietal pleural membrane lines the inner surface of the chest wall. There is a narrow space between the two pleurae called the pleural cavity, which is filled with 10–20 ml of pleural fluid. This fluid ensures the two pleural membranes are held tightly together by surface tension in the same way that a thin layer of water would stick two sheets of glass together. This adherence is essential for breathing (ventilation) since it ensures that when the rib cage expands during inspiration, the elastic tissues of the lungs also expand. The pleural fluid also acts as a lubricant to prevent abrasion to the outer surface of the delicate lung tissue. Unfortunately, if bacteria gain access to the pleural cavity, they can grow rapidly in the pleural fluid, leading to a painful condition called pleurisy.

Pneumothorax, chest drain and underwater seal

If air is introduced between the pleural membranes, the attractive force (surface tension) between them is disrupted, and the elastic recoil of the lung causes the lung to pull away from the chest wall and deflate (collapse). This is called a pneumothorax and is a life-threatening emergency. A pneumothorax may be caused by a penetrating chest wound, or during or following thoracic surgery. To further your understanding of pneumothorax, attempt Activity 4.1.

Activity 4.1   Pneumothorax – evidence-based practice and research

John, a 23-year-old man, was taken to his local A&E after a mugging in which he was stabbed in the left side of his chest. Within minutes of the injury, John was experiencing severe chest pain, dyspnoea (difficulty breathing) and tightness in the chest, and had a heart rate of 125. What would be the treatment required to relieve John's symptoms?

There are some possible answers to all activities at the end of the chapter, unless otherwise indicated.

Now that you have a good understanding of the respiratory tract structure, we will examine the process of breathing

Pulmonary ventilation (breathing)

Breathing involves cycles of inspiration and expiration, where air enters and leaves the lungs.

Ventilation relies predominantly on respiratory muscles which facilitate the mechanical processes of inspiration and expiration. The diaphragm is a dome-shaped sheet of skeletal muscle that separates the thoracic cavity from the abdominal cavity, while the intercostal muscles are found between the ribs. There are two major groups of intercostals: the external intercostal muscles are found on the outer side of the ribcage, while the internal intercostal muscles are located on the inner surface of the ribcage.

A bit of simple physics

To fully comprehend the mechanics of inspiration and expiration, two simple principles of physics need to be understood (no mathematics needed).

1. Volume is inversely proportional to pressure: This is known as Boyle's law and can be explained very easily. If you take a bag (a crisp bag would be perfect) and scrunch up the end, when you squeeze the bag, you reduce its volume, which increases the pressure inside. Conversely, if you stop squeezing the bag, its volume increases and the pressure inside decreases. This is what we mean when we say volume is inversely proportional to pressure: in plain English, when you reduce the volume of a container, the pressure increases, and when you increase the volume of a container, the pressure decreases (Figure 4.7).

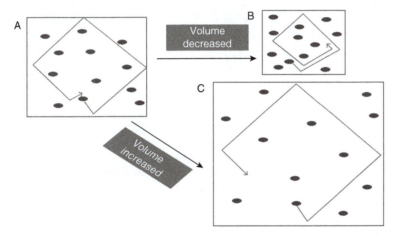

Figure 4.7   Boyle's law in action

© Nikki Williams

2. Air moves from regions of high pressure to regions of low pressure: We know this intuitively, and the concept is very easy to demonstrate with a bicycle pump. If you put your finger over the end of the pump and push in the plunger, the pressure builds up inside; when you take your finger off the end of the pump, the air will rush out of the pump into the atmosphere. You have just demonstrated the simple principle that air moves from regions of high pressure to regions of low pressure.

To help you understand these principles, attempt Activity 4.2.

Activity 4.2   Understanding Boyle's law

Read through physics principle 2 above. Why would pushing the plunger into a pump increase the pressure inside?

Now that you have learnt these two simple physical principles, you will be able to understand the mechanics of inspiration and expiration (Figure 4.8).

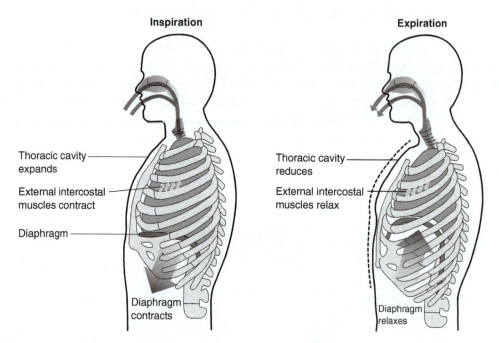

Figure 4.8   Mechanics of inspiration and expiration

Source: OpenStax (2013) *Anatomy and Physiology*. Rice University. Available at: https://openstax.org/books/anatomy-and-physiology/pages/1-introduction

Inspiration

Inspiration is an active process that requires energy. During inspiration, the diaphragm contracts and moves downwards while the external intercostal muscles contract, lifting the ribcage upwards and outwards. This increases the volume of the thoracic cavity, decreasing the pressure within (remember, volume is inversely proportional to pressure). Eventually, the pressure inside the thorax falls below that of the atmosphere, and air rushes into the respiratory tract, inflating the elastic lung tissue (remember, air flows from regions of high pressure). The process of lung expansion and inflation is aided by the pleural membranes which attach the lungs to the inner wall of the thorax. The pleural membranes ensure the elastic lungs expand as the volume of the thorax increases.

Expiration

Expiration can be regarded as the opposite process to inspiration. At rest, expiration is primarily a passive process with minimal energy expenditure. During expiration the diaphragm relaxes and moves upwards into the thorax; this is aided by the recoil of the abdominal organs such as the stomach, liver and intestines. Simultaneously the internal intercostal muscles contract to pull the ribcage downwards and inwards. These events reduce the volume of the thoracic cavity, increasing the pressure inside (volume is inversely proportional to pressure).

Eventually, the pressure inside the thorax rises above that of the atmosphere, and air rushes out of the lungs which deflate (air moves from regions of high pressure to regions of low pressure). Again, the pleural membranes are essential to this process since their firm attachment to the lungs ensures that when the volume of the thorax is reduced during expiration, the lungs are squeezed. This helps increase the pressure within the bronchial tree, forcing air out.

Accessory muscles of respiration

When breathing becomes laboured, e.g. during high-intensity exercise or in the presence of significant lung disease, the diaphragm and intercostal muscles may require additional support to ensure adequate airflow into and out of the lungs. The muscles of the neck, shoulders and upper chest, such as the scalenes, sternocleidomastoids and pectoral muscles, can all help with expanding the thorax during the active phase of inspiration.

Lung volumes and capacities

Lung function can be tested using a variety of devices including spirometers and peak flow meters. Spirometry can be used to assess lung volume capacities (a capacity is calculated by adding two or more lung volumes together) (Figure 4.9). During normal breathing, when in a relaxed state, around half a litre (500 ml) of air is inspired into and expired from the lungs. Since this volume of air is continually coming in and out of the respiratory tract, it is referred to as the tidal volume. If a patient is asked to inhale as much air as possible after a normal tidal inhalation, this volume is known as the inspiratory reserve volume (IRV), and in health this is around 2–3 litres (2000–3000 ml).

Conversely, the expiratory reserve volume (ERV) is the amount of air that can be exhaled following a normal tidal exhalation, and in health this is normally between 0.8 and 1.1 litres (800–1100 ml). If the IRV and ERV are added together, the resulting value is called the vital capacity (VC), and this can vary between 3 and 5 litres (3000–5000 ml). Since it is impossible to fully exhale all of the air within the lungs, a certain amount of air will remain following a full forced expiration; this remaining air is called the residual volume (RV) and is usually around 1.2 litres (1200 ml). If the IRV, ERV and RV are added together, the resulting value is the total lung capacity, and this typically ranges between 4 and 6 litres (4000–6000 ml).

Lung volumes and capacities are commonly assessed as one of the best indicators of overall lung and respiratory health. Such assessments are routinely carried out to monitor chronic lung diseases such as COPD and asthma.

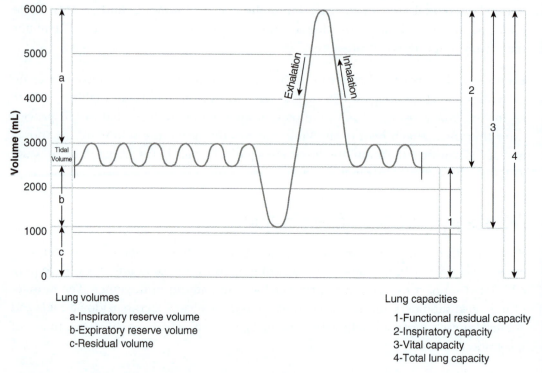

Figure 4.9 Lung volumes and capacities

Gas exchange

Gas exchange is the primary function of the alveoli, and the alveolar structure is perfectly adapted to this role. Each alveolus is surrounded by a tight network of extremely thin-walled capillaries allowing inspired air and blood to be brought into close proximity. This facilitates the efficient diffusion of gases; remember, the thickness of the alveolar wall is comparable to the wall of a soap bubble, ranging between only 0.2 μm and 2.5 μm in thickness. The total surface area of all the alveoli that are in contact with the alveolar capillaries is approximately 100 m² (half the area of a singles tennis court). Oxygen from inspired air diffuses rapidly across the alveolar wall into the blood, circulating through the alveolar capillaries, while simultaneously carbon dioxide diffuses from the blood into the alveoli to be expired.

Oxygen transport

Oxygen is not very soluble in the aqueous medium of the blood, so only around 1.5 per cent oxygen is transported dissolved in the plasma. As much as 98.5 per cent of oxygen diffuses into the erythrocytes (red blood cells) circulating through the alveolar capillaries and binds to haemoglobin. Haemoglobin is a dark cherry-red protein containing four haem groups, each of which contains an iron ion (Fe^{2+}). Oxygen molecules (O_2) bind to the haem groups resulting in bright cherry-red oxyhaemoglobin. Since there are four haem groups, each haemoglobin molecule is capable of binding to four oxygen molecules. As described in Chapter 3, oxygenated blood flows around the systemic circulation, constantly delivering oxygen to the tissues. Gas exchange between the blood and the cells which form our tissues is often referred to as internal respiration.

Pulse oximetry

Nurses routinely use a device which clips onto a finger called a pulse oximeter to give a non-invasive estimate of blood oxygen saturation, known as SpO_2. In health, an SpO_2 value of 98 per cent would be typical and indicates that 98 per cent of the haemoglobin molecules in the blood have the full complement of four oxygen molecules. These devices shine a light through the skin and effectively measure the colour of the blood to derive their readings (remember, haemoglobin is dark cherry-red while oxyhaemoglobin is a much brighter cherry-red colour). Patients with respiratory disease or heart disease may have a low SpO_2 (below 95 per cent), and readings may also be reduced in a variety of other diseases such as anaemia and kidney disease.

To help you understand the use of pulse oximetry in clinical practice, attempt Activity 4.3.

Activity 4.3   Oxygen therapy – evidence-based practice and research

Jamilla is a 75-year-old lady living with chronic obstructive pulmonary disease (COPD) after many years of heavy smoking. She has been admitted to a respiratory ward with an infective exacerbation of her COPD. While in otherwise healthy people, an oxygen saturation level (SpO_2) of 95–100 per cent is normal, in people with severe COPD, SpO_2 of between 88 and 92 per cent is not uncommon. In order to maintain this value, Jamilla is prescribed 24 per cent oxygen via nasal cannulae in accordance with British Thoracic Society Guidelines (O'Driscoll et al., 2017). Use textbooks and other resources to explain how oxygen therapy works to improve SpO_2 levels.

Carbon monoxide (CO) poisoning

Carbon monoxide (CO) combines with haemoglobin in the same way as oxygen. It is, however, a poisonous gas, colourless, odourless and tasteless. It can be released into the environment from the combustion of fossil fuels such as coal and gas, and is also found in car exhaust fumes and cigarette smoke. Once in the lungs, CO diffuses into deoxygenated erythrocytes, where it combines with haemoglobin to form carbonmonoxyhaemoglobin. The affinity of haemoglobin for carbon monoxide is about 250 times greater than that for oxygen. Thus, carbon monoxide binds more readily and less reversibly to haemoglobin than oxygen does, and depending upon levels of exposure, inhibits the ability of the blood to transport oxygen to body tissues.

With chronic low-dose exposure (e.g. smoking) the reduced oxygen availability can cause hypoxia, resulting in an increased production of red cells. This in turn may raise plasma viscosity and BP, causing vasoconstriction in the pulmonary capillaries and possible lung damage. A high dose of CO (e.g. attempted suicide by exposure to car exhaust) may be fatal or cause permanent damage to the regions of the brain with the highest metabolic demands, such as the cortex and the basal ganglia. In mothers who smoke during pregnancy, the inhalation of CO may cause intra-uterine growth retardation of their babies.

Carbon dioxide transport

In the tissues

Carbon dioxide (CO_2) is produced as the major metabolic waste product by cells during cellular metabolism. The transport of carbon dioxide in the blood is more complex than oxygen and is one of the concepts of physiology that students often struggle with.

There are three major ways of transporting CO_2. CO_2 is more soluble than oxygen in the aqueous medium of the blood. This allows approximately 8 per cent of the total CO_2 to be transported dissolved in the plasma. A further 20 per cent of CO_2 crosses into the erythrocytes and binds to haemoglobin to form carbaminohaemoglobin.

By far, the greatest proportion of CO_2, i.e. the remaining 72 per cent, is transported in the form of bicarbonate ions (HCO_3^-). Erythrocytes contain an enzyme called carbonic anhydrase which links a molecule of CO_2 to a molecule of water (H_2O) to form carbonic acid (H_2CO_3). This weak acid is unstable and rapidly breaks down (dissociates) into hydrogen ions (H^+) and bicarbonate ions (HCO_3^-). As you can see, the single atom of carbon and the two atoms of oxygen which originally formed the CO_2 molecule are now incorporated in the bicarbonate ion (HCO_3^-).

$$CO_2 + H_2O \xrightarrow{\text{Carbonic anhydrase}} H_2CO_3 \longrightarrow HCO_3^- + H^+$$

$$\text{carbon dioxide + water} \qquad \text{carbonic acid} \qquad \text{bicarbonate ion + hydrogen ion}$$

In the alveoli

As blood passes through the alveolar capillaries, the CO_2 that has been transported dissolved in the plasma will diffuse rapidly across into the alveoli. Similarly, the CO_2 transported in the form of carbaminohaemoglobin will dissociate from its haemoglobin vehicle before diffusing across the alveolar wall.

The carbonic anhydrase reaction highlighted above is reversible, so when blood rich in bicarbonate ions (HCO_3^-) reaches the alveoli, the dissociated hydrogen ions (H^+) and bicarbonate ions (HCO_3^-) re-associate to form carbonic acid (H_2CO_3). The erythrocyte enzyme carbonic anhydrase then splits the carbonic acid (H_2CO_3) into water (H_2O) and CO_2, allowing the free CO_2 to diffuse into the alveoli.

The CO_2 from all three modes of transport can then be exhaled from the lungs.

The respiratory system and acid base balance

Respiratory acidosis

Since CO_2 combines with water to form carbonic acid which then dissociates to give hydrogen ions (H^+) and bicarbonate ions (HCO_3^-), any rise in the CO_2 level will increase the acidity of the blood (lowering its pH). Normal arterial blood pH is around 7.35–7.45. Increased CO_2 is commonly seen in lung diseases which decrease respiratory function, reducing the clearance of CO_2. Since increased CO_2 increases blood acidity, this is known as a respiratory acidosis. In health increased blood CO_2 and acidity would normally be detected by specialised chemoreceptors (see below), and the respiratory rate would be increased to 'blow off' the excess CO_2 and normalise the pH of the blood.

However, with chronic lung diseases such as COPD, this may not be possible. Acidosis is usually defined as an arterial blood pH of less than 7.35. If this is caused by a respiratory acidosis, then the kidneys will usually attempt to compensate by retaining alkaline compounds such as bicarbonate ions (HCO_3^-) to bring the arterial pH to back within its normal limits.

We have just examined the nature of respiratory acidosis; in the case study in Activity 4.4, we have the opposite situation. Read through Sian's history and explain how hyperventilation could lead to a respiratory alkalosis.

Activity 4.4   Hyperventilation and respiratory alkalosis – evidence-based practice and research

Sian suffers from anxiety and during episodes of extreme stress often hyperventilates. This is due to the body's response to adrenaline which prepares the body for 'flight or fight' by increasing oxygen intake to power our muscles in order to deal with the danger. However, unless the stress can be dealt with in a physical way, hyperventilation can cause unpleasant symptoms such as dizziness or breathlessness. You are asked to accompany Sian to a CT scan which has made her extremely anxious, and as she enters the X-ray department, she has a panic attack and begins to hyperventilate.

How can you help Sian regain control of her breathing?

We have just seen from Sian's case study that the breathing rate can significantly influence the pH of the blood. Pulmonary ventilation and gas exchange need to be tightly regulated to ensure sufficient O_2 is available for normal cellular respiration and CO_2 levels and arterial blood pH are maintained within acceptable limits.

Control of ventilation

The respiratory centres in the medulla oblongata are connected to the major respiratory muscle groups. The phrenic nerve innervates the diaphragm, while the intercostal muscle groups are innervated by the intercostal nerves (Figure 4.9). Two major respiratory areas are located within the medulla. The dorsal respiratory group (DRG) is located at the back of the medulla and controls normal restful breathing by acting as a respiratory pacemaker. The DRG typically sets the baseline respiratory rate at approximately 15 to 20 breaths per minute and appears to be primarily involved in driving inspiration.

To the front of the medulla is the ventral respiratory group (VRG), which tends to activate when more forceful breathing is required. The VRG seems to have a more dominant role in controlling the process of expiration and in particular forced expiration. The third respiratory group is called the pontine group because of its location in the pons of the brain stem (Chapter 6); it plays a role in regulating both the respiratory rate and the depth of breathing.

Peripheral and central chemoreceptors

Two major groupings of chemoreceptors monitor blood gas concentrations and pH, continually relaying real-time information to the respiratory centres. The peripheral chemoreceptors consist of the carotid bodies within the carotid sinuses of the carotid arteries and the aortic bodies within the aortic arch. A second group of chemoreceptors are found on the surface of the medulla oblongata. Since these are close to the midline of the body, they are called central chemoreceptors. When the peripheral and central chemoreceptors detect an increase in acidity, which is typically associated with elevated CO_2, the respiratory centres respond by increasing the breathing rate and depth.

Modifications to the normal breathing pattern

When necessary, the normal breathing pattern can be interrupted to allow protective mechanisms such as the coughing and sneezing reflexes to be initiated. Simple everyday tasks such as speaking or blowing up a balloon also require interruption of normal breathing.

Throughout the lung tissue, there are large numbers of stretch receptors which continually monitor lung inflation and feed information back to the respiratory centre to limit over-inflation. This is a well-understood reflex response known as the Hering-Breuer reflex and is particularly important in neonates, where the ribcage is more flexible and the lungs more susceptible to hyperinflation.

Now you have completed this chapter, test your acquired knowledge by attempting the short series of multiple-choice questions in Activity 4.5.

Activity 4.5 Multiple-choice questions

1. Which of the following regions of the airway is *not* part of the upper respiratory tract?

   a) The nasal cavity
   b) The carina
   c) The oropharynx
   d) The turbinate bones

2. The paranasal cavities are air-filled cavities in which bones?

   a) Sphenoid, ethmoid, frontal and turbinate bones
   b) Turbinate, sphenoid, ethmoid and frontal bones
   c) Sphenoid, turbinate, frontal and maxilla bones
   d) Sphenoid, ethmoid, frontal and maxilla bones

3. The functional unit of the lung is known as the

   a) Acinus
   b) Acetate
   c) Acronyx
   d) Actin

4. Which of the following is *not* true of the alveoli?

   a) Alveoli are thin-walled, sac-like structures composed of type I and type II alveolar cells
   b) Type I cells are flat and make up approximately 95 per cent of the alveolar wall
   c) Particulate material is cleared by type I cells
   d) Type II cells make surfactant

(Continued)

(Continued)

5. During inspiration

    a) The thoracic volume increases

    b) The pressure inside the thorax increases

    c) The thoracic volume decreases

    d) The diaphragm relaxes and moves upwards

6. Which of the following are the accessory muscles of respiration?

    a) Diaphragm, scalenes, sternocleidomastoids

    b) Scalenes, sternocleidomastoids, pectoral

    c) Scalenes, diaphragm, pectoral

    d) Pectoral, sternocleidomastoids, diaphragm

7. The law that states that volume is inversely proportional to the pressure is:

    a) Charle's law

    b) Gay-Lussac's law

    c) Avagadro's law

    d) Boyle's law

8. When fully saturated, haemoglobin can carry

    a) Four oxygen molecules

    b) Eight oxygen molecules

    c) Two oxygen molecules

    d) One oxygen molecule

9. The process by which oxygen moves from the alveoli into the pulmonary capillaries is

    a) Osmosis

    b) Active transfer

    c) Passive transfer

    d) Simple diffusion

10. The percentage of CO_2 carried in the blood as the bicarbonate ion (HCO_3^-) is

    a) 8 per cent

    b) 20 per cent

    c) 72 per cent

    d) 100 per cent

Chapter summary

The respiratory system is divided into the upper and lower respiratory tracts. The upper respiratory tract is primarily concerned with conditioning inhaled air by humidification and warming the air nearer to the core temperature. The upper respiratory tract also begins the process of trapping and removing particulates. The lower respiratory tract is primarily concerned with gaseous exchange. Air is initially passed along the conduction zones of the branching tracheobronchial tree to the respiratory zone and acini, which are functional units of the lungs which contain the alveolar air sacs.

During inspiration, the thoracic cavity expands and the pressure inside drops, allowing air to rush in and inflate the lungs. Expiration involves reducing the thoracic volume, increasing the pressure inside the thorax and forcing air from the lungs. Gas exchange takes place within the respiratory zone of the airway, predominantly in the alveolar air sacs. Oxygen rapidly diffuses into the blood with most transported to the tissues bound to haemoglobin. Carbon dioxide is the major waste product of respiration; the majority of carbon dioxide is transported to the lungs for elimination in the form of bicarbonate ions.

The process of ventilation is controlled by the respiratory centres of the brain stem; these receive sensory input from the central and peripheral chemoreceptors and are able to modify the breathing rate and pattern. The respiratory system can influence the pH of the blood and in conjunction with the kidneys helps maintain acid base balance.

Activities: Brief outline answers

Activity 4.1: Pneumothorax – evidence-based practice and research (page 94)

The treatment for a significant pneumothorax is a chest drain with an underwater seal. A sterile tube is inserted between the ribs, and negative pressure is applied to the tube to drain the air from the pleural cavity, which allows the lung to re-inflate and re-adhere to the chest wall. Once sealed, the rate of re-absorption of air in the pleural space is 1.24 per cent of the volume of the pneumothorax in each 24 hours, so recovery can take 20 days for a pneumothorax that occupies 25 per cent of the pleural cavity (Choi, 2014).

Activity 4.2: Understanding Boyle's law (page 95)

When the plunger is pushed into the pump, the volume of the pump chamber decreases and in accordance with Boyle's law the pressure inside rises (remember, volume is inversely proportional to pressure).

Activity 4.3: Oxygen therapy – evidence-based practice and research (page 99)

The air we breathe is a gas mixture composed of approximately 78.05 per cent nitrogen, 20.94 per cent oxygen and 0.04 per cent carbon dioxide, plus very small amounts of argon and other inert gases. At sea level, the pressure of air (atmospheric pressure) is around 101 kPa or 760 mmHg; this is the total pressure exerted by air on the surface of the Earth. We can calculate the partial pressure of any of the individual gases in air using the following formula: Partial pressure of gas = (% of gas/100) in air × the total pressure of the air. So, the partial pressure of oxygen in the air we breathe (at sea level) is (20.94/100) × 760 mmHg = 159.14 mmHg, or (20.94/100) × 101 kPa = 21.14 kPa.

Oxygen therapy works by increasing the partial pressure of oxygen entering the patient's respiratory system, which increases the partial pressure gradient between the alveoli and pulmonary capillary blood. Oxygen therapy is delivered using a reservoir of 100 per cent oxygen, from a piped oxygen system in a hospital setting, a cylinder of oxygen or an oxygen concentrator in the patient's home, which is delivered to the patient via a face mask or nasal cannula. The partial pressure of oxygen delivered to the patient having oxygen therapy is called the fractional inspired concentration, FiO2. This is determined by the flow rate of oxygen and the type of interface (mask or cannula) used. Typically, the FiO2 given during oxygen therapy is 0.24, 0.28, 0.35 or 0.60, which equates to increasing the partial pressure of oxygen in the air from 21 per cent to 24 per cent, 28 per cent, 35 per cent or 60 per cent.

Activity 4.4: Hyperventilation and respiratory alkalosis – evidence-based practice and research (page 101)

It is important to support Sian in regaining control of her breathing. You should talk to her gently and reassure her. If possible, take her somewhere private and quiet. Breathing through the nose rather than the mouth will encourage slower, deeper and calmer breathing. If this doesn't help, it might be helpful to encourage Sian to breathe out through pursed lips. It's harder to hyperventilate when you breathe through your nose or pursed lips because you can't move as much air.

Abdominal or diaphragmatic breathing can also help. Help Sian to sit or lie down and ask her to place one hand on her abdomen and the other on her chest. Sian should breathe in deeply through her nose so that the breath pushes against the hand on her abdomen. As Sian breathes out, she should be able to feel her hand fall. Her chest should not move. Ask Sian to focus on doing this and repeat until she feels calmer. Counting to four during each breath in and each breath out will slow her breathing down.

Activity 4.5: Multiple-choice questions (pages 103–4)

1) b, 2) d, 3) a, 4) c, 5) a, 6) b, 7) d, 8) a, 9) d, 10) c

Further reading

Kenny BJ, Ponichtera K Physiology, Boyle's Law. In: StatPearls [Internet]. Treasure Island (FL): StatPearls Publishing; 2020 Jan-. Available from: https://www.ncbi.nlm.nih.gov/books/NBK538183/

Spicuzza L, Caruso D and Di Maria G (2015) Obstructive sleep apnoea syndrome and its management: Therapeutic advances in chronic disease, 6(5): 273–85.

Useful websites

http://sleepeducation.org/essentials-in-sleep/sleep-apnea

This website provides accessible information on sleep apnoea from the American Academy of Sleep Medicine.

www.msdmanuals.com/en-sg/professional/pulmonary-disorders/symptoms-of-pulmonary-disorders/hyperventilation-syndrome#v911280

Online medical resource highlighting features of hyperventilation.

Chapter 5 The endocrine system

Chapter aims

After reading this chapter, you will be able to:

- explain how hormones act as blood-borne chemical signals;
- describe the nature of peptide and steroid hormones;
- highlight the overlap between the endocrine and nervous systems;
- identify the major endocrine glands and their location;
- explain how the major hormones exert their physiological effects;
- describe how hormones play a crucial role in maintaining homeostasis.

Introduction

Case study: Sharma – hypothyroidism

Sharma has noticed that for the last few years she has gradually accumulated an extra 32 pounds (14.5 kg) of body weight. Since she is 48, she assumed this weight gain was due to approaching the menopause, which she also blames for her increasing lack of get-up-and-go and feelings of total exhaustion. For the last few years she has noticed that her heating bills have increased and her family are complaining that she has the central heating set too high, but she can never seem to get warm and frequently wakes up in the morning with cold feet and hands.

Sharma visited her GP because she has noted significant hair loss which has left her with small patches of scalp visible. She has also admitted to feelings of anxiety and depression. After doing a thorough examination, her GP arranged for a blood sample to be taken, and a week later Sharma was diagnosed with hypothyroidism and was immediately prescribed levothyroxine, which has gradually alleviated most of her symptoms.

Endocrine disorders such as the hypothyroidism experienced by Sharma and diabetes mellitus diagnosed in Ian (Chapter 2) are very prevalent and require careful assessment and management. The endocrine system consists of several glands which release their secretions, called hormones, directly into the blood. The cardiovascular system therefore plays a key role in circulating these hormones, most of which are either dissolved in the plasma or transported bound to plasma proteins such as albumin. Hormones act as simple chemical messengers which are able to interact with receptors at target cells and tissues which may be distant from their site of origin. The endocrine system, together with the nervous system, plays a crucial role in integrating the activities of the major organ systems, ensuring that the homeostatic balance essential to health and survival can be maintained.

This chapter will begin by providing an overview of the general features of endocrine glands before exploring the structure of peptide and steroid hormones. Once you have an understanding of the nature of hormones and their role as chemical signals, we will then examine the structure and function of each of the major endocrine glands, working from the top to the bottom of the body. The physiology of key hormones will be explored, including their site of synthesis, target organs and tissues and the major effects they exert. Throughout the chapter, we will consolidate key information by exploring endocrine pathologies commonly encountered in clinical practice.

Overview of the endocrine system

Most glands in the human body, such as sweat glands or salivary glands, release their secretions into a central duct which acts to carry the secretion to its site of action. Endocrine glands (Figure 5.1) differ in that they do not have ducts (ductless) but are highly vascular, allowing hormones to be secreted directly into the blood and transported to their target organs and tissues.

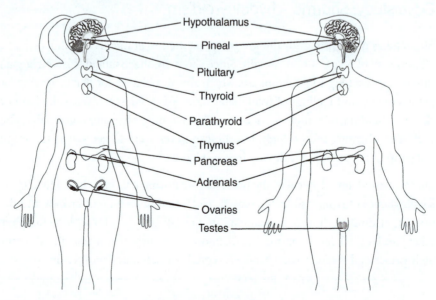

Figure 5.1 Glands and organs of the endocrine system

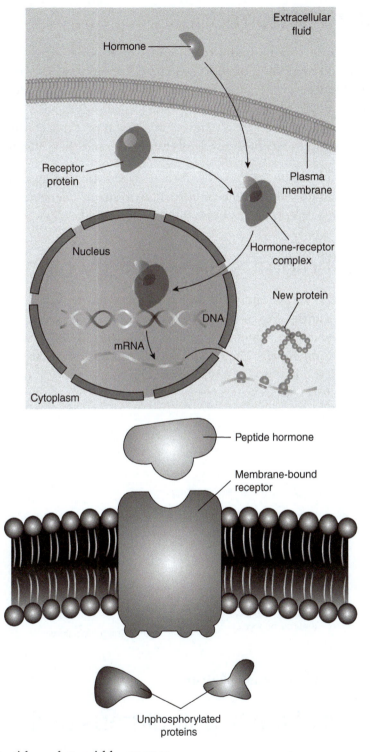

Figure 5.2   Peptide and steroid hormones

Source: Zifan, A (2016) Regulation of gene expression by steroid hormone receptor. Available at: https://
commons.wikimedia.org/w/index.php?search=steroid+hormones&title=Special%3ASearch&go=Go&ns0
=1&ns6=1&ns12=1&ns14=1&ns100=1&ns106=1#/media/File:Regulation_of_gene_expression_by_steroid_
hormone_receptor.svg

The nature of hormones

Hormones are broadly divided into two major classes. Peptide hormones are proteinaceous in nature and composed of short sequences of amino acids, and usually exert their effects by binding to receptors which are located on the outside of the plasma membrane (Figure 5.2). Steroid hormones such as testosterone are synthesised from cholesterol. Since steroids are lipids, they are able to diffuse through the plasma membrane and usually bind to receptors inside of the cell to exert their effects (Figure 5.2).

Some hormones fall outside of these two broad classes; for example, adrenaline is a simple hormone synthesised from the amino acids tyrosine or phenylalanine. Hormones are specific to their receptors and slot into the receptor site like a key going into a lock.

The hypothalamus and pituitary gland

The hypothalamus is an almond-sized region of the brain typically weighing around 4 g. As well as being a vital area of the brain (Chapter 6), the hypothalamus is also a key component of the endocrine system and is responsible for producing several hormones essential to human physiology. The hypothalamus extends downwards into the posterior pituitary, which is composed of neural tissue and can be thought of as an extension of the hypothalamus (Figure 5.3).

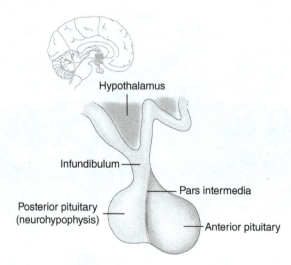

Figure 5.3   The hypothalamus and pituitary

Hormones of the hypothalamus and posterior pituitary

The hormones produced by the hypothalamus are synthesised in the cell bodies of the hypothalamic neurons (nerve cells) before being concentrated and stored in the posterior pituitary prior to release.

Antidiuretic hormone (vasopressin)

As described in Chapter 3, antidiuretic hormone (ADH) is released from the posterior pituitary gland when there is a drop in blood pressure or increase in the plasma solute concentration. As suggested by its name, the primary function of ADH is to reduce urine output, and this hormone plays a key role in fine-tuning the volume of urine produced by the kidneys to maintain effective water balance. The mechanism of action of ADH is explained in detail in Chapter 11.

To help you understand the importance of ADH in water balance, read through Paul's case study.

Case study: Paul – diabetes insipidus

Paul is a 27-year-old scaffolder who had an accident at work and fell approximately 3 m, sustaining a head injury. He was rushed to the hospital and admitted to the neurology intensive care unit. The following day, it was noticed that his urine output over the previous 24 hours was in excess of 3500 mls and that his urine was pale in colour. Doctors suspected that Paul's posterior pituitary gland was damaged and was no longer releasing ADH, resulting in diabetes insipidus (the release of copious, dilute urine). Paul was initially given 100 µg of desmopressin (a drug that mimics ADH) three times daily to manage his increased diuresis. Gradually, as Paul recovered, his posterior pituitary resumed ADH secretion, and the desmopressin was discontinued.

Paul's case study highlights how important it is for nurses to fastidiously monitor urine output; otherwise, Paul would not have received such a swift diagnosis and treatment.

Oxytocin

The second major hormone produced by the hypothalamus and concentrated, stored and released from the posterior pituitary is oxytocin. This is the hormone that initiates labour (parturition) and its role was discussed in Chapter 2.

Origin of the anterior pituitary

While the posterior pituitary is composed of neural tissue, the anterior pituitary is formed from the roof of the oral cavity. During early human development, the epithelial tissue forming the roof of the mouth bulges upwards (invaginates) into the skull to create a small bubble called Rathke's pouch. This bubble fuses with the posterior pituitary gland to form the anterior pituitary gland (Figure 5.3).

In most individuals, during early development, Rathke's pouch closes, sealing off the roof of the mouth from the cranial cavity; however, in some babies, this closure may be incomplete, potentially leading to clefts and cysts. The mature pituitary gland is typically around 8 mm wide (often described as the size of a large garden pea) and weighs approximately 500 mg.

Hormones of the anterior pituitary

The anterior pituitary produces several 'stimulating hormones' which are involved in regulating the activity of other distant endocrine glands; for this reason, the pituitary is often referred to as 'the master gland'. However, the activity of the anterior pituitary is itself regulated by the hypothalamus, which produces a variety of releasing hormones. Ultimately the hypothalamus governs the function of many of the major endocrine glands and forms a critical crossover point that bridges the activities of the central nervous system and endocrine system.

The anterior pituitary and somatotropin

Somatotropin (growth hormone) is a small protein consisting of 191 amino acids. Its primary role is in promoting bone growth and this role is explored in detail in Chapter 8. Somatotropin also stimulates the growth of most internal organs and increases lean muscle mass.

The pars intermedia and melanocyte-stimulating hormone (MSH)

The pars intermedia is the inner portion of the anterior pituitary gland and corresponds to the zone where the anterior pituitary fuses with its posterior portion. It is the source of melanocyte-stimulating hormone (MSH) which helps regulate the activity of the pigment-producing cells (melanocytes) present in the lower layer of the epidermis of the skin (Chapter 7). Melanocytes respond to MSH by releasing the dark-black pigment melanin, which protects the skin from damaging ultraviolet radiation.

MSH secretion usually increases during pregnancy, and together with the effects of oestrogen and progesterone, this causes a darkening (hyperpigmentation) of skin around the nipples (areolae) and sometimes the appearance of a vertical dark line along the midline of the abdomen (linea nigra). Many pregnant women also notice a darkening around their eye sockets, cheekbones, upper lip, nose and forehead; this hyperpigmentation of the face is termed melasma or the 'mask of pregnancy' (Handel et al., 2014).

The thyroid gland

The thyroid is a small bilobed gland typically weighing around 14–16 g. It is positioned just below the larynx and consists of two major cell types. Follicular cells are typically cube-shaped and synthesise hormones that regulate metabolism, while parafollicular cells are diamond-shaped cells which synthesise the hormone calcitonin, involved in calcium homeostasis. The posterior portion of the thyroid gland has four small areas of glandular tissue embedded within. These are the parathyroid glands (Figure 5.4) which synthesise parathyroid hormone (PTH), which functions as the natural antagonist of calcitonin.

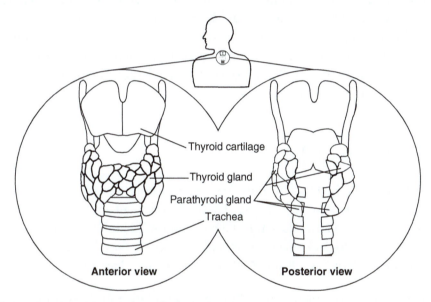

Figure 5.4   The thyroid and parathyroid glands

The thyroid gland and metabolism

The energy required to power the biochemical processes necessary for life is derived from the food we consume. Although carbohydrates, proteins and fats can all be used as substrates to release energy, the preferred primary fuel for human cells is glucose. During cellular respiration, energy is released from glucose and used to synthesise the energy storage molecule ATP. This process occurs within the cytoplasm and mitochondria of our cells (Chapter 1). The rate at which food is utilised as fuel during cellular respiration is referred to as the metabolic rate and this is regulated predominantly by the thyroid gland.

The follicular cells of the thyroid synthesise two iodine-containing hormones; triiodothyronine (T3) has three atoms of iodine and tetraiodothyronine (T4), which is also known as thyroxine, has four. Iodine is obtained through the diet with the major sources in the UK currently coming from dairy products and eggs, with seafood including fish and shellfish being particularly rich sources of this mineral. Non-animal sources of iodine include seaweed, potato skins, watercress, kale, green beans and strawberries.

The recommended daily intake of iodine for adults is 150 µg (micrograms – a microgram is 1 millionth of a gram), rising to 200 µg in pregnant or breastfeeding women (The UK Iodine Group, 2019).

Although the dietary requirement for iodine is relatively low, many people in the UK are mildly deficient in this mineral, and prolonged iodine deficiency can lead to a swelling of the thyroid referred to as goitre. Both T3 and T4 are essential in regulating the metabolic rate; typically 80 per cent of secretion is in the form of T4, with the remaining 20 per cent being T3, which is approximately three to four times as potent as T4.

The secretion of T3 and T4 is under the control of the anterior pituitary gland which releases thyroid-stimulating hormone (TSH); this travels in the blood to the thyroid before binding to receptors on the follicular cells to initiate T3 and T4 secretion. The release of TSH is itself controlled by the hypothalamus which is continually monitoring T3 and T4 levels in the blood. When concentrations begin to fall, the hypothalamus releases the thyrotropin-releasing hormone.

Role of T3 and T4

T3 and T4 circulate in the blood with the vast majority bound to plasma proteins such as albumin and thyroxine-binding globulin (TBG). Only a small amount of T3 and T4 are actually free within the plasma (around 0.03 per cent for T4 and 0.3 per cent for T3) and able to exert a physiological effect; for this reason, when assessing thyroid function in patients, it is the levels of free T3 and T4 that are of greatest diagnostic significance.

Free T3 and T4 cross the plasma membranes of target cells and exert their effects by binding to receptors within the nucleus of the cell. Following uptake by target cells, most T4 is rapidly converted into the more biologically active T3. Virtually all cells and tissues are able to respond to free T3 and T4, which exert a variety of diverse physiological effects which are summarised in Table 5.1.

Hypothyroidism and hyperthyroidism

Hypothyroidism is most frequently associated with autoimmune destruction of the T3- and T4-producing follicular cells of thyroid, resulting in Hashimoto's thyroiditis. The exact cause of Hashimoto's thyroiditis is unclear, but antibodies are produced which bind to the follicular cells and initiate progressive destruction and inflammation of the thyroid tissue. Age itself is associated with an increase in circulating autoantibodies that react with the thyroid gland (Calsolaro et al., 2019), which may contribute to reductions in the basal metabolic rate as we grow older. As we have seen with Sharma's case study at the beginning of this chapter, reduced secretion of T3 and T4 (hypothyroidism) is associated with a slowing of the metabolic rate that often leads to weight gain and a reduction in thermogenesis (heat production), resulting in reduced body temperature.

Hypothyroidism is also associated with thinning of the hair and a depressed mood, both of which were also experienced by Sharma prior to treatment.

Conversely, hyperthyroidism is associated with an increased metabolic rate and significant weight loss through the catabolic breakdown of glycogen, fat and lean muscle mass. Increased metabolism also enhances thermogenesis, increasing body temperature, with patients frequently complaining of heat intolerance (not being able to tolerate warm ambient conditions). Individuals with hyperthyroidism also have an increased heart rate, partially as a result of increased activity of the sympathetic nervous system (see Table 5.1). The most common cause of hyperthyroidism is Grave's disease, which is an autoimmune disease where antibodies are generated which bind to the same receptors as TSH, thereby stimulating the increased release of T3 and T4.

When hyperthyroidism is severe, fatty tissue begins to accumulate behind the eyeball, leading to a pronounced bulging of the eyes termed exophthalmos. As with most autoimmune diseases, Grave's disease disproportionately affects females, with typical ratios quoted being between 5 and 10 females affected for every male. The cause of Grave's disease is currently unknown, although smoking is thought to be a significant modifiable risk factor (NHS, 2019b).

Table 5.1   Physiological effects of T3 and T4

Organs/tissues	Effect
Virtually all cells and tissues	Regulates metabolic rate. Increased T3 and T4 secretion increases the number and activity of mitochondria enhancing food metabolism and synthesis of ATP. Speeding up the metabolic rate increases thermogenesis, raising body temperature. T3 and T4 are also essential for the catabolic breakdown of protein and fats with increased secretion associated with loss of fat and muscle mass
Cardiovascular system	Increases heart rate and cardiac output. Since increased T3 and T4 secretion increases the basal metabolic rate, more heat is produced, necessitating vasodilation and increased blood flow to the skin to facilitate heat loss
Respiratory system	Increases breathing rate – essential to ensure increased oxygen availability for increased aerobic respiration
Reproductive system	Thickening of the endometrium in females with low levels of T3 and T4 associated with reduced fertility in both sexes
Central nervous system	Essential for brain development; increases or decreases in the secretion of T3 and T4 are associated with changes in mental state. Enhances activity of catecholamines such as adrenaline, increasing activation of the sympathetic branch of the autonomic nervous system contributing to increased heart rate. Increased or decreased secretion is also associated with abnormal sleep patterns, with increased time spent sleeping seen in both hyper and hyposecretion
Muscular system	Increased secretion of T3 and T4 can promote the catabolic breakdown of lean muscle tissue, while decreases are associated with sluggish muscular responses, slower relaxation of major muscle groups and decreased heat production during muscular activity

To help you understand the importance of diet to thyroid function, attempt Activity 5.1.

Activity 5.1   Communication

Kaiden has been a vegetarian since he was 17, and three years ago he switched to a totally vegan lifestyle. Kaiden recently noticed a swelling developing in his neck and was worried that this might be cancer. Kaiden visited his GP who immediately referred him to an endocrinologist, where it was established that he was deficient in iodine.

Based on what you have learnt in this chapter, what dietary advice would you offer to Kaiden to help normalise his iodine levels while still being able to maintain his vegan lifestyle?

There are some possible answers to all activities at the end of the chapter, unless otherwise indicated.

Now that we have examined the role of the thyroid in regulating metabolism, we will examine its role in regulating plasma calcium levels.

The thyroid and parathyroid roles in calcium homeostasis

The parafollicular cells of the thyroid are also known as C-cells because they secrete the hormone calcitonin. As the name implies, calcitonin is a hormone involved in regulating plasma levels of ionic calcium (Ca^{++}). Calcium is essential for a diverse range of physiological processes including the maintenance of bone and tooth density, contraction of muscles, cell division, transmission across nerve synapses and clotting of blood. For all of these physiological processes to be carried out efficiently, calcium must be maintained within a narrow normal range within the plasma of between 2.2 and 2.6 mmol/l.

The parafollicular cells continually monitor plasma calcium levels and release calcitonin when an increase is detected (hypercalcaemia), e.g. drinking a pint of milk. Calcitonin is a small peptide hormone and has several major effects that reduce plasma calcium, including:

1. Inhibiting the activity of osteoclasts; the cells that are continually breaking down bone (Chapter 8). By inhibiting osteoclasts, the bone-forming cells of the skeleton called osteoblasts are able to deposit the excess calcium into the bone matrix without this deposition being offset by osteoclast activity.

2. Reducing the re-absorption of calcium by the kidney nephrons, thereby enhancing the elimination of excess calcium in the urine. In people with high-calcium diets this can increase the risk of renal calculi (kidney stones).

3. Inhibiting calcium absorption in the GI tract.

The parathyroid glands

The parathyroid glands are located within the posterior portion of the thyroid gland (Figure 5.4) and produce parathyroid hormone (PTH), which can be thought of as the natural antagonistic hormone to calcitonin.

PTH is a peptide hormone released when plasma calcium levels fall (hypocalcaemia). PTH acts predominantly by enhancing osteoclast activity, increasing bone breakdown and the release of calcium into the plasma; this helps to restore calcium to within its normal range. PTH also increases calcium re-absorption in the distal convoluted tubules and collecting ducts of kidney nephrons, further increasing plasma concentrations. Within the kidney, PTH initiates activation of vitamin D, which is essential to allow efficient absorption of calcium and phosphate from food within the GI tract.

Hypocalcaemia usually occurs when there is insufficient dietary intake of calcium and is particularly common in people who have eliminated dairy products from their diet. Hypocalcaemia is also frequently seen during pregnancy as the developing foetus progressively absorbs calcium from the mother's blood to build its own skeleton. This means that PTH levels are often high during pregnancy, which can encourage bone and tooth demineralisation, increasing the risk of bone fracture and tooth loss. This is one of the reasons why free dental care is offered to all pregnant women in the UK (NHS, 2019c).

The thymus gland

The thymus is a small bilobed gland that sits on the superior portion of the heart and is located behind the sternum. In young children, it is relatively large at around 5 cm long and between 2.5 and 5 cm wide. At puberty, it undergoes atrophy in response to sex hormones with its glandular structure gradually replaced with fatty tissue. In older adults the thymus becomes a vestigial organ weighing as little as 5 g (Zdrojewicz et al., 2016).

In addition to being a component of the endocrine system, the thymus is one of the two primary lymphoid organs and plays a crucial role in the development of immune cells and modulation of immune responses. The role of the thymus as an endocrine gland is still poorly understood; it is known to produce several hormones including thymosin, thymulin and thymopoietin, all of which play a role in the maturation of key immune cells called T helper cells (Chapter 9).

117

The endocrine pancreas: the islets of Langerhans

The pancreas is a vital accessory organ of the GI tract with its exocrine portion producing alkaline pancreatic juice, which is essential to the processes of chemical digestion. Scattered throughout the pancreas are small islands of endocrine tissue known as the islets of Langerhans (Figure 5.5). Each islet has several cell types present which are highlighted in Table 5.2.

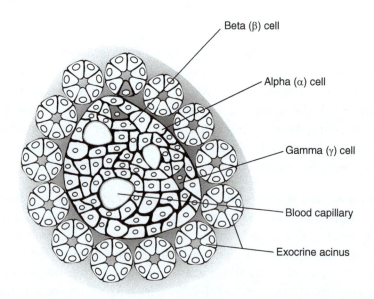

Figure 5.5   The islets of Langerhans

The hormones of the pancreas can be broadly divided into two antagonistic pairs; ghrelin and pancreatic polypeptide are involved in regulating appetite, while insulin and glucagon play key roles in controlling the blood glucose concentration.

The pancreas and appetite

In most people secretion of the hunger hormone ghrelin peaks just before the major meals of the day, with spikes corresponding to breakfast, lunch and the evening meal. Ghrelin is a peptide hormone and, once released from the epsilon cells and mucosal lining of the stomach, circulates in the blood before binding to receptors in the hypothalamus to induce sensations of hunger. Ghrelin also activates dopamine-based reward pathways leading to food cravings (Perello and Dickson, 2015).

Pancreatic polypeptide is a peptide hormone released from the PP cells of the pancreas following a meal. Foods rich in protein and fat induce the greatest secretion, with

Table 5.2 Cells types of the pancreatic islets of Langerhans and their hormones

Cell type	%	Hormone	Function
Beta cells (β cells)	70%	Insulin	Promotes glucose uptake into cells, reducing the blood glucose concentration
		Amylin	Slows emptying of the stomach to help allow gradual absorption of nutrients and prevent sudden spikes in blood glucose
Alpha cells (α cells)	20%	Glucagon	Promotes glycogenolysis, the breakdown of glycogen, particularly in the liver to release glucose and increase the blood glucose concentration
Delta cells (δ cells)	< 10%	Somatostatin	Slows digestion; inhibits the release of pancreatic juice and the pancreatic hormones insulin and glucagon. Inhibits the release of somatotropin (growth hormone) and thyroid-stimulating hormone (TSH) from the anterior pituitary
Epsilon cells (ε cells)	< 1%	Ghrelin	Promotes feelings of hunger and activates and reinforces reward pathways in response to food
PP cells (γ cells)	< 5%	Pancreatic Polypeptide	Promotes feelings of satiety (feeling satisfied) after food

carbohydrate-rich foods initiating less release. Pancreatic polypeptide is an important satiety hormone, although currently its exact mechanism of action is not fully understood. Individuals with Prader-Willi syndrome, a genetic disorder that predisposes to overeating, are known to produce little or no pancreatic polypeptide; indeed, infusions of pancreatic polypeptide are known to curb food intake in these patients, highlighting the pivotal role played by this hormone in promoting satiety and switching off hunger (Williams, 2014).

The pancreas and blood glucose

The normal fasting blood glucose range is between 3.9 and 5.4 mmol/l (Diabetes UK, 2019a).

Control of blood glucose is complex, with multiple hormones, including somatotropin, adrenaline, cortisol and glucagon, all increasing blood glucose concentrations. Insulin is unique in that it is the only major hormone that can antagonise the hyperglycaemic effects of these other hormones to normalise the blood glucose concentration. Unsurprisingly, if insulin is no longer produced or can no longer exert its influence, the end result is pronounced hyperglycaemia and a diagnosis of diabetes mellitus (DM).

The insulin response

Following consumption of a carbohydrate-rich meal, e.g. a plate of pasta, the starch component is quickly digested into glucose, and the blood glucose concentration rises outside of its normal physiological range, triggering the release of insulin.

Insulin is a small peptide hormone and circulates throughout the body before binding to insulin receptors, which are found on the surface of most human cells. Binding of insulin to its receptor initiates movement of glucose transporter proteins (Gluts) from inside the cytoplasm towards the plasma membrane. These Gluts are inserted into the plasma membrane, forming channels which allow glucose to rapidly diffuse into cells to be used as fuel for metabolism. This insulin response reduces the concentration of glucose in the blood to within its normal physiological range. There are many different types of glucose transporter proteins; the form that responds to insulin is called Glut-4 (Figure 5.6).

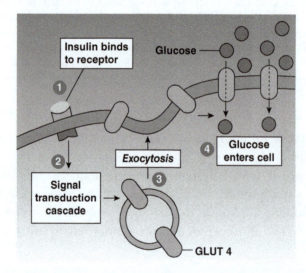

Figure 5.6   The role of insulin and glucose transporters (Gluts) in promoting glucose uptake

Since glucose is soluble in the aqueous environment of the cell, it exerts an osmotic effect, attracting water into cells. For this reason, cells can only take up a limited amount of pure glucose. To get around this problem a secondary effect of insulin is to induce the production of the enzyme glycogen synthase in cells (particularly in liver and muscle tissue). This enzyme joins (polymerises) the glucose molecules into a long branching chain consisting of thousands of individual glucose molecules. This molecule is glycogen, which is also known as animal starch. Glycogen is an important energy storage molecule, and small amounts are stored in many cell types. Unlike glucose, glycogen is insoluble in water and cannot exert an osmotic effect, and therefore does not attract water into the cells in which it is stored.

The human body can only store a limited amount of glycogen with only around 600 g stored in the entire body. If a high carbohydrate intake is maintained when glycogen stores are full, insulin promotes the conversion of glucose into fat, which is stored in the subcutaneous and visceral adipose tissues. Insulin is the principal hormone that promotes fat deposition in humans; furthermore, it also inhibits the breakdown (lipolysis) of stored fat. Developed countries with diets rich in highly refined carbohydrates unsurprisingly have higher numbers of people that fall into the obese category.

In addition to promoting the uptake of glucose, insulin also promotes the uptake of amino acids into cells and is generally regarded as an anabolic hormone capable of enhancing muscle growth. Unfortunately, this reputation has led to insulin being abused by bodybuilders and athletes as a quick method of 'bulking up' before events and competitions; this form of insulin abuse has led to many cases of hypoglycaemic shock, coma and even death (Heidet et al., 2019).

We have just explored the role played by insulin in glucose homeostasis. To further your understanding of the importance of this hormone, read through Lucy's case study.

Case study: Lucy – type I diabetes mellitus (DM)

Lucy is a seven-year-old girl with a six-week history of polydipsia (exceptional thirst). She also complained of polyuria (excessive urine output), and recently she had started to wet the bed. Lucy felt constantly tired, and her teachers mentioned to her mother that she was having trouble concentrating in school. Lucy's mum attributed this to her waking up in a wet bed and being unable to settle again afterwards. Lucy was a slight child who had lost weight recently. Lucy and her mum visited their GP. A urine sample taken in the surgery showed glucose +++ and the presence of ketones. The GP strongly suspected type I DM and suggested a blood glucose test.

Lucy refused to allow the practice nurse to take a capillary blood sample, so she was referred to the local hospital where a venous blood sample could be taken under the supervision of a play therapist who could distract and soothe Lucy during the procedure. A referral was made to a consultant paediatrician, and following diagnosis, insulin therapy was commenced.

Lucy's case study highlights perfectly that when young children show excessive thirst and increased urination, diabetes should always initially be suspected. Type I diabetes is routinely encountered by child-branch nurses, and although this condition usually manifests in childhood, nurses should be aware it can, more rarely, arise in adolescents and adults.

Diabetes mellitus (DM)

It has been estimated that 4 million people in the UK have either been diagnosed with DM or are living with the disease undiagnosed; this equates to around 6 per cent of the UK population (Diabetes UK, 2019b). DM arises as a result of an impaired or absent insulin response. Two major types of DM are recognised, with each form thought to be a distinct disease: type I DM is also referred to as insulin-dependent DM and is an autoimmune disorder most frequently seen in children and young adults. It is the rarer of the two major forms of DM, affecting around one in ten people with diabetes in the UK.

Patients with type I DM have had their insulin-producing beta cells destroyed by auto-immune attack and have lost the ability to produce insulin. To survive, these patients must inject insulin regularly, usually following main meals. This exogenous insulin replaces the insulin that the pancreas would normally produce and allows the glucose from food to enter the cells as fuel for metabolism. Type II DM is far more common than type I and is estimated to account for around nine in ten patients with diabetes in the UK. Even following decades of research, the causes of type II DM are still poorly understood, with many different theories currently being investigated. Whatever the exact cause, type II DM is associated with 'insulin resistance'.

Most people with type II DM can still produce insulin, but it no longer seems to exert its physiological effects. It has been speculated that this may be due to structural changes to the insulin receptor or interference with the ability of insulin to bind to its receptor in the usual manner. Without a normal insulin response glucose begins to accumulate in the blood, leading to hyperglycaemia, which is the defining clinical feature of DM.

Activity 5.2   Evidence-based practice and research

We have just explored how patients with DM become hyperglycaemic. In many type II patients, the progression to hyperglycaemia can be quite slow, and patients may not initially experience any apparent symptoms. Using textbooks or online resources, identify the symptoms that are most commonly associated with undiagnosed DM. Which of these symptoms most frequently lead the patient to seek medical advice from their GP or other healthcare professionals?

Now that we have examined the nature of the insulin response and explored the pathophysiology associated with DM, we will examine the role played in regulating blood glucose by glucagon, a hormone which functions as the natural antagonist to insulin.

Glucagon: the between-meals hormone

As with the insulin-producing beta cells, the alpha cells of the pancreas are continually monitoring the blood glucose concentration. When no carbohydrate-rich food has been consumed for a couple of hours or following a bout of prolonged activity, blood glucose levels usually begin to fall, and the alpha cells secrete their glucagon directly into the blood. Glucagon is a peptide hormone and circulates in the blood to its major target organ, the liver. Glucagon binds to receptors on liver hepatocytes (the major cells of the liver) and stimulates the synthesis of the enzyme glycogen phosphorylase. This enzyme begins to remove individual glucose subunits from glycogen molecules, releasing them into the blood and increasing the blood glucose concentration to ensure it remains within its normal range.

This process of promoting glycogen breakdown is termed glycogenolysis. When glycogen stores have been depleted, glucagon can also promote gluconeogenesis (the formation of new glucose) from stores of fat and even via catabolism of lean muscle mass to release amino acids, which can then be converted readily into glucose. Glucagon release is essential when we are sleeping to ensure that blood glucose concentrations are maintained throughout the night when our body is resting. Since glucagon is so effective in raising the blood glucose concentration, it is often used in emergency care to treat patients who are hypoglycaemic, commonly as a result of injecting too much insulin. It is of particular use in treating unconscious patients where administration of oral glucose may be difficult.

The adrenal glands

The adrenal glands are so named because of their position above the kidneys (adrenal means above the kidney). The adrenal glands are around 5 cm long and 3 cm wide, with each weighing around 4–6 g. The right adrenal gland is usually triangular in shape (Figure 5.7), while the left is more flattened with a crescent or semicircular appearance. Each adrenal gland has two distinct regions: the adrenal medulla (inner portion towards the middle of the gland) and the adrenal cortex (outer portion).

The adrenal medulla

The adrenal medulla is the location of chromaffin cells which secrete the catecholamines: adrenaline (around 80 per cent total) and noradrenaline (around 20 per cent total). Both catecholamines are synthesised from the amino acid tyrosine before being released directly into the blood following activation of the sympathetic branch of the autonomic nervous system. Adrenaline and noradrenaline are usually released when there is a

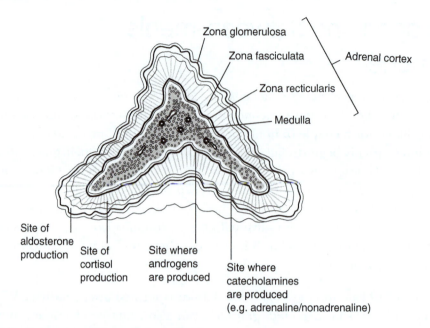

Figure 5.7 Structure of the adrenal glands

perceived threat or in an exciting, stressful or dangerous situation; for this reason they are often called the 'fight-or-flight' hormones. The catecholamines have multiple effects throughout the body, which generally involve preparing the body for immediate activity.

The major physiological effects experienced during an adrenaline rush are centred around the cardiovascular system, with a significant increase in heart rate readily perceived by most people (see Chapter 3 for further detail). Additionally, adrenaline increases blood pressure and the breathing rate, dilates the airway, increases blood glucose, enhances sensory perception and decreases pain perception. All of these effects improve responsiveness and performance in a fight-or-flight situation. Increased heart rate, blood pressure, breathing and blood glucose all enhance the performance of the major muscle groups, while increased sensory acuity improves response times.

Decreases in pain perception theoretically allow pain to be endured longer during a fight or during a period of high-intensity sprinting to escape from a threat. Unfortunately, catecholamines, particularly adrenaline, are often released at high concentration in response to relatively non-threatening situations such as a public speaking engagement or an exam, and in these scenarios the effects of a fight-or-flight response can be counterproductive and reduce performance.

The adrenal cortex

The cells of the adrenal cortex are continually absorbing cholesterol to synthesise a variety of steroid hormones. Structurally the adrenal cortex consists of three distinct bands of tissue (Figure 5.7), which are highlighted in Table 5.3.

Table 5.3 Hormones of the adrenal cortex

Region of cortex	Hormones secreted	Physiological function
Zona glomerulosa	Mineralocorticoids (aldosterone)	Regulation of plasma sodium and potassium concentration
Zona fasciculata	Glucocorticoids (cortisol)	Long-term stress hormone that is anti-inflammatory and promotes gluconeogenesis (production of new glucose usually from proteins and the glycerol component of fats)
Zona reticularis	Androgens, e.g. dehydroepiandrosterone (DHEA)	Testosterone-like hormones which are particularly important in females during puberty. Promote the growth of axial (armpit) and pubic hair and increase libido (Chapter 12)

The anterior pituitary and the release of glucocorticoids

The principal glucocorticoid hormone is cortisol, which functions as the primary long-term stress hormone. Cortisol is synthesised in the zona fasciculata of the adrenal cortex; its release is regulated by adrenocorticotrophic hormone (ACTH), a peptide hormone secreted by the anterior pituitary. The release of ACTH is itself regulated by the hypothalamus which releases corticotropin-releasing hormone (CRH) in response to long-term stress. CRH is a peptide hormone that quickly initiates ACTH release from the anterior pituitary, which then initiates cortisol release from the zona fasciculata.

Levels of cortisol are continually monitored by the hypothalamus, with increased cortisol secretion leading to inhibition of CRH release via negative feedback. This complex system involving a cascade of several hormones is referred to as the hypothalamic–pituitary–adrenal axis (HPA axis); the major steps are summarised in the flow diagram below.

Overview of the HPA axis

Long-term stressors

↓

Release of corticotropin-releasing hormone (CRH) from the hypothalamus

↓

Release of adrenocorticotrophic hormone (ACTH) from the anterior pituitary

↓

Release of cortisol from the zona fasciculata of the adrenal cortex

CRH is also released in response to stress, with increased release occurring when we are deprived of food (starvation), suffer a physical injury or are exposed to psychological stressors such as suffering bereavement, changing job or moving house. All such stressors ultimately lead to activation of the HPA axis and enhanced secretion of cortisol.

Physiological actions of cortisol

Cortisol has a multitude of physiological roles and is particularly important in helping to ensure suitable substrates are available to fuel metabolism and in regulating immune responses.

Cortisol, metabolism, appetite and fat deposition

When food intake is reduced (e.g. when dieting) the HPA axis is activated, initiating the release of cortisol. If carbohydrates are in limited supply, cortisol initially promotes the release of glucagon from the alpha cells of the pancreatic islets, initiating glycogenolysis in the liver and releasing glucose into the blood (see glucagon section above). When food is unavailable in the longer term, glycogen stores quickly become depleted, and cortisol promotes gluconeogenesis, the biochemical process by which new glucose is created from fat and protein sources such as lean muscle mass.

While this is a useful strategy for survival in the short term when starvation becomes prolonged, e.g. in people with eating disorders such as anorexia nervosa, it can lead to significant muscle wastage (sarcopaenia). Since the heart is also a muscle, elevated cortisol can eventually initiate myocardial thinning, potentially leading to heart failure, which is a significant cause of death in anorexic patients.

Since cortisol secretion increases when we are deprived of food, unsurprisingly cortisol is also associated with sensations of hunger, which is thought to lead us to seek out highly palatable foods that are high in fats and sugars (Chao et al., 2017). The sensations of hunger associated with increased cortisol secretion are thought to be at least partially mediated through the hunger hormone ghrelin (see above), with ghrelin secretion rising in response to elevated plasma cortisol (Azzam et al., 2017). Since cortisol secretion is also enhanced following psychological stress, its powerful effect in stimulating appetite is thought to partially explain the phenomenon of comfort eating, for example bingeing on cakes and chocolate when preparing for an exam or after splitting up with a partner.

Clearly, long-term exposure to elevated cortisol can promote overeating, with preferences skewed in favour of calorie-dense foods which are high in refined carbohydrates and fats (junk food). More worryingly, when an excess of calories is consumed, increased levels of cortisol promote visceral fat deposition in the abdominal region; this leads to increased central obesity, which is frequently associated with high blood pressure, increased levels of cholesterol and type II diabetes mellitus (Van Rossum, 2017). These clinical features are collectively referred to as metabolic syndrome, which is a growing problem in developed countries and significantly increases the risk of major cardiovascular diseases including myocardial infarction (MI) and stroke (cerebrovascular accident).

Cortisol and immune responses

Cortisol has potent anti-inflammatory effects within the body, and when secreted at normal concentrations this hormone plays an essential role in keeping inflammatory immune responses in check. However, when cortisol secretion increases, it can lead to progressive and general immunosuppression, which has been shown to increase the risk of infection. Chronic exposure to elevated cortisol can result in the immune system becoming resistant to its anti-inflammatory effects, and this can result in an increased risk of inflammatory autoimmune diseases and even certain cancers (Bae et al., 2019).

In addition to the naturally produced glucocorticoid hormone cortisol, many people are prescribed steroid medications to treat a variety of inflammatory disorders such as rheumatoid arthritis or inflammatory bowel disease. Many of these steroids, such as prednisone, mimic the effects of cortisol and interact with the same receptors. Such drugs have to be used with care since they can increase the risk of infection and, as with naturally produced cortisol, can increase blood glucose concentrations. Long-term use of corticosteroids can result in chronic hyperglycaemia; this may lead to insulin resistance and steroid-induced diabetes, which is similar in nature to type II diabetes mellitus. When corticosteroids are discontinued, blood glucose control usually begins to normalise (Carter, 2019).

Although cortisol concentrations are usually tightly regulated via the HPA axis, disease can lead to overproduction of this key hormone. To further your understanding of how excess cortisol can adversely affect human physiology, read through Cathy's case study.

Case study: Cathy – Cushing's syndrome

Cathy is a 33-year-old female who had a baby nine months ago. Her periods didn't resume after the delivery, and she was reassured that it was only a matter of time before 'things got back to normal'. After she stopped breastfeeding her baby, Cathy's periods still did not resume. She also noticed that her hair had become thinner, and she started to develop facial hair and acne. Initially, Cathy's GP suspected polycystic ovary disease, but this was ruled out following an abdominal ultrasound scan.

(Continued)

(Continued)

Over the next few months, Cathy's weight continued to increase, with fat being distributed primarily around her abdomen and between her shoulders ('buffalo hump') and stretch marks on her arms, legs and abdomen. Her GP suspected Cushing's syndrome and referred Cathy to an endocrinologist. A 24-hour urine collection showed an elevated cortisol level, while an MRI scan revealed a 7.5 × 5 mm tumour on the left side of Cathy's pituitary gland. Cathy underwent successful surgery to remove the tumour mass and her cortisol levels normalised.

Cathy's case study reveals the complexity of diagnosing many endocrine disorders. Although the symptoms of Cushing's syndrome are associated with overproduction of cortisol by the adrenal cortex, in Cathy the ultimate cause is a tumour in her pituitary. The tumour was causing increased release of ACTH, which was stimulating the enhanced secretion of cortisol responsible for Cathy's symptoms. Nurses should be aware that Cushing's syndrome can also arise from tumours within the adrenal glands or even from excessive use of steroidal drugs such as prednisone, which can act to mimic cortisol.

Aldosterone and sodium/potassium homeostasis

Aldosterone is released primarily in response to a decreased plasma sodium (Na^+) concentration and increased plasma potassium (K^+) concentration. Na^+ and K^+ ions are essential to nerve conduction (Chapter 6) so it is vital that these ions are maintained within their normal physiological ranges.

Since most human cells have a sodium-potassium pump which pumps K^+ ions into cells and Na^+ ions out, most Na^+ ions are found outside cells and eventually accumulate in the plasma of the blood. This explains why the normal range for Na^+ in the plasma is high, at around 135–145 mmol/l, and since most K^+ ions are being actively pumped into cells, the normal range for plasma K^+ is low at around 3.5–5.0 mmol/l.

Aldosterone is released from the zona glomerulosa during episodes of hyponatraemia (low blood sodium), e.g. because of a lack of dietary salt intake. Its primary effect is to enhance Na^+ re-absorption in nephrons, specifically acting on the distal convoluted tubule and collecting duct, thereby increasing plasma Na^+ concentrations towards their normal physiological range. Aldosterone is also thought to promote salt cravings in patients, thus encouraging the consumption of salty foods, further boosting plasma Na^+.

Conversely, when plasma Na^+ levels are high (hypernatraemia), e.g. as a result of a bout of watery diarrhoea or simply consuming too much salt, the secretion of aldosterone is inhibited and little or no Na^+ re-absorption occurs in the nephrons, allowing excess Na^+ ions to be eliminated in the urine.

Homeostatic control of plasma K^+ concentrations via aldosterone is effectively the opposite of Na^+. During periods of hyperkalaemia (high blood potassium), which frequently occur following the consumption of too much potassium-rich food (e.g. several bananas), aldosterone is secreted from the zona glomerulosa and triggers the secretion of K^+ ions into the kidney nephrons, with excess K^+ accumulating in the renal filtrate before being eliminated in the urine. Hyperkalaemia is also frequently seen in patients following major trauma such as crush and burn injuries where widespread tissue damage and cell death occur. Cellular death usually results in lysis (bursting of cells) which liberates the concentrations of K^+ ions that were previously accumulated within cells via the $Na^+ K^+$ pump. Severe hyperkalaemia is potentially life-threatening since it can trigger dangerous ventricular arrhythmias, some of which can result in cardiac arrest.

Hypokalaemia is most frequently seen in patients who are prescribed diuretic medications which are commonly used to treat high blood pressure and the oedema associated with heart failure. Common non-potassium-sparing diuretics such as furosemide can cause hypokalaemia by progressively 'flushing out' K^+.

During hypokalaemia, secretion of aldosterone is inhibited and tubular secretion of K^+ into kidney nephrons ceases, resulting in the retention of K^+ in the plasma which begins to normalise the blood K^+ concentration. Patients who experience hypokalaemia as a result of diuretics are usually switched to more expensive potassium-sparing diuretics such as amiloride, which offer the benefits of lowering blood pressure and reducing the complications of heart failure, particularly leg oedema, without significant losses of K^+.

Now you have completed the chapter, attempt the multiple-choice questions to assess your learning.

Activity 5.3   Multiple-choice questions

1. ADH is released from the posterior pituitary gland

    a) When patients are over-hydrated
    b) When blood pressure increases
    c) When the concentration of the blood increases
    d) When body temperature increases

    (Continued)

(Continued)

2. Somatotropin

   a) Increases brain mass

   b) Reduces muscle mass

   c) Helps regulate growth

   d) Delays the development of internal organs

3. Which of these statements is untrue?

   a) Shellfish is a valuable source of iodine

   b) Iodine requirements increase during pregnancy and breastfeeding

   c) Iodine deficiency contributes to pyrexia (fever)

   d) Mild iodine deficiency is common in the UK

4. Hypothyroidism is associated with

   a) Loss of hair and weight gain

   b) Anabolic breakdown of glycogen, fat and lean muscle

   c) Catabolic breakdown of protein, fat and lean muscle

   d) Anabolic breakdown of protein, fat and lean muscle

5. Hyperthyroidism is associated with increased metabolic rate, resulting in

   a) Weight loss and heat intolerance

   b) Weight gain and heat intolerance

   c) Weight loss and reduced body temperature

   d) Weight gain and reduced body temperature

6. Which of these statements is untrue?

   a) PTH enhances osteoclast activity

   b) PTH reduces the re-absorption of calcium by the nephrons

   c) PTH increases calcium re-absorption by the nephrons

   d) PTH initiates activation of vitamin D

7. The thymus gland is responsible for producing

   a) Thymosin, thyroxine and thymopoietin

   b) Thymosin, thymulin and thymopoietin

   c)   Thyroxine, thymulin and thymopoietin

   d)   Thymosin, thymulin and thyroxine

8.   Which of the pancreatic cells releases the hunger hormone ghrelin?

   a)   Alpha cells

   b)   Beta cells

   c)   Delta cells

   d)   Epsilon cells

9.   Glycogenolysis is

   a)   The formation of new glucose

   b)   The promotion of glycogen breakdown

   c)   The release of glycogen into the muscles

   d)   The conversion of amino acids into glucose

10.   An increased concentration of plasma potassium is known as

   a)   Hypernatraemia

   b)   Hyponatraemia

   c)   Hyperkalaemia

   d)   Hypokalaemia

Chapter summary

The endocrine system consists of a complex array of ductless glands which secrete chemical signals called hormones directly into the blood. These hormones are distributed to their target organs and tissues, exerting their effects by binding to specific receptors. The hypothalamus is a major crossover point between the nervous system and the endocrine system; it synthesises important hormones such as oxytocin and ADH, together with a variety of releasing hormones which regulate the activity of other endocrine glands. The pituitary gland consists of a posterior portion which can be thought of as an extension of the hypothalamus; this serves to concentrate hormones produced by the hypothalamus prior to release.

(Continued)

(Continued)

The anterior pituitary gland produces several hormones including somatotropin, which regulates growth, and TSH, which is involved in regulating the activity of the thyroid gland. The pars intermedia marks the point where the posterior pituitary is fused with its anterior portion; this thin band of tissue releases MSH, which influences skin pigmentation. The thyroid gland produces the iodine-containing hormones T3 and T4 which regulate metabolism and calcitonin, which together with parathyroid hormone regulates plasma calcium levels. The thymus gland produces several hormones which are involved in coordinating immune responses and the development of immunologically active cells. The islets of Langerhans form the endocrine portion of the pancreas; each islet consists of several cell types which secrete hormones that regulate blood glucose levels and help control appetite.

The adrenal glands are located above the kidneys with each gland having two regions. The adrenal medulla is located in the centre of each adrenal gland and produces adrenaline and noradrenaline which play a key role in the fight-or-flight responses. The adrenal cortex is the outer portion of each adrenal gland and produces steroid hormones. These include cortisol, which is the major long-term stress hormone, androgens, which are testosterone-like hormones, and aldosterone, which regulates plasma sodium and potassium concentrations.

Activities: Brief outline answers

Activity 5.1: Communication (page 116)

Kaiden should be advised to increase his intake of foods that are rich in iodine. Usually, this would involve suggesting eating more eggs, dairy products, fish and shellfish. Since Kaiden is a vegan, he should try to eat more green vegetables such as kale and green beans. Since seaweed is so rich in iodine, he could consider incorporating small amounts in his dishes. Certain fruits, particularly strawberries, also contain iodine. Kaiden should also think of purchasing an iodine supplement (vegan-friendly options are available). Use of iodised salts should be kept to a minimum to avoid excessive intake of sodium.

Activity 5.2: Evidence-based practice and research (page 122)

Increased thirst (polydipsia), increased urination (polyuria), ketoacidosis (build-up of ketone bodies in the blood), increased hunger (polyphagia) and occasionally weight loss and blurred vision are all common symptoms of undiagnosed diabetes. Of these, it is polydipsia and poluria (increased urine production) that frequently result in patients seeking advice from their GP, particularly when sleep patterns are disturbed by constant visits to the toilet; indeed, many patients complain of feeling totally exhausted in the run-up to seeking advice.

Activity 5.3: Multiple-choice questions (pages 129–31)

1) c, 2) c, 3) c, 4) a, 5) a, 6) b, 7) b, 8) c, 9) b, 10) c

Further reading

Boore J et al. (2016) Chapter 7: The endocrine system – Control of essential functions, in *Essentials of Anatomy and Physiology for Nursing Practice*. London: SAGE Publications Ltd.

A textbook to develop your knowledge of human anatomy and physiology that is aimed specifically at nurses.

Tortora G and Derrickson B (2017) *Tortora's Principles of Anatomy and Physiology* (15th edition). New York: John Wiley & Sons.

In-depth coverage of human anatomy and physiology.

Useful website

www.yourhormones.info/endocrine-conditions

An overview of the common endocrine disorders.

Chapter 6　The nervous system

Zubeyde Bayram-Weston

Chapter aims

After reading this chapter you will be able to:

- specify the divisions of the nervous system;
- identify the major cell types of the nervous system;
- describe the nature of nerve impulses (action potentials);
- describe the structure of the brain and spinal cord;
- list cranial nerves and describe their function;
- compare and contrast the sympathetic and parasympathetic divisions of the autonomic nervous system;
- describe the structure and function of the eye and ear.

Introduction

Case study: Ahmed – subarachnoid haemorrhage

Ahmed is a 52-year-old builder and has been working all day at a construction site. Suddenly, Ahmed experiences a sharp pain in his head and loses his balance before collapsing to the floor, unconscious. When the paramedics arrive, he is still unconscious with a pulse of 55 and blood pressure of 195/100. He is rapidly transferred to hospital where CT scans reveal he has suffered a subarachnoid haemorrhage.

Nurses routinely encounter acute neurological emergencies such as Ahmed's stroke. Indeed, there are around 32,000 stroke-related deaths in England each year, with many more strokes resulting in permanent disability. In addition, chronic neurological conditions such as Parkinson's disease, multiple sclerosis and Alzheimer's disease also require long-term nursing care. This chapter will begin by highlighting the divisions and subdivisions of the nervous system before exploring the diverse cell populations from which

134

the nervous system is constructed. We will then examine the nature of nerve conduction and explore how nerve cells interact and connect via structures called synapses.

Since a detailed working knowledge of the central nervous system is essential to nursing practice, we will explore the structure and function of the brain and spinal cord and examine how these regions are protected. Finally, we will examine the special senses, highlighting the key anatomical and physiological features of the eye and ear. To reinforce the key points throughout this chapter, we will explore the nature of some of the common pathologies affecting the nervous and sensory systems.

Overview of the nervous system

The nervous system allows the body to rapidly respond to changes in both the external and internal environment. This ability to respond quickly is essential to our survival, allowing us to escape from unpleasant environmental stimuli and ensuring that our internal homeostatic balance can be maintained.

Anatomically, the nervous system (Figure 6.1) is divided into two major divisions: the central nervous system (CNS) and the peripheral nervous system (PNS).

- The CNS consists of the brain and the spinal cord.
- The PNS is all the remaining nerves that reside outside of the brain and spinal cord, consisting predominantly of the cranial and spinal nerves.

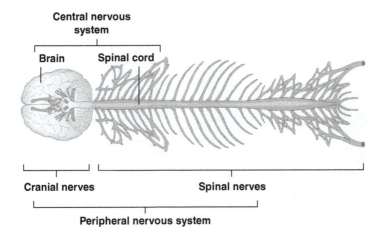

Figure 6.1   The CNS and PNS

A common mistake in assessments is to focus too heavily on learning the role of the CNS at the expense of the PNS. Knowledge of the PNS is essential to nursing practice, and so before we look in more detail at the CNS, we will examine the PNS and its subdivisions.

The PNS has two primary divisions (Figure 6.2).

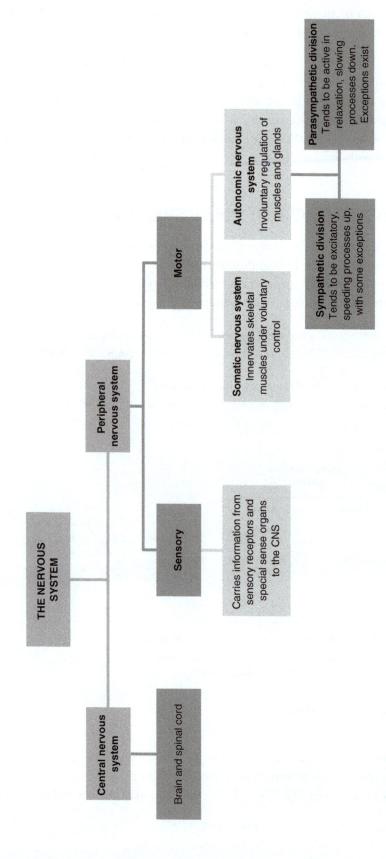

Figure 6.2   Divisions of the nervous system

Divisions of the PNS

The sensory division

Sensory organs and receptors monitor both internal variables in the body and external stimuli in the environment. These include highly specialised sensory organs such as the eyes and ears which are responsible for detecting light and sound waves and maintaining our sense of balance. Simpler chemical receptors are responsible for our sense of taste and smell (olfaction), while mechanical receptors are essential for sensations of touch. Additionally, specialised receptors called nociceptors detect painful stimuli such as a burn or a cut.

As we have seen in Chapter 2, there are a multitude of internal variables which need to be maintained within narrow physiological ranges to ensure homeostatic balance and health. Consequently, throughout the body a variety of receptors monitor key parameters such as temperature, blood pressure and blood pH, and continually feed this information to the integrative control centres of the brain. Sensory information is rapidly relayed towards the CNS along specialised sensory neurons, most of which are located in the PNS.

The motor division

Once a control centre within the brain has decided how to respond, effector organs need to be activated, and this is most frequently achieved by sending nerve impulses along motor nerves. For example, if our blood oxygen concentration falls, this will be detected by chemoreceptors and information relayed via sensory nerves to the respiratory centre, which will respond by sending nerve impulses via motor nerves to the major breathing muscles (diaphragm and intercostals) to increase the breathing rate and raise the blood oxygen concentration.

The motor division of the PNS is itself subdivided into two branches (Figure 6.2):

The somatic nervous system (SNS) (soma = body)

The SNS is responsible for conscious voluntary control and is associated with motor nerves that connect to skeletal muscles. The SNS allows us to perform the conscious physical movements necessary for our day-to-day activities such as walking, dressing ourselves or preparing a meal.

The autonomic nervous system (ANS)

As suggested by the name, the autonomic nervous system controls most of those vital life support functions that we don't need to think about such as heart rate, blood pressure and digestion. The ANS also has two subdivisions (Figure 6.2):

137

The sympathetic division: This generally up-regulates physiological processes (e.g. increasing heart rate and sweat production). Simply put, the sympathetic branch can be regarded as being responsible for gearing the body for immediate activity.

The parasympathetic division: This is generally antagonistic to the sympathetic nervous system and regulates our vegetative (sedate/resting) functions, and is often referred to as being responsible for 'rest and digest'.

Once we have explored the brain and spinal cord, we will return to the autonomic nervous system and examine its structure and function in greater detail.

Cells of the nervous system

The nervous system consists of two principal cell types: neurons, which are the cells that conduct electrical signals called action potentials, and neuroglial cells, which provide protection support and nourishment to the neurons.

Neurons

Structurally, each neuron has two distinct regions (Figure 6.3):

The cell body: This is easy to identify as it is the location of the nucleus, which is usually centrally located and has a granular cytoplasm which consists predominantly of Nissl bodies (granules). Nissl bodies are actually collections of prominent rough endoplasmic reticulum (ER) which is the region of a cell responsible for protein synthesis (Chapter 1). Neurons are metabolically very active, generating nerve impulses and synthesising chemicals called neurotransmitters, which are responsible for communication between neurons and other tissues and organs. Unlike most other cells in the human body, most neurons are not capable of cell division, lacking the centrioles necessary for chromosome segregation (Chapter 14).

The axon: The cell body can be drawn out into two kinds of extensions (or processes). Dendrites (dendritic = branch or tree-like) are short, branching extensions that facilitate interconnection with neighbouring neurons. Additionally, each neuron has a much longer extension known as an axon which can be anything from a fraction of a mm to 1.5 metres in length. Axons can be thought of as being similar to a piece of electrical wiring and function to carry electrical signals throughout the body. Just as electrical wiring usually has a layer of insulation wrapped around it, the axons of most neurons are insulated by special neuroglial cells (see below) containing a fatty-like material called myelin.

These myelin-containing cells wrap around the axon in a spiral manner to provide insulation. This myelin sheath is not continuous; along the length of the axon there are tiny gaps between each myelin-containing cell. These are called the nodes of Ranvier

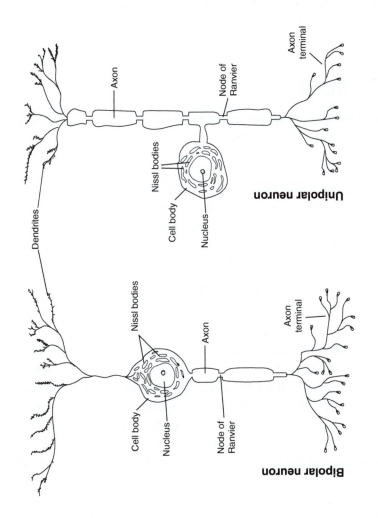

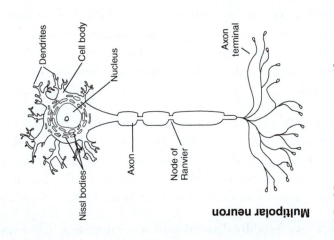

Figure 6.3 Neuron structure and type

and play a key role in efficient, rapid nerve conduction (see below). While the axons of most neurons are myelinated, some neurons lack a myelin sheath and are referred to as non-myelinated or unmyelinated neurons.

Types of neuron

There are structurally three major types of neuron. A good tip to help remember these is to first identify the cell body and then count how many processes are extending from it.

Multipolar neurons: These have multiple dendrites and a single axon extending from the cell body. This is the dominant cell type found within the brain, with each neuron capable of forming multiple connections (synapses) with its neighbouring cells. In this way the multipolar neurons of the brain can form intricate neural networks necessary for complex tasks and abstract thinking.

Bipolar neurons: These have two extensions: one dendrite and one axon extending from the cell body. They are found in many locations such as sensory organs including the eyes, ears and nose.

Unipolar neurons: These have a single short extension which quickly divides into a single axon and a single dendrite. These types of neuron are usually very long and most often located in the PNS, where they extend into sensory organs often connecting to receptors directly or via intermediary bipolar neurons. Since these types of neuron are not strictly unipolar (since the short extension splits quickly into axon and dendrite), some textbooks and neurophysiologists refer to them as pseudounipolar neurons. It is wise to learn both terms since they are often used interchangeably.

Neuroglial cells

There are multiple cell types in the nervous system which do not conduct electrical signals but play a crucial role in protecting, supporting and nourishing electrochemically active neurons. The word glia originates from Greek and means 'glue' since initially it was thought the dominant role of these cells was to hold the neurons together and anchor them in position.

Today we know that glial cells are very diverse in terms of structure and function and carry out many essential functions within the nervous system. Unlike most neurons, many of the glial cell types can divide. Unfortunately, that means these cells are susceptible to malignancy and the vast majority of cancers that affect the nervous system are gliomas, which are tumours formed from uncoordinated glial cell division.

Neuroglial cells can be broadly divided into two categories based on their location (Figure 6.4).

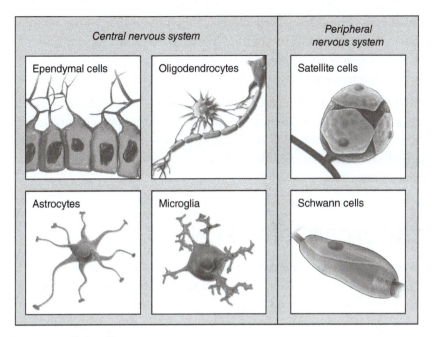

Figure 6.4 Neuroglial cells

Neuroglial cells of the CNS

Astrocytes: These are most abundant glial cells of the CNS and, as implied by their name, they are star-shaped. Astrocytes have several functions within the CNS; they act as supporting cells for neural tissue, forming a scaffold-like structure to help anchor neurons in place. The fine extensions of these cells (called foot processes) wrap around the small blood vessels of the brain, forming a physical barrier between the blood and neurons. This so-called blood-brain barrier (BBB) is a selective barrier that protects the brain from toxins in the blood while allowing free movement of small molecules such as oxygen, carbon dioxide and glucose.

Lipid-soluble materials such as alcohol also pass across this barrier easily, whereas many larger organic molecules including many drugs cannot cross over. Knowledge of the BBB is essential to nurses since it will influence the choice of drugs such as antibiotics and analgesics. Astrocytes also play an important role in regulating electrolytes such as potassium, which are essential to nerve conduction (see below).

Ependymal cells: These are cuboidal epithelial cells found lining the hollow cavities of the brain (ventricles). Their major role is to produce cerebrospinal fluid (CSF) which fills the ventricles and surrounds the brain and spinal cord. Some ependymal cells have cilia on their surface which assist the movement and circulation of CSF. This fluid acts as a cushion to help protect the brain and spinal cord; unfortunately, it also forms an ideal medium for microbial growth which may lead to serious infections such as meningitis.

Microglial cells: These are the smallest and least numerous of the neuroglial cells and function primarily to protect the CNS from infection. In response to injury, infection or inflammation, microglial cells can increase in size and become actively phagocytic to remove pathogens.

Oligodendrocytes: These are the myelin-containing cells of the CNS and are densely arranged compact cells. Each oligodendrocyte has several extensions capable of wrapping around and insulating multiple axons. This capability is essential in the CNS where billions of neurons are packed together in close proximity.

Neuroglial cells of the PNS

Schwann cells: These are the myelin-containing cells of the PNS. Like oligodendrocytes, these cells wrap around and insulate axons, but these are much larger cells and are only found wrapped around a single axon.

Satellite cells: These are found surrounding and intimately associated with the cell bodies of neurons in sensory and autonomic ganglia (see below). Satellite cells perform a similar role to astrocytes in the CNS, adjusting the micro-environment and limiting exposure to toxic materials.

To help consolidate your understanding of the key cells of the nervous system, attempt Activity 6.1.

Activity 6.1   Reinforcing key information

Knowledge of neuron and neuroglial structure and function is commonly assessed in nursing exams. To help reinforce the information you have learnt above, take a blank piece of paper and draw a sketch of each of the three major types of neuron and the six major types of neuroglial cells. Next to each diagram briefly outline the major roles and location of these cells.

When you have completed this exercise, score yourself based on the information provided in this section of the chapter.

There are some possible answers to all activities at the end of the chapter, unless otherwise indicated.

Now that you understand the structure of neurons and neuroglial cells, we will examine how electrochemical signals are generated and conducted in the nervous system.

Action potentials (nerve impulses)

Neurons communicate with each other and with other organs and tissues using electrochemical signalling. These cells have the ability to move charged atoms called ions across their cell membranes to generate small electrical currents called action potentials. Our ability to perceive our surroundings, carry out complex mental activities and respond favourably to various stimuli is dependent on the ability to generate these electrical signals and conduct them efficiently.

The sodium potassium pump and resting potential

Most human cells including neurons have the ability to actively pump potassium ions (K^+) across their cell membranes into their cytoplasm, while simultaneously pumping sodium ions (Na^+) out. Therefore in health the majority of Na^+ inside the body is found outside of our cells and the majority of K^+ is found inside our cells.

When neurons are resting (not conducting an action potential), they are said to be polarised. The distribution of Na^+ ions outside the cell and the K^+ ions inside the cell gives resting neurons an overall voltage of around -70 mV (millivolts; a millivolt is 1 thousandth of a volt). Since the neuron is resting, this -70 mV is referred to as its resting potential (Figure 6.5).

Action potentials

Along the length of a neuron's axon are tiny Na channels which are closed while the cell is resting. As soon as a nerve cell is activated (e.g. a sensory nerve ending in the skin is touched), the Na channels immediately open, allowing Na^+ ions to flood into the axon. Since Na^+ ions have a positive charge associated with them, this depolarises the neuron, changing the voltage from the resting potential of -70 mV to +30 mV. This voltage of +30 mV is called an action potential.

It is important to notice that we have now gone from a negative resting potential to a positive action potential; for this reason, this process is often referred to as depolarisation. Remember that neurons have an active sodium potassium pump and so Na^+ ions are quickly pumped back out of the neuron to restore the resting potential (Figure 6.5).

To help you understand how the action potential passes along the axon, a good analogy is to think of the nerve axon as a row of people who are going to perform a Mexican wave. When you activate the neuron, this is like the first person putting up their hands; everyone else follows behind until the nerve end is reached (the end of the line). Effectively each segment of the axon undergoes its own action potential.

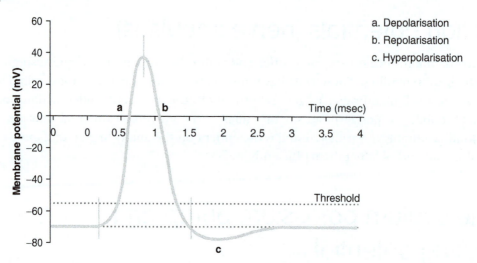

a. Depolarisation
b. Repolarisation
c. Hyperpolarisation

Figure 6.5 Resting potential and generation of an action potential

The role of the myelin sheath

Earlier in this chapter we discussed the nature of the myelin sheath and mentioned that this layer of insulation is not continuous, with small gaps called the nodes of Ranvier existing between adjacent cells of the myelin sheath. Rather than having to travel through the entire length of the axon (like the Mexican wave described above), in myelinated neurons the action potential can leapfrog from one node of Ranvier to the next, greatly speeding up nerve conduction (Figure 6.6).

This leapfrogging from one node to the next is termed saltatory conduction (the word saltatory literally means to leapfrog) and is essential to a healthy, efficient and optimally functioning nervous system. Unfortunately, there are many diseases that can damage the myelin sheath, slowing or preventing saltatory conduction. Unsurprisingly, such diseases can be devastating, since the ability to coordinate physical movement can be compromised and mental acuity may decline.

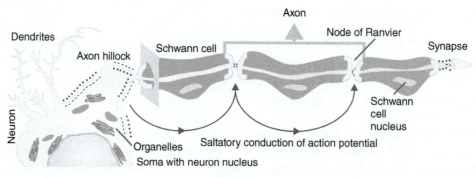

Figure 6.6 Saltatory conduction along myelinated axon

Synapses and synaptic transmission

When action potentials reach the branching ends of an axon, they eventually reach the bulb-like synaptic boutons (also known as synaptic knobs or presynaptic terminals). These are typically in close proximity to the dendrite of an adjacent neuron and separated by a tiny gap called the synaptic cleft. These junctions, where neurons connect to each other or other structures such as muscles or glandular tissues, are called synapses.

Electrical and chemical synapses

In some synapses in the brain the synaptic cleft between two neurons is so small (gap junctions) that the action potential can be transmitted directly onto the next neuron. However, most synapses require a chemical called a neurotransmitter to carry the signal across the synaptic cleft; synapses that utilise neurotransmitters are called chemical synapses (Figure 6.7).

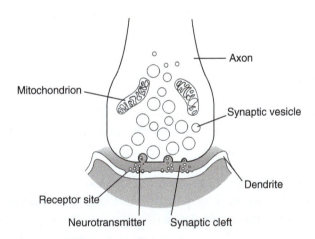

Figure 6.7 Structure of a chemical synapse

Neurons stockpile neurotransmitters which are continually transferred along the length of the axon and stored in the presynaptic terminals in secretory vesicles. When an action potential arrives at a presynaptic terminal, calcium channels open, allowing calcium ions to flood inside. This calcium influx stimulates the secretory vesicles to fuse with the presynaptic membrane and release their stockpiled neurotransmitter into the synaptic cleft. Neurotransmitters rapidly diffuse across the aqueous environment of the synaptic cleft before binding to specific receptors on the postsynaptic membrane. This binding of neurotransmitter to its receptor may stimulate or inhibit the generation of an action potential in the postsynaptic cell.

There are many different kinds of neurotransmitters including acetylcholine and norepinephrine, serotonin, dopamine and γ (gamma) aminobutyric acid (GABA). Neurotransmitters do not usually remain in the synaptic cleft for very long. Most are either rapidly broken down by enzymes or recycled by being transported back into the presynaptic terminal. Many drugs can modify or even block the action of a neurotransmitter at the synapse.

For example, the class of drugs termed beta blockers block the neurotransmitter noradrenaline (norepinephrine) from binding to its receptor. Noradrenaline is a key neurotransmitter in the sympathetic branch of the autonomic nervous system, so a beta blocker may be of use, for example, to slow a patient's heart rate (Chapter 3).

Brain structure and function

The brain is a large organ located within the cranial cavity and surrounded and protected by three protective membranes called the meninges. A typical adult brain weighs between 1.3 and 1.5 kg and consists of around 10 billion interconnected neurons. Structurally, the brain is divided into four major regions (Figure 6.8): the brain stem, the cerebellum, the diencephalon and the cerebral cortex, which consists of the two cerebral hemispheres.

The brain stem

This part of the brain is evolutionarily the oldest and plays a key role in many of the processes that are essential to survival. It is continuous with the spinal cord and consists of three distinct regions: the midbrain, pons and medulla oblongata.

These regions have diverse roles that can often be described as 'primitive' in nature, including behaviours that are necessary for survival and reproduction. The brain stem also provides pathways for the nerve fibres that connect the higher centres of the cerebral cortex with the lower brain regions, as well as housing the origins of 10 of the 12 pairs of cranial nerves.

The medulla oblongata

Frequently abbreviated to the medulla, this is the most inferior portion of the brain stem, extending from the pons above and continuous with the spinal cord below. It is about 2.5 cm in length and positioned just above the foramen magnum, the large opening in the skull where the spinal cord exits into the spinal canal. The ventral surface of the medulla is characterised by two longitudinal ridges called pyramids which form the corticospinal and corticobulbar tracts, which are prominent nerve pathways descending from the motor cortex that subsequently decussate (cross over) within the medulla.

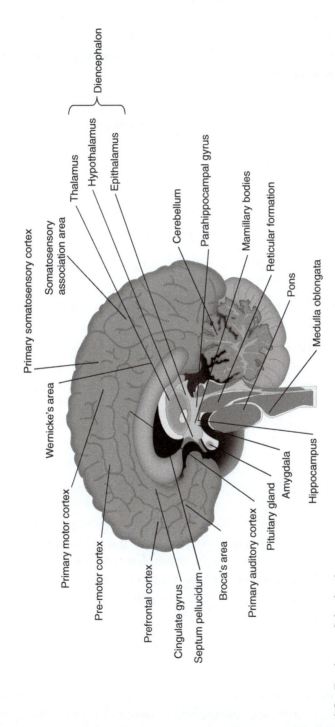

Diencephalon

Thalamus

Hypothalamus

Epithalamus

Cerebellum

Parahippocampal gyrus

Mamillary bodies

Reticular formation

Pons

Medulla oblongata

Primary somatosensory cortex

Somatosensory association area

Wernicke's area

Primary motor cortex

Pre-motor cortex

Prefrontal cortex

Cingulate gyrus

Septum pellucidum

Broca's area

Primary auditory cortex

Pituitary gland

Amygdala

Hippocampus

Figure 6.8 Regions of the brain

The dorsal medulla contains the ascending sensory tracts which relay somatic sensory information from the spinal cord to the somatosensory cortex. Like the fibres that relay motor information from the motor cortex, these sensory fibres also decussate (cross over) within the medulla. This 'crossing over' of fibres relaying motor and sensory movement ensures the activity of the cerebral hemispheres is contralateral in nature, with the right cerebral hemisphere responsible for sensation and movement on the left side of the body and the left cerebral hemisphere responsible for sensation and movement on the right side of the body.

This is essential information for nurses to learn and understand since it allows regions of brain disease and injury to be identified based on the symptoms experienced by the patient. For example, if a patient has a stroke and experiences numbness/paralysis on the right side of their body, it is highly likely that the event has taken place in the left hemisphere.

The medulla is the location of many of the brain's most vital autonomic centres that are essential to health and survival, including in particular:

The cardiac centre: Also known as the cardioregulatory centre, this controls the heart rate and adjusts the force of myocardial contraction (Chapter 3).

The vasomotor centre: Controls the diameter of blood vessels to regulate blood pressure (Chapter 3).

The respiratory centres: The dorsal respiratory group (DRG) and ventral respiratory group (VRG) control the rate and depth of breathing and, in conjunction with the pneumotaxic centre in the pons, maintain respiratory rhythm (Chapter 4).

In addition, there are other reflex centres which regulate vomiting, hiccupping, swallowing, coughing and sneezing.

The pons

The pons is situated immediately above the medulla oblongata and anteriorly to (in front of) the cerebellum. It is mainly composed of tracts which run vertically to complete the pathways between the cerebral hemispheres and the spinal cord. The pons contains a specialised respiratory area called the pneumotaxic centre which works synergistically with the respiratory groups of the medulla to control the respiratory rate and breathing pattern (Chapter 4).

The midbrain

The midbrain is the most superior portion of the brain stem and contains large bundles of motor nerves on its ventral side which descend towards the spinal cord. The midbrain has specialised regions called the superior and inferior colliculi which play a key role in coordinating head and eye movements.

Cerebellum

The word cerebellum literally means 'little brain'. This region is located posteriorly to the pons and medulla. It consists of two hemispheres separated by a narrow midline called the vermis. Its major role is to process information from the somatic motor cortex, various brain stem nuclei and sensory receptors throughout the body to provide the accurate timing necessary for smooth, coordinated and balanced movements.

Recently the cerebellum has also been shown to play a role in understanding language, mental imagery and learning of new motor skills (muscle memory). Unsurprisingly, damage to the cerebellum (e.g. following a stroke) results in clumsy, uncoordinated muscular movements as seen in ataxia disorders, and these may be associated with speech problems and difficulties with language.

Diencephalon

The diencephalon is relatively centrally located within the brain and connects the cerebral cortex and brain stem. It consists of three distinct regions:

Thalamus

Sensory information from all parts of the body converge on the thalamus. In addition, virtually all other inputs ascending to the cerebral cortex funnel through the thalamus. The role of the thalamus is to 'sort out' and 'edit' information. Therefore it effectively acts as the gateway to the cerebral cortex. There are two special areas of the thalamus. These are the lateral geniculate nuclei (LGN) and the medial geniculate nuclei (MGN).

The LGN provides a relay centre for information passing from the eyes to the brain. The optic nerves end here and synapse with the nerves that will travel to the visual cortex in the occipital lobes of the cerebral cortex. The MGN has a similar role, but for auditory information coming from the cochlea via the vestibulocochlear nerve to the auditory cortex in the temporal lobes.

Hypothalamus

The hypothalamus is a small but vital structure. It is located just below the thalamus with its base connected to the pituitary gland by a thin stalk called the infundibulum (Chapter 5).

The hypothalamus is the main visceral control centre and essential to homeostasis, since it functions as a bridge between the nervous system and the endocrine system. Its many diverse roles include:

Autonomic control: The hypothalamus controls the brain stem and spinal nuclei responsible for ANS activity. It will therefore affect blood pressure, heart rate and force of myocardial contraction, digestive tract motility, and respiratory rate and depth.

Emotional responses: The hypothalamus is a major component of the 'limbic system' (the emotional part of the brain). Nuclei involved in pleasure, fear, rage and biological rhythms and drives (such as the sex drive) are centred in or around the hypothalamus.

Body temperature regulation: The hypothalamus is the location of the thermoregulatory centre which functions as the body's thermostat, receiving and acting upon information from thermoreceptors located throughout the skin, brain and other regions (Chapter 2).

Regulation of food intake: Ultimately it is the hypothalamus that regulates sensations of hunger and satiety (fullness) in response to levels of certain nutrients such as glucose and hormones such as insulin. The hypothalamus also has receptors for the hunger hormone ghrelin.

Regulation of water balance and thirst: Special osmoreceptors are activated by changes in blood plasma concentrations, allowing the amount of antidiuretic hormone (ADH) released from the posterior pituitary to be adjusted (Chapter 11). Hypothalamic neurons in the thirst centre also influence water balance by affecting the urge to drink water.

Regulation of sleep/wake cycles: The hypothalamus works together with other brain regions to regulate sleep. It is the location of the suprachiasmatic nucleus (our biological clock) which sets the timing of the sleep cycle in response to daylight/darkness cues as perceived via the visual pathways.

Control of the endocrine system: The hypothalamus acts as a regulator of the endocrine system by producing several releasing hormones, which directly control secretion of hormones by the anterior pituitary and indirectly regulate the secretion of hormones from several other endocrine glands (Chapter 5).

Epithalamus

The epithalamus is the third region of the diencephalon and contains a pine cone-shaped structure called the pineal gland. This tiny pea-sized endocrine structure secretes the hormone melatonin (a sleep-inducing signal), which helps regulate the sleep/wake cycle and some aspects of mood.

Cerebral cortex

The cerebrum is the largest part of the brain consisting primarily of the left and right hemispheres. Its surface has a highly convoluted appearance with prominent folds called gyri (and grooves of varying depth called sulci). Each gyrus and each sulcus greatly increase the surface area of the cerebral cortex, allowing a greater number of neurons to be packed in. The two hemispheres are separated by a deep crevice called the central fissure (Figure 6.9).

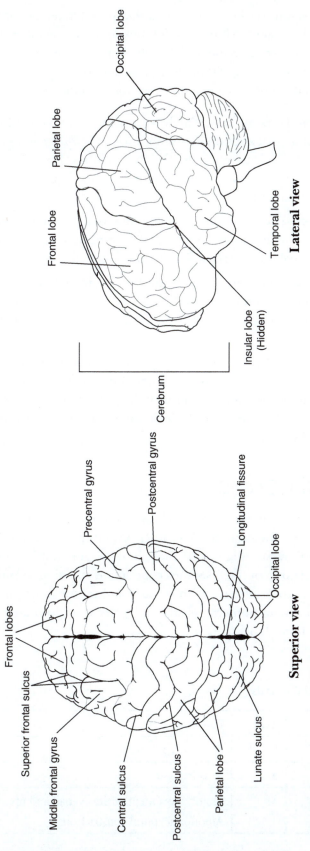

Figure 6.9 The cerebral hemispheres

Each hemisphere has four distinct lobes called the frontal lobe, parietal lobe, temporal lobe and occipital lobe (Figure 6.9b). A useful trick to help remember these is to realise that their names are derived from the names of the bones of the skull which overlie them. Each of the four lobes has its own distinct functions, although in reality there are intimate connections between the lobes, meaning that they work together and not in isolation.

The frontal lobes: These sit immediately behind the frontal bone (forehead). The somatic motor cortex resides in this location; it is this region of the brain that initiates conscious motor movements. The frontal lobes also have a multitude of other functions, being involved in memory, motivation, aggression, mood and the sense of olfaction (smell).

The parietal lobes: These are found beneath the parietal bones (top of the skull). Here resides the somatosensory cortex which is important to receiving most sensory input, including real-time information relating to touch, pain and temperature.

The occipital lobes: These are found behind the occipital bones (back of skull) and receive visual input from the eyes via the optic nerves. It is the occipital lobes that take the raw visual information and actually interpret this to create the picture of the world around us.

The temporal lobes: These are located beneath the temporal bones at the side of the skull (temples). The temporal lobes are intimately connected to the other three lobes and have diverse functions including olfaction, memory and personality traits. The temporal lobes are also the location of the auditory cortex responsible for our sense of hearing.

The cranial nerves

There are 12 pairs of cranial nerves which are denoted by roman numerals in the order they emerge from the brain from its anterior to its posterior portion. The cranial nerves are peripheral nerves that can be thought of as the brain's equivalent of spinal nerves (see below). As part of the PNS, they conduct information to and from the brain and may be sensory, motor or have both sensory and motor functions. In addition to being denoted by a roman numeral, each cranial nerve is given a name that is often indicative of its function (Table 6.1).

Table 6.1 The cranial nerves

Name and number	Type	Function
Olfactory (I)	S	Sensory: sense of smell
Optic (II)	S	Sensory: vision
Oculomotor (III)	M, P	Motor: movement of the eyeball and upper eyelid Autonomic: pupil constriction

Trochlear (IV)	M	Motor: movement of the eyeball
Trigeminal (V)	S, M	Sensory: general sensation from face, scalp, cornea, nasal and oral cavities Motor: chewing
Abducens (VI)	M	Motor: movement of the eyeball
Facial (V)	S, M, P	Sensory: taste Motor: facial expression Autonomic: secretion of tears and saliva
Vestibulocochlear (III)	S	Sensory: hearing and balance
Glossopharyngeal (IX)	S, M, P	Sensory: taste and touch to back of tongue Motor: swallowing and speech Autonomic: secretion of saliva
Vagus (X)	S, M, P	Sensory: taste and sensation from epiglottis and pharynx Motor: swallowing and speech Autonomic: muscle contraction of organs in the thorax and abdomen, and secretion of digestive fluids
Accessory (XI)	M	Motor: head movement
Hypoglossal (XII)	M	Motor: movement of the tongue muscle
S, sensory; M, motor; P, parasympathetic		

Sensory, motor and parasympathetic functions of the cranial nerves

There are two general categories of cranial nerve function: sensory and motor. Motor functions are further subdivided into somatic motor and parasympathetic (Table 6.1). Three cranial nerves (I, II and VIII) are sensory only. Four cranial nerves (IV, VI, XI and XII) are considered somatic motor, although these nerves also have a proprioception (positional awareness) sensory function. The oculomotor nerve (III) is somatic motor and parasympathetic, while the remaining nerves all have sensory, somatic motor and parasympathetic functions.

Knowledge of cranial nerves in clinical diagnosis

Head injuries, strokes or tumours frequently damage one or more of the cranial nerves, producing characteristic symptoms which reflect their loss of function. For example, injury of the optic nerve (II) may result in vision loss, and injury of the abducens nerve (VI) may cause the eye to turn inwards, whereas injury of the vestibulo-cochlear nerve (III) may lead to deafness or problems with balance.

To help you learn and retain key information relating to the cranial nerves, attempt Activity 6.2.

Activity 6.2   Designing learning tools

Nurses are expected to know the names of the 12 cranial nerves and their major functions.

It is often useful to use memory aids such as mnemonics to remember sequential information such as this for quick recall in exams and in clinical practice. Design your own mnemonic to remember the correct sequence of cranial nerves as highlighted in Table 6.1. This will be time well spent since knowledge of this area of human anatomy and physiology is frequently assessed in nursing exams and is essential to effective nursing practice.

A sample answer is given at the end of the chapter, although you will have to design your own mnemonic to use as a memory aid.

Now that you have a good understanding of the 12 cranial nerves, we will examine further the structure of the brain and spinal cord.

Physical structure of the cerebral cortex

If the gross anatomy of the cerebral hemispheres is viewed in cross-section then regions of grey matter and white matter are visible. The grey matter is made up of billions of neuron cell bodies, dendrites and unmyelinated axons, together with their associated neuroglial cells. The white matter corresponds to the bundles of myelinated neurons that are relaying information to and from different parts of the brain and spinal cord. Unfortunately, with increasing age there is a progressive loss of neural tissue, which results in brain shrinkage. During this ageing process the sulci (grooves) of the cerebral cortex become deeper, which gives the gyri (folds) a more prominent appearance.

Spinal cord and spinal nerves

The second region of the CNS is the spinal cord, which can be thought of as an elongated, almost cylindrical extension of the brainstem. It is contained and protected by the vertebral column. The spinal cord provides a line of communication between the brain and the rest of the body below the head. Sensory and motor information travels along the neurons of the PNS, passing to and from the cord via the spinal nerves which exit the cord at regular intervals.

There are 31 pairs of spinal nerves and they emerge from the spinal cord as indicated below:

8 pairs from cervical segments

12 pairs from thoracic segments

5 pairs from lumbar segments

5 pairs from sacral segments

1 pair from coccygeal segments

Unlike the cranial nerves, the spinal nerves do not have special names but are identified by a letter and number which signifies their longitudinal position. For example, L1 indicates the nerve that emerges from the first segment of the lumbar portion of the spinal cord. After emerging from the spinal cord, the spinal nerves branch into smaller peripheral nerves which extend into the body.

Spinal cord structure

The internal portion of the spinal cord consists of grey matter. Like the grey matter of the brain, it is composed of nerve cell bodies, dendrites, synapses, unmyelinated axons and glial cells. The outer region is primarily composed of white matter which consists of densely arranged bundles of myelinated axons (Figure 6.10).

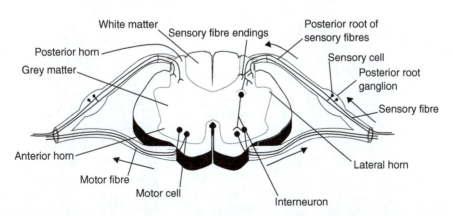

Figure 6.10 Internal structure of the spinal cord

Ascending and descending information

Sensory nerves enter the spinal cord at the dorsal (posterior) horn, while motor nerves exit on the ventral (anterior) horn. Interneurons within the grey matter communicate directly between sensory and motor fibres in the spinal reflexes. They also relay information up to and from the higher centres. These ascending and descending fibres run in discrete columns, some sensory, some motor.

Dermatomes and referred pain

In the skin, sensory nerve endings detect touch, pressure, temperature and pain. Information about detected changes in the external and internal environment is transmitted to the CNS via sensory spinal nerves. Each spinal nerve innervates a consistent area of skin called a dermatome (Figure 6.11). Understanding dermatomes is essential to nurses for use in clinical diagnosis. Patients frequently complain of pain in the skin or region of skin which overlies a damaged or inflamed internal organ.

Since there is no actual damage or inflammation in the skin itself, this type of pain is called referred pain. This sensation happens because the skin and the damaged internal organ are innervated by sensory neurons that supply information to the same area of the somatosensory cortex. Therefore, the brain cannot distinguish between two sources of painful stimuli. Common examples of referred pain are highlighted in Figure 6.11.

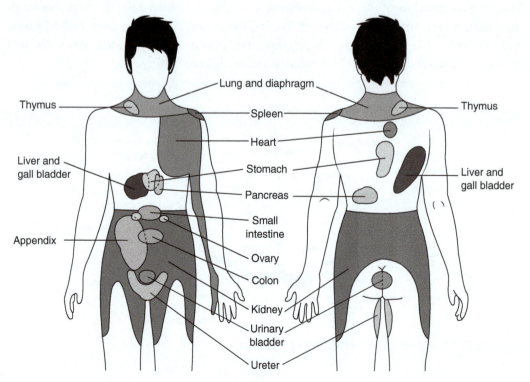

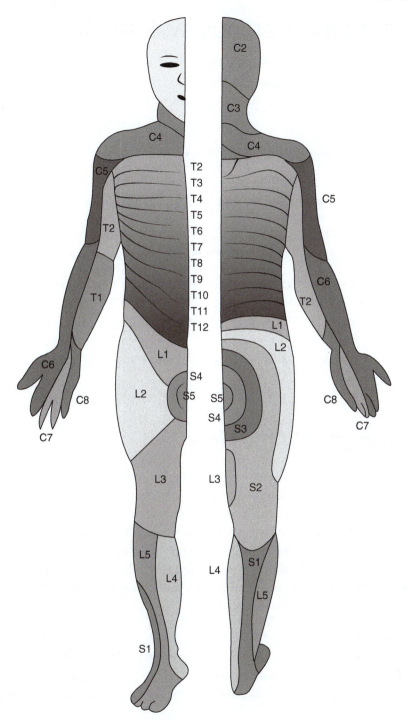

Figure 6.11 Dermatomes and map of referred pain

Source: OpenStax (2013) *Anatomy and Physiology*. Rice University. Available at: https://openstax.org/
books/anatomy-and-physiology/pages/1-introduction

The autonomic nervous system (ANS)

Earlier in this chapter we explained that the ANS consists of two main divisions known as the sympathetic and parasympathetic branches (Figure 6.12). The autonomic motor nerves transmit information from the brain stem or spinal cord to the following types of effector tissues:

Cardiac muscle in the myocardium of the heart.

Smooth muscle – found in multiple places throughout the body including the airways, GI tract, blood vessels and attached to hair follicles in the skin.

Glandular tissues – including endocrine glands (ductless glands) which produce hormones and exocrine glands (glands with ducts), such as digestive and sweat glands.

The motor neurons of the ANS have axons that terminate at structures termed ganglia (discrete collections of neural tissue found outside of the CNS). Since these autonomic neurons are positioned before the ganglia, they are called preganglionic neurons. Exiting from the ganglia are a second set of neurons called postganglionic neurons which, as the name suggests, conduct action potentials from the ganglia to their effector organs (Figure 6.12).

The sympathetic division

The ganglia of the sympathetic nervous system run parallel to the spinal cord in chains (Figure 6.12). This means that the preganglionic neurons are relatively short since they only have to travel a small distance from the spinal cord. Most of these exit the spinal cord in the thoracic and lumbar regions. The sympathetic postganglionic neurons conduct action potentials to distant regions of the body, including the smooth muscles layers of blood vessels, sweat glands and the arrector pili muscles that are attached to hair follicles in skin. For this reason, although their preganglionic neurons are short, their postganglionic neurons can be very long.

The sympathetic division of the ANS is activated during emergency situations where the body needs to be rapidly prepared for immediate action. We can think of these as the 'E situations': exercise, excitement, emotions. Table 6.2 summarises the major sympathetic responses which are often collectively referred to as the fight-or-flight response.

By referring to this table you can see that the key physiological effects of sympathetic activation are an increase in heart rate and peripheral vasoconstriction to increase blood pressure and ensure rapid blood flow to key organs such as the muscles, heart and lungs. Simultaneously, blood vessels in skeletal muscle dilate, enhancing blood flow further. This is essential in fight-or-flight situations where a steady supply of oxygenated blood is vital to prevent oxygen debt and early muscle fatigue; this could mean

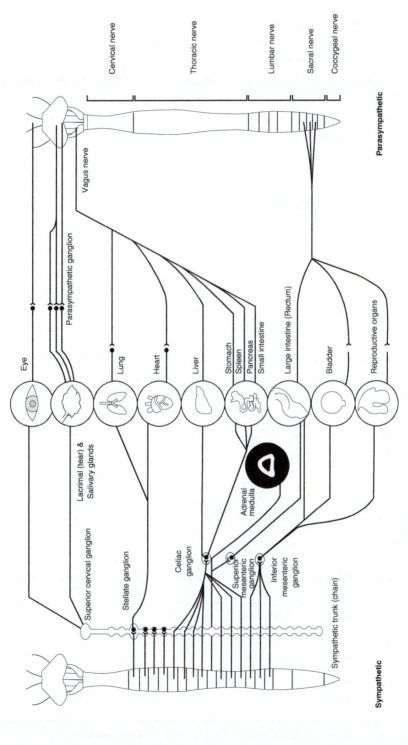

Figure 6.12 Neural pathways in the sympathetic and parasympathetic branches of the ANS

the difference between life and death. Activation of sweat glands helps prevent over-heating during bouts of extreme muscular activity where lots of heat is generated.

The liver is stimulated to release glucose into the blood to ensure a steady supply of fuel to our muscles and to our brain to enhance alertness. The adrenal glands are stimulated to release adrenaline (our fight-or-flight hormone), which further activates the sympathetic branch of the ANS, amplifying its response. Sympathetic activation also inhibits physiological processes that are non-essential in an emergency situation such as digestion. The human body needs these preparations when facing a threat. Either we resist (fight) the threat or remove ourselves (flight) from the situation as quickly as possible.

The parasympathetic division

Unlike the sympathetic nervous system, the ganglia of the parasympathetic nervous system are found in close proximity to their effector organs or tissues. This means that the preganglionic neurons are generally much longer than their sympathetic counterparts, while the parasympathetic postganglionic neurons are generally much shorter. The motor neurons of the parasympathetic nervous system exit the CNS either in the cranium or the sacral area of the spinal cord (craniosacral).

The parasympathetic division of the ANS is largely antagonistic to the sympathetic branch and tends to be active when the body is at its most relaxed. For this reason, the parasympathetic nervous system is regarded as controlling many of our so-called vegetative functions which are frequently summarised as 'rest and digest'. Its key roles are summarised in Table 6.2 and include slowing of the heart rate (Chapter 3) and enhancing digestion by increasing the secretion of digestive enzymes and increasing gut motility.

Table 6.2 Physiological effects associated with activation of sympathetic and parasympathetic nervous systems

Effector (target)	Effect of sympathetic stimulation	Effect of parasympathetic stimulation
Eyes	Dilates pupil, relaxes ciliary muscle	Constricts pupil, contracts ciliary muscle
Salivary glands	Inhibits secretion of saliva	Stimulates secretion of saliva
Lungs	Dilates bronchioles	Constricts bronchioles
Heart	Increases heartbeat	Decreases heartbeat

Blood vessels	Peripheral vasoconstriction Increases blood pressure Vasodilation in muscle	No effect
Liver	Conversion of glycogen to glucose and release into the blood	No effect
Stomach and intestinal wall	Decreases motility	Increases motility
Adrenal gland	Secretes adrenaline	No known effect
Glands of digestive system	Decrease secretion of digestive enzymes and insulin	Increases secretion of digestive enzymes and insulin
Bladder	Delays emptying (relaxes muscle, constricts sphincter)	Empties bladder (contracts muscle, relaxes sphincter)
Sweat gland	Secretes sweat	No known effect

Protection of the CNS

Since the CNS is so vital in coordinating human physiological processes, it is very well protected. It is primarily shielded from physical trauma by the bones of the cranium which surround the brain and the individual bones (vertebrae) of the vertebral column, which enclose the spinal cord (Chapter 8). Additional protection is afforded by three membranes called the meninges which surround the brain and spinal cord.

The meninges

The meninges are often referred to as the 'three protective mothers' because they enclose and protect the delicate tissues of the CNS (Figure 6.13).

> **The dura mater (tough mother):** This outer fibrous membrane is often simply known as the dura and is found attached to the periosteum lining the inner surface of the cranial vault. As the dura passes into the vertebral column, a small gap is present between the dura and the spinal canal. This small space is called the epidural space and is a common site for introducing local anaesthetics for pain relief, e.g. during childbirth or to allow surgical procedures to be carried out.

> **The arachnoid mater (spider-like mother):** This forms the middle of the three membranes and has a soft, wispy appearance that is said to resemble a spider's web.

> **The pia mater (small mother):** This is the innermost of the meninges and is a thin membrane that resembles a thin sheet of cling-film, and is found permanently attached to the surface of the brain and spinal cord.

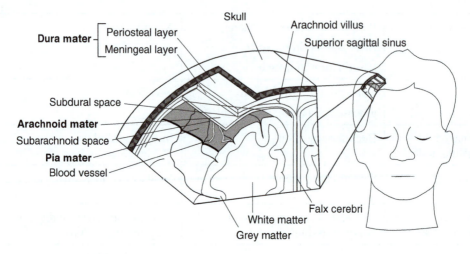

Figure 6.13 The meninges

The subarachnoid space, CSF and lumbar puncture

Between the pia and arachnoid mater lies the subarachnoid space. This space contains the cerebrospinal fluid (CSF) which is produced by the choroid plexuses that line the ventricles of the brain and are composed of ependymal cells (see above). In health there is typically around 80–150 ml of CSF, which is usually clear and colourless and drains into the subarachnoid space of the spinal column through a small duct called the aqueduct of Sylvius.

The CSF continually circulates throughout the subarachnoid space. You may recall that this circulation is aided by the movements of cilia, which are present on the surface of some of the ependymal cells. The CSF acts as a third layer of protection, with the brain and spinal cord effectively floating in this fluid, which acts as a cushion (see Activity 6.3).

Occasionally it is necessary to take samples of CSF to look for evidence of pathology. This is normally achieved via a process called a lumbar puncture (spinal tap). During this procedure a needle is carefully inserted into the subarachnoid space in the lumbar region and fluid is withdrawn. CSF collected by lumbar puncture may have bacterial or viral contamination, possibly together with pus and inflammatory mediators, which may be indicative of meningitis. Sometimes blood may be present, which could be indicative of a cerebral haemorrhage.

To help you understand the protective role of CSF, attempt Activity 6.3.

Activity 6.3   Assessing the cushioning effect of CSF

Fill a jam jar with water, add an intact uncooked egg and close the lid tightly. Shake the jar vigorously; what happens to the egg? From what you have just learnt, try and relate this experiment to the protective role of the cerebral spinal fluid. What would happen to the egg if you repeated this experiment without the water? (Hint: don't try this unless you fancy an omelette!)

From Activity 6.3 you should now have a good appreciation of how CSF acts as an effective cushion to protect the brain and spinal cord; however, this fluid and the membranes that surround and protect the brain are susceptible to infection. This is explored in Claire's case study.

Case study: Claire – meningitis

Claire is a 27-year-old school teacher who has gone home early from work with what she thought were severe flu-like symptoms. Claire had previously experienced a severe headache before coming into work that morning but took some ibuprofen and the pain had eased. On her return, her mother noticed that Claire was feeling nauseated and in great pain, and worryingly had begun to develop a skin rash. Her mother immediately took Claire to the local A&E where CSF obtained via a lumbar puncture was sent for analysis. She was immediately placed on intravenous antibiotics and given pain relief. The CSF results revealed Claire was suffering with bacterial meningitis, which fortunately responded well to antibiotic therapy and Claire was able to return home after five days of treatment.

Now that you have a good understanding of the CNS, PNS and some of the pathologies associated with the nervous system, we will examine the two most advanced sensory organs in the body: the eyes and the ears.

The special senses

Vision

Like many animals, humans are equipped with stereoscopic binocular vision which not only provides a real-time visual representation of our surroundings but also allows us to effectively judge distances and orientate ourselves in our environment. Each eyeball is located within its eye socket (orbital cavity) within the skull and is attached to several skeletal muscles, which allow it to be moved to change the visual field without the need for moving the head.

Accessory structures of the eye

Each eye has several accessory structures which play important roles in ensuring optimal eye health. The eyebrows are involved in non-verbal communication and are also thought to function to direct sweat away from the eyes. The eyelashes are attached to the eyelids (palpebras) and help prevent dust and other particulates from making contact with the surface of the eye. When closed or during blinking, the eyelids cover the front of the eyeballs and help ensure an even distribution of watery lacrimal secretions to help prevent the eyes from drying out. The eyelids can also close over the eyes to prevent mechanical damage from debris or photo damage from excessively bright light sources.

A lacrimal gland is found above the upper lateral corner of each eye socket. The lacrimal glands produce tears which, in addition to moistening the eye and preventing desiccation, also contain antimicrobial chemicals such as the enzyme lysozyme which breaks open bacterial cell walls on contact. The lacrimal secretions are continually passing over the surface of the eyeball, aided by blinking. These secretions drain into small ducts in the medial corner of the eyes before eventually draining into the nasal cavity. If the eyes are irritated or a person is emotionally upset, the lacrimal glands can increase their secretions, significantly overwhelming the ability of the drainage system, resulting in an over-spilling of tears into the corners of the eyes.

Structure of the eye

Each eyeball can be thought of as a fluid-filled sphere consisting of two cavities (Figure 6.14). The anterior cavity is filled with a watery fluid called aqueous humour, while the posterior cavity is filled with a jelly-like material called vitreous humour. The front surface of the eyeball is covered by a thin, delicate protective membrane known as the conjunctiva, which extends around the inner surface of the eyelids. Since the conjunctiva is exposed to the external environment when the eyes are open, it is susceptible to infection which commonly results in either viral or bacterial conjunctivitis (literally inflammation of the conjunctiva).

The wall of the eyeball consists of three distinct layers. The outer layer is called the sclera or sclerotic coat and consists of tough, collagen-rich connective tissue. The sclera corresponds to the white of the eye and is responsible for maintaining the shape of the eyeball. Underneath the sclera is a thin layer called the choroid; this is usually a dark-black colour because of the presence of large numbers of melanin-secreting melanocytes. This dark-black layer is essential to prevent internal reflection of light within the eye.

The innermost layer of the eyeball is the delicate photosensitive layer known as the retina. Here reside specialised light-sensitive receptor cells known as rods and cones. Rods

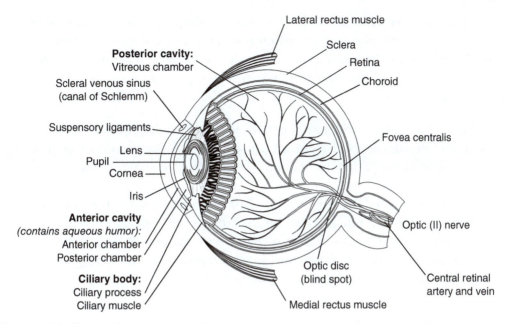

Figure 6.14 Internal structure of the eye

are important in detecting different levels of light intensity and are particularly important for night vision. Cones tend to be concentrated at high density in a small region of the retina called the fovea centralis. This is the portion of the retina where light is focused and the cones in this region are responsible for colour vision.

The cornea is the transparent, curved front portion of the eyeball which begins the process of focusing light within the eye. The amount of light entering the eye is controlled by the iris, which is a ring of smooth muscle under the control of the autonomic nervous system. In dark conditions the iris relaxes and its aperture, known as the pupil, dilates to let more light into the eye. Conversely, in brighter conditions the smooth muscle of the iris contracts, constricting the pupil and limiting the entry of light. The iris is usually pigmented with melanin to give the eye its colour; more pigment results in darker-brown-coloured eyes, while less pigment is associated with green- and blue-coloured eyes. The genetic condition albinism results in irises that lack pigmentation and usually have a pinkish or violet colour.

Iris responses and pupil dilation are useful tools for nurses when looking for potential neurological damage in their patients. The lens is immediately behind the iris and attached by tiny suspensory ligaments to a structure called the ciliary body, which is largely composed of smooth muscle. The lens is responsible for final focusing of light within the eye via a process called accommodation. When viewing distant objects, the smooth muscle of the ciliary body is relaxed and the suspensory ligaments pull tight against the lens, ensuring that it is thin and flat for optimal focus at a distance. When looking at objects up close, e.g. as you are doing now reading this textbook, the smooth muscle of the ciliary body contracts, loosening the tension on the suspensory ligaments and allowing the lens to adopt a thicker, fatter shape, which is optimal to focus at near.

Unfortunately, as we grow older the lens loses its elasticity, and its ability to adopt a thicker, fatter appearance is progressively lost. This means that by our mid-40s most of us will have difficulty focusing on objects close up, which can make reading difficult; this is why from middle-age onwards reading glasses become a necessity for most people.

When light is focused onto the fovea centralis of the retina the photosensitive cones are activated and depolarise to generate an action potential. Action potentials from both eyes are relayed to the occipital lobes of the brain along the optic nerves (cranial nerve II). It is important to realise that the image we perceive is actually constructed within the occipital lobes based on the raw input from the optic nerves. The visual system is not infallible; indeed, a quick search on the Internet for optical illusions will reveal just how easy it is to fool our visual sense. Similarly, diseases such as schizophrenia and certain forms of epilepsy are frequently associated with very convincing visual hallucinations which may feel completely real to the patient.

Hearing and balance

Our senses of hearing and balance are very closely linked as they are associated with organs located in close proximity within the inner ear.

Structure of the ear

The ear has three major regions (Figure 6.15). The outer (external) ear consists of the pinna (also known as the auricle). This is composed of elastic cartilage covered in skin and serves to collect sound waves and funnel them into the external auditory meatus. This final portion of the outer ear ends at the tympanic membrane (ear drum) and is lined by skin that is rich in a specialised type of sweat gland called a ceruminous gland. These are found in huge numbers and produce a thick modified type of sweat called cerumen, which is more commonly known as earwax. Cerumen is antiseptic in nature and has antimicrobial compounds which help prevent ear infection.

The ears are often described as 'self-cleaning' and, left alone, the cerumen secretions will gradually make their way out of the auditory meatus, collecting in the inferior portions of the pinna. Unfortunately, many people regard earwax as unsightly and the use of cotton buds is widespread. However, the use of buds often serves to push the cerumen secretions up against the tympanic membrane where they can progressively harden, impairing hearing and potentially resulting in conductive deafness. Hardened earwax commonly requires the use of wax softeners and subsequent ear syringing or micro-suction.

Sense of hearing

Sound waves that have been funnelled along the auditory meatus strike the tympanic membrane, causing it to vibrate in harmony. The inner surface of the ear drum is connected to the malleus (hammer), which is the first of three tiny bones collectively known

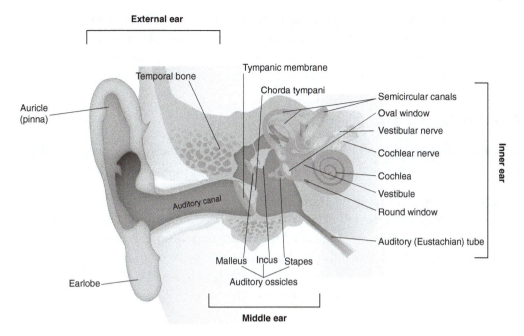

Figure 6.15 Regions of the ear

as the auditory ossicles. Sound waves are transmitted to the malleus and then onto the incus (anvil) and finally the stapes (stirrup). The role of the auditory ossicles is to conduct and amplify the sound waves across the air-filled chamber of the middle ear (Figure 6.15).

The middle ear is connected to the back of the pharynx (throat) by a small passage-way called the Eustachian or auditory tube. Its role is to ensure that there is equal air pressure on both sides of the eardrum. Unfortunately, because of its location, bacteria that reside in the pharynx, perhaps as the result of a sore throat, can travel up the Eustachian tube and cause an infection of the middle ear. Such infections are very common and known as otitis media. These infections can increase the pressure within the middle ear, potentially damaging and even rupturing the ear drum, which is only around 100 μm (0.1 mm) thick. Middle-ear infections are not only painful but may also reduce hearing acuity and lead to dizziness and vertigo.

The stapes is the final of the three ossicles and conducts sound waves into the inner ear. This tiny bone rests in a small aperture called the oval window which leads into a coiled fluid-filled structure called the cochlea. Within the cochlea are specialised sensory cells called hair cells, which are so named because they have hair-like cilia protruding from their membranes. When sound waves exit the stapes, they are transferred via the oval window into the fluid medium within the cochlea. Sound waves in the fluid of the cochlea cause the cilia on the sensory hair cells to bend and depolarise to produce action potentials.

These are relayed to the auditory cortices within the temporal lobes via the vestibulo-cochlear nerve (cranial nerve III), where they are decoded into recognisable sounds that we can interpret. Unfortunately, the hair cells within the cochlea are very delicate, and when exposed to loud sounds (particularly over extended periods), the tiny cilia can snap off and the hair cells can no longer depolarise and generate an action potential. This can lead to permanent neurological deafness or increase the risk of tinnitus, where sounds are perceived when not actually present in the external environment.

Sense of balance (equilibrium)

In addition to the cochlea, the inner ear contains two other sensory regions called the vestibule and semicircular canals. These are the regions responsible for our sense of balance.

> **The vestibule:** This region is primarily involved in static equilibrium which can be defined as our sense of balance when the body is standing still. The vestibule consists of two distinct regions called the utricle and saccule. Both regions contain hair cells, with their cilia embedded in a slab of jelly-like material known as the otolithic membrane. This jelly is given extra weight by small inclusions of calcium carbonate called otoliths, which are embedded in its structure.

When the body position is changed (e.g. leaning to the right or left) the weight of the gelatinous otolithic membranes shifts within the utricle and saccule, bending the cilia of the hair cells, which depolarise to generate an action potential. Action potentials are relayed along the vestibulocochlear nerve (cranial nerve III) to the vestibular nuclei which are found within the brain stem; these decode the raw signals to establish the current bodily position.

> **The semicircular canals:** There are three of these to detect movement in three different planes. These regions of the inner ear are responsible for dynamic equilibrium, which can be defined as the ability of the body to balance itself when moving, e.g. when walking, running or dancing. Like the cochlea, each of the semicircular canals is filled up with fluid which undergoes movement depending on how the body is moving. At the distal end of each semicircular canal is a bulbous expanded cavity termed the ampulla.

Each of the three ampullae contain a triangular gelatinous mass called a cupula, which shifts in harmony with any fluid movements. Each ampulla has a population of sensory hair cells which have their cilia embedded into the gelatinous structure of the cupula. During periods of physical movement, the shifting fluid within the semicircular canals shifts the cupulas, bending the cilia of the attached hair cells. This leads to hair cell depolarisation and the generation of an action potential which is relayed along the vestibulocochlear nerve (cranial nerve III) to the vestibular nuclei to be decoded into real-time information about the current position of the body.

Now that you have completed this chapter, attempt Activity 6.4 to assess your understanding.

Activity 6.4   Multiple-choice questions

1. Which of the following neuroglial cells can be regarded as having primarily an immune function?

   a) Microglial cells

   b) Schwann cells

   c) Ependymal cells

   d) Astrocytes

2. Which of the following is not controlled by the autonomic nervous system?

   a) Cardiac muscle

   b) Exocrine glands

   c) Skeletal muscle

   d) Endocrine glands

3. The sympathetic division of the autonomic nervous system is responsible for

   a) Initiating digestion

   b) Conscious control of skeletal muscles

   c) Slowing the heart rate

   d) Gearing the body up for action

4. The parasympathetic division of the autonomic nervous system

   a) Mediates the body's response to stress

   b) Has relatively long preganglionic fibres

   c) Has numerous collateral ganglia

   d) Has short preganglionic fibres

5. The human nervous system contains how many pairs of spinal nerves?

   a) 35

   b) 28

   c) 33

   d) 31

(Continued)

(Continued)

6. The cerebellum plays a key role in

    a) Sleep and wakefulness

    b) Balance, coordination and posture

    c) Higher intellectual process

    d) Emotion, mood and sensation of pain/pleasure

7. The region of the brain primarily responsible for regulating body temperature is

    a) The vasomotor centre

    b) The cardiac centre

    c) The hypothalamus

    d) None of the above

8. The outermost layer of the meninges is the

    a) Periosteum

    b) Pia mater

    c) Arachnoid mater

    d) Dura mater

9. The photosensitive portion of the eye is known as the

    a) Retina

    b) Choroid

    c) Sclera

    d) Iris

10. The final of the three auditory ossicles that transmits sound waves into the cochlea is called the

    a) Malleus (hammer)

    b) Stapes (stirrup)

    c) Incus (anvil)

    d) Hyoid

Chapter summary

The nervous system is divided into the central nervous system (CNS), which consists of the brain and spinal cord, and the peripheral nervous system (PNS), which consists of all the remaining nerves external to the CNS. The nervous system contains two major categories of cells. Neurons are the specialised cells that conduct electrochemical signals called action potentials. Neuroglial cells are involved in protecting and supporting the neurons. These include astrocytes which form the blood-brain barrier, ependymal cells which produce cerebrospinal fluid, microglial cells which protect against infection and myelin-containing cells called Schwann cells and oligodendrocytes which increase the speed of action potential conduction.

The major regions of the brain are the brain stem which is continuous with the spinal cord and the location of key autonomic regions such as the respiratory and vasomotor centres. The cerebellum is found behind the brain stem and is essential to balance and coordination of physical movements, while the diencephalon is located immediately above the brain stem and is the location of the hypothalamus. The cerebral hemispheres are responsible for sensation and movement and have a contralateral relationship with the body, with the left hemisphere largely responsible for sensation and movement on the right-hand side of the body, and vice versa.

The brain and spinal cord are surrounded and protected by three membranes termed the meninges. The eyes focus light from the external environment onto the retina which contains specialised photosensitive cells called rods, which detect light intensity, and cones, which are responsible for colour vision. The ears collect sound waves from the environment; the cochlea within the inner ear is responsible for detecting sound. The inner ear also contains the vestibular apparatus and semicircular canals, which are responsible for the sense of equilibrium (balance).

Activities: Brief outline answers

Activity 6.2: Designing learning tools (page 154)

Mnemonic for cranial nerves:

Oh Oh Oh To Touch And Feel Very Green Vegetables AH

Olfactory **O**ptic **O**culomotor **T**rochlear **T**rigeminal **A**bducens **F**acial **V**estibulocochlear **G**lossopharyngeal **V**agus **A**ccessory **H**ypoglossal

Activity 6.4: Multiple-choice questions (pages 169–70)

1) a, 2) c, 3) d, 4) b, 5) d, 6) b, 7) c, 8) d, 9) a, 10) b

Further reading

Colloby SJ, Cromarty RA, Peraza LR, Johnsen K, Jóhannesson G, Bonanni L, Onofrj M, Barber R, O'Brien JT and Taylor JP (2016) Multimodal EEG-MRI in the differential diagnosis of Alzheimer's disease and dementia with Lewy bodies. *Journal of Psychiatric Research*, 78: 48–55.

The use of medical scans in detecting dementia.

Crossman AR and Neary D (2015) *Neuroanatomy: An Illustrated Colour Text.* London: Churchill Livingstone.

A more detailed overview of neuroanatomy.

Serlin Y, Shelef I, Knyazer B and Friedman A (2015) Anatomy and physiology of the blood-brain barrier. *Seminars in Cell & Developmental Biology*, 38: 2–6.

A more detailed overview of the nature and role of the blood-brain barrier.

Vander H and Gould D (2015) *Nolte's The Human Brain: An Introduction to Its Functional Anatomy.* St Louis, MO: Mosby.

A detailed overview of brain function.

Useful websites

www.gov.uk/government/news/new-figures-show-larger-proportion-of-strokes-in-the-middle-aged

An overview of the risk of stroke in the middle aged population.

www2.estrellamountain.edu/faculty/farabee/biobk/BioBookNERV.html

An overview of the components of the nervous system including nerve conduction.

www.mstrust.org.uk/a-z/central-nervous-system-cns

A nice basic overview of the spinal nerves.

Chapter 7   The skin

Chapter aims

After reading this chapter, you will be able to:

- identify the major anatomical layers of the skin;
- describe the key functions of the epidermis, dermis and hypodermis;
- explain how the skin acts as a physical barrier;
- provide an overview of the sensory functions of the skin;
- explain the importance of skin integrity and common disorders affecting the skin.

Introduction

Case study: Rema – infected surgical wound site

Rema is a 72-year-old lady who underwent a laparotomy and excision of a tumour in her colon. Three days postoperatively, nurses found that her wound was red and inflamed and decided to keep a close eye on it. By day 5, Rema was feeling hot, and the level of pain in the wound had increased. When the sutures were removed on day 7, the lower 5 cm of the wound opened and purulent fluid drained out. A wound swab was saved, and *Staphylococcus aureus* was cultured. Rema was commenced on Flucloxacillin.

Nurses routinely encounter skin problems in their patients, ranging from infected lesions such as that seen in Rema's case study through to pressure ulcers and skin malignancies. This chapter will begin by reviewing the structure and function of the epidermis, dermis and underlying hypodermis. The role of the skin as a sensory organ will then be examined, together with its role as a physical barrier to infection. We will take a look at the importance of skin integrity, linked with clinically relevant examples.

Overview of the skin

The skin is the body's largest organ, covering the entire body with a surface area of approximately 1.67 square metres and weighing about 4–5 kg for an average adult. It is continuous with the mucous membranes of the body and is a malleable, tough structure surrounding and holding in all the body contents, but also multi-tasking on a range of other vital functions: it acts as a barrier to the outside environment, and prevents invasion from microorganisms, chemical assailants and mutation of cells exposed to ultraviolet light. It offers protection from rapid and excess water loss from our body and plays a key role in thermoregulation. The skin is also the largest sensory organ and can react to external physical stimuli such as cold, heat, touch and pressure. Without it, we would quickly succumb to water loss, heat loss and pathogen invasion.

Skin structure and function

Structurally, skin consists of two main parts: the epidermis and the dermis. Below these two layers is an innermost layer of subcutaneous tissue, the hypodermis, which lies with the fascia surrounding the muscles (Figure 7.1). The thickness of these layers varies depending on the location on the body. For example, the eyelid has the thinnest layer of epidermis, measuring less than 0.1 mm, whereas the palms of the hands and soles of the feet have the thickest epidermal layer, measuring approximately 1.5 mm (James et al., 2015).

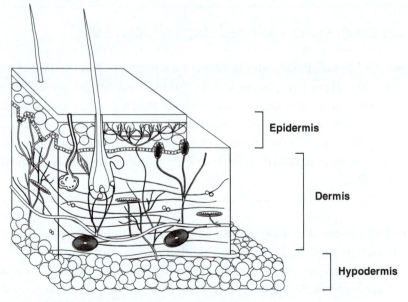

Figure 7.1 Layers of the skin

The epidermis

The top layer of skin is the epidermis. Although there is no blood supply here, the epidermis provides vital functions and protects the underlying skin layers from the outside environment, mainly through cells which have an abundance of a tough protein, keratin, and form an outer barrier of dead skin cells (stratum corneum). The epidermis also contains three other specialised cells: melanocytes, Langerhans cells and Merkel cells.

Keratinocytes

The majority of the epidermis consists of eight to fifteen layers of keratinocytes, a specific constellation of cells which function to synthesise keratin, a long, threadlike substance which enables the skin to have a waterproof quality. Keratin strengthens cells and provides a barrier against microbes. Around 80 per cent of cells in the epidermis are keratinocytes (Kolarsick et al., 2011).

Keratinocytes are formed in the bottom (basal) layer of the epidermis but continually migrate upwards from the constantly replicating basal layer, accumulating more and more keratin as they travel upwards to the skin surface. It is only the lowest three layers that are living, nucleated cells. The journey from the bottom to the top of the epidermis can take between 25 and 45 days. During the last phase of keratinisation, cellular organelles degenerate within keratinocytes, which eventually die. The outermost layer of the skin is therefore made of dead cells which constantly and continuously slough off – indeed, house dust is mainly dead, sloughed-off keratinocytes!

The epidermis is divided into layers according to keratinocyte morphology and position, representing different stages of maturation in the epidermis (Figure 7.2).

Stratum basale (basal/germinal cell layer)

The stratum basale comprises actively dividing cells and is the deepest layer of the epidermis. Here, there is a single layer of columnar keratinocytes with interspersed melanocytes and Merkel cells (see later). The keratinocytes of the basal layer undergo continuous mitotic division, with each cell resulting in the production of daughter cells; one of these migrates up through the layers while the other remains in the stratum basale for further division and expansion.

Epidermal cells travel away from the dermis to reach the top and make up the superficial layer of the skin, providing the protective barrier that skin offers. Blood vessels in the dermis extend only to the cells in this germinal layer via a basement membrane to which the cells are attached. This leaves the remaining layers of the epidermis malnourished and avascular. The cells here begin to lose most of their water content, become infused with keratin and get pushed progressively upwards towards the surface.

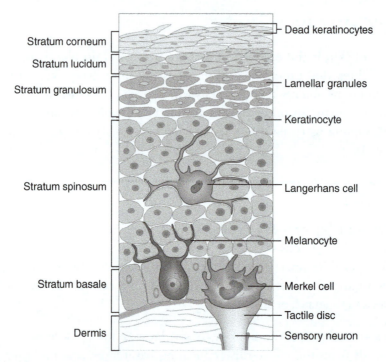

Stratum corneum	Dead keratinocytes
Stratum lucidum	
Stratum granulosum	Lamellar granules
	Keratinocyte
Stratum spinosum	Langerhans cell
	Melanocyte
Stratum basale	Merkel cell
	Tactile disc
Dermis	Sensory neuron

Figure 7.2   Epidermal layers in stages of maturation

Generally, the cells of the basal layer progress slowly through the upper layers but under certain conditions, such as wounding, these cells are stimulated to divide and increase the number of cycling cells in the epidermis.

Abnormal growth of dividing cells may give rise to epithelial tumours. Malignant change of the cells of the basal layer is known as basal cell carcinoma. More seriously, the pigment-producing cells of the basal layer called melanocytes may become malignant and this is explored in Isabel's case study later.

Stratum spinosum (squamous cell layer)

The second layer immediately above the stratum basale is made up of about five to ten rows of cells stacked upon one another and is known as the stratum spinosum. Adjacent keratinocytes here are bridged by tight junctions called desmosomes, providing resistance to physical stresses, increasing tensile strength and flexibility of the epidermis. This layer gets its name because of the spine-like appearance of these numerous desmosomes along cell margins (Chu, 2008).

Between skin cells (intercellular substance)

The cells of the epidermis are supported by a lipid-rich intercellular fluid. Lipid-soluble substances dissolve in this and pass through the skin. Certain lipid-soluble medicines, such as oestrogens for hormone replacement therapy, are absorbed here and can be administered as skin patches.

If a malignant change occurs in cells above the basal layer, squamous cell carcinoma arises. This is more common in the sun-exposed skin of older people. Fortunately, this type of skin cancer has a good prognosis if treated by prompt surgical excision. Non-malignant tumours, such as sebaceous cysts, senile warts or keratoses, can also arise.

Stratum granulosum (granular cell layer)

The last layer of living cells of the epidermis is the stratum granulosum, which generally contains about three to five layers of keratinocytes. However, this granular layer can vary in thickness, often being almost ten times thicker, for example, under the palms of the hands (Kolarsick et al., 2011). The keratinocytes in this layer begin to lose their nucleus and all metabolic functions. They become progressively flattened as they travel upwards.

In certain parts of the body, there are additional layers of flattened keratinocytes present between the stratum granulosum and stratum corneum. This layer is known as stratum lucidium, a thin translucent layer present in areas where the skin needs to be thicker, like the fingertips or the soles of the feet. Cells of the stratum lucidium do not show distinct boundaries and are filled with eleidin, an intermediate form of keratin. They provide an additional buffer of cells to help waterproof the skin, especially in areas where water can quickly be lost from the body (Figure 7.1).

A very thin or absent stratum granulosum layer can lead to abnormal maturation of cells with retention of nuclei of keratinocytes as they move into the stratum corneum. This occurs in certain conditions such as psoriasis (see later).

Stratum corneum (outer cornified or horny layer)

The stratum corneum is composed of dozens of layers of flattened keratinocytes. These large, polyhedral-shaped cells are rich in protein and low in lipids. They have lost their nuclei and maximised their keratin content, and are considered dead. Deeper layers of stratum corneum cells are densely compact and display a greater attachment than the more superficial layers which will eventually be exposed to the outside world. In this layer, desmosomes connecting keratinocytes undergo proteolytic degradation as the cells progress outward, contributing to the shedding of clumps of these cells, a process known as desquamation. If an area such as the heel or palm is exposed to consistent friction (e.g. ill-fitting shoes), abnormal thickening of the stratum corneum occurs, resulting in calluses and corns.

Melanocytes

The epidermis also has a smaller population of other cells. The cells that contain melanin, the dark pigment that gives skin its colour, are known as melanocytes and lie mainly at the junction of the dermis and epidermis. Melanocytes make up about one in six cells in this basal layer of the epidermis and have long projections that extend upwards into other cell layers. Each projection contains granules of the protective pigment melanin, which are transferred to the surrounding keratinocytes. Melanin is produced particularly in response to specific stressors (such as ultraviolet (UV) radiation).

This response results in tanning of the skin. In darker-skinned people, a greater number of granules are present in melanocytes, which are also transferred more quickly to keratinocytes than they are in fair-skinned people (Kolarsick et al., 2011). Once melanin granules have infiltrated a keratinocyte, they gather around the nucleus, protecting the DNA from UV radiation and other stressors.

Malignant melanomas can arise from melanocytes. It is essential to regularly check moles for changes that might be due to cancer. Inflammation, bleeding, itching or crusting of a mole should be investigated. The ABCDE approach is also a useful guide:

A – Asymmetry

B – Border: ragged or blurred edge

C – Colour: uneven in colour or becoming darker

D – Diameter: cancerous moles are usually > 6 mm in diameter

E – Elevation: raised above the surface of the surrounding skin.

(NHS, 2017)

Case study: Isabel – malignant melanoma

Isabel is a 47-year-old red-headed woman who has pale skin and freckles. She loves to travel but because of her pale skin she often suffers from sunburn. Isabel has had several moles on her body since she was a teenager and thought nothing of them until she noticed that a mole on her left thigh was itching and looked slightly larger than before. Isabel's GP made an urgent referral to a consultant dermatologist who took a biopsy and confirmed a diagnosis of malignant melanoma.

Malignant melanoma is the second most common cause of cancer in the under-50s. It is most common in those who are fair-skinned, burn in the sun, don't tan easily and have freckles and moles. Exposure to ultraviolet light either through sunbeds or sunlight is the leading cause of skin cancer. Treatment will depend on the stage of cancer but will initially require surgical excision of the tumour and may be followed by biological therapy, chemotherapy or radiotherapy, depending on the stage of cancer (Cancer Research UK, 2016).

In Isabel's case study one of the treatment options following excision of Isabel's cancerous mole is chemotherapy to target the rapidly dividing malignant cells. However, most forms of chemotherapy are indiscriminate and will kill actively dividing cells throughout the body. For this reason, chemotherapies used to treat many cancers will damage the germinal cells in the basal layer of the epidermis. With reduced cell division, the skin becomes thinner and more fragile, and the risk of abrasions and pressure ulcers increases.

Radiotherapy can also cause damage to the skin and may result in red, sore skin at the site of treatment and may feel like sunburn. Any soreness will usually feel better within two to four weeks of treatment, but the skin may always be slighter darker (rather like a tan). Radiotherapy may also cause hair loss two to three weeks after commencement of treatment. The hair will usually return, but the colour and texture may be slightly different.

Merkel cells

Merkel cells are specialised oval-shaped cells which function as sensory receptors located in sites of high tactile sensitivity in the skin. Merkel cells are found densely packed in some regions of the body, like the lips, fingers and toes, and make direct contact with specialised structures known as Merkel discs. Any small deformation of nearby keratinocytes stimulates a signal to the brain, resulting in a sensation of being touched.

Langerhans cells

Also present are Langerhans cells, specialised, sentinel immune dendritic cells, which form the front door of the immune system in the epidermis, providing immunity against bacteria and other foreign invaders by recognising antigens, microbes and toxins. Microscopically, Langerhans cells appear prickly because of their tree-like (dendritic) projections extending out of the cells. These are mainly distributed among the squamous and granular layers, with fewer cells in the basal layer. They act as (foreign) antigen-presenting cells to other vital immune cells, the T-cells. T-cells are then able to mount an appropriate response to defend the skin from pathogens.

The basement membrane

The epidermal layer of the skin relies on the dermis to provide oxygen. The interface between the epidermis and dermis is formed by a porous basement membrane that holds the two layers together and functions as a semipermeable barrier between them. This structure is unique in its hills-and-valleys undulations and ensures distribution of nutrients and mediators to the epidermis across the basement membrane from the vascular dermis lying underneath it.

Sweat glands

Various ducts and glands originate from the epidermis, including eccrine and apocrine sweat glands:

Eccrine sweat glands

Eccrine sweat glands help the body to regulate heat. They are most abundant on the forehead, palms and soles of the feet and least abundant on the back. Sweat is released initially as an isotonic solution, but sodium ions become actively re-absorbed from sweat, resulting in an extremely hypotonic and watery fluid that is emitted out of the duct onto the skin surface. In this way, the body conserves sodium but still undergoes cooling.

Apocrine sweat glands

Apocrine glands are primarily involved in scent release and are found mainly in regions such as the axillae (armpits) and groin and perineum (the skin between the anus and genitals). Apocrine glands do not open directly to the skin surface but instead into nearby hair follicles. These sweat glands are triggered by hormones to become active just before puberty. Their proteinaceous, viscous secretion has a distinct, individual and often unpleasant odour since it provides an ideal environment for bacterial growth.

Skin accessory structures

In addition, modified epithelial cells present in the epidermis give rise to associated structures such as hair follicles, skin glands and nails. Even though these structures are derived from epithelial tissue, their anatomical origin is deep within the basal layer of the epidermis, extending into the dermis.

Hair

Hair plays a significant role in our lives. Its absence, presence and appearance have important psychosocial functions. It also protects skin and underlying tissue from the elements and is involved in thermoregulation.

Hair structure

Hair consists of two distinct parts: the follicle or root, which is the living part located under the surface of the skin, and the hair shaft, which is dead and fully keratinised and projects above the skin surface (Figure 7.3). Hairs can vary considerably in size and shape, depending on their location on the body. The hair follicle is wider at its base where it forms the hair bulb. Here, cells divide and grow to build the hair shaft nourished by blood vessels, which deliver hormones that can modify hair growth and structure at different times of life. Hair bulbs serve as a reservoir for melanocytes and epithelial stem cells, and if this area is destroyed, hair cannot regrow.

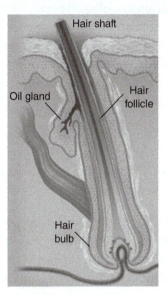

Figure 7.3   Hair follicle showing bulb and hair shaft

Each hair follicle has an accompanying sebaceous gland which adds an oily secretion called sebum to hair as it grows upwards out of the follicle. In some skin regions, apocrine glands also open into the follicle. Along the same side of the follicle below the sebaceous gland is the arrector pili muscle which can contract in the cold to allow hair to 'stand on end' and trap a layer of air to increase insulation (creating goosebumps).

The hair bulb contains melanocytes that synthesise granules and transfer them to the keratinocytes of the bulb, so hair colour is determined by melanin granules in the hair shaft.

Typically, approximately 100 scalp hairs are shed every day. Hair grows in a cyclical manner. The hair growth cell cycle is composed of three stages:

1. Anagen (the active growth stage): each hair spends several years in this phase. For scalp hair, this can typically last three to five years, during which time hairs grow at a rate of about 0.33 mm per day. The length of this phase decreases with age and decreases dramatically in individuals with baldness (alopecia).

2. Catagen (the transitional, die-back phase): this usually lasts about two weeks. Hair growth slows down, and the hair follicle shrinks.

3. Telogen (the resting and shedding phase): lasting three to five months on the scalp, hair growth stops, and the old hair detaches from the hair follicle, pushed out by a new hair shaft. Other sites on the body tend to have shorter growth phases and longer resting phases so that most body hair is shorter than scalp hair and does not fall out so frequently.

Many hormones influence hair growth, including oestrogens, thyroid hormones and growth hormone. The most dramatic effect is seen by testosterone, which increases the size of hair follicles on the face and mandibular areas during puberty. Later in life, these hormones may cause shrinkage of follicles in the scalp, resulting in male pattern baldness. Hair loss can also occur because of other traumas such as surgery, severe stress, anaemia, malnutrition, administration of oestrogen and certain drugs such as warfarin.

Anagen hair follicles are highly susceptible to cytotoxic agents. Consequently, one of the major causes of hair loss is chemotherapy. Hair loss usually starts a week or more after the first administration of the relevant medication. In most cases, the hair will grow back on completion of treatment, but in some cases baldness may be permanent.

Scalp cooling by applying a cold gel cap or refrigerated cooling system (preferred method) to the head can reduce or prevent loss of hair on the head during the administration of some chemotherapy medication. It works by decreasing the blood flow to the scalp and is indicated for all patients with solid tumours receiving chemotherapy.

Scalp cooling is continuously applied 20–45 minutes before, during and 20–150 minutes after a chemotherapy infusion (Komen et al., 2016). Patients occasionally complain of headaches or feeling cold, but scalp cooling is usually well tolerated (Nangia et al., 2017; Rugo et al., 2017). The role of the nurse is vital in the care of patients undergoing scalp cooling. Careful fitting of the cap to avoid air pockets will maximise its effect and support patients to cope with the cold.

Sebaceous glands

Oil-secreting sebaceous glands produce the oil in the skin which keeps it from drying out. The oil also helps to soften hair and kill bacteria that get into the skin's pores. These glands are all over the body, found in their highest numbers on the face and scalp, but also present in many locations of the body except on the palms of the hands and the soles of the feet. Cells of the sebaceous glands contain abundant lipid droplets in their cytoplasm. This secretion is known as sebum and has important lubrication properties to keep skin and hair pliable. Even though there are protective antimicrobial properties of sebum, overproduction may cause hair follicles to block and cause trapped bacteria to initiate an inflammatory response.

Teenage spots can impact greatly on self-image, and this is highlighted in Ali's case study.

> ## Case study: Ali – acne
>
> Ali is a 15-year-old schoolboy. When he was about 13, he began to develop spots, whiteheads and blackheads on his face, neck, back and chest. Ali became increasingly embarrassed by the appearance of his skin and changed from being an outgoing, happy child into a quiet, reserved teenager who shunned company. Ali's parents bought over-the-counter skin products aimed at reducing spots, but they had no impact.
>
> Eventually Ali was persuaded to see the Advanced Nurse Practitioner at the local medical centre. He explained to Ali and his family that puberty triggers the release of hormones that caused the sebaceous glands to produce excessive oil. This oil creates an ideal environment in which a bacterium, *Cutibacterium acnes*, thrives. This causes inflammation and spots to develop. In addition, cells lining the pores of the skin are not shed properly and combine with the excess oil and inflammatory exudates to create blackheads and whiteheads.
>
> Initially, Ali was prescribed a cream known as nicotinamide, which contains vitamin B3, but Ali's acne failed to respond so he was then prescribed oral erythromycin, an antibiotic he took for six months, which resulted in a significant improvement. As the condition of his skin improved, Ali became happier and began to socialise with his friends more often.

Ali's case study reveals perfectly that although teenage acne is seen in virtually all adolescents, there are effective treatments available to manage this condition.

Nails

Fingernails are toughened, keratinised structures which enhance sensation and provide protection to the fingertips. The nail plate is formed from matrix keratinocytes, and the underlying nail bed contains blood vessels and nerves. Fingernails can grow at a rate of 0.1 mm per day, two to three times faster than the rate of toenail growth. Any abnormal pressure or excessive physical activity may distort growth, resulting in ingrowing toenails.

Skin microbes

The epidermis is covered with a normal flora of staphylococci, micrococci and *Cutibacterium acnes*, formerly known as *Propionibacterium acnes*. These bacteria produce metabolites which control the pH of the skin and prevent the growth of other potentially harmful microorganisms.

Resident organisms reside and multiply on the skin. They cannot be entirely eliminated from the skin during hand washing, but in the majority of cases, they are harmless. However, when patients are vulnerable because of immunosuppression or if a wound is present, these organisms can result in infection. In addition to the resident microorganisms, we constantly pick up transient microorganisms during contact with each other and the environment. These organisms are frequently the cause of healthcare-associated infection and are easily transmitted from person to person. The good news is that they can be readily removed by thorough hand hygiene. In 2005 (revised 2009), the World Health Organization issued the five moments for hand hygiene, and it is essential that all healthcare professionals follow the five moments to minimise cross-infection.

Activity 7.1 asks you to reflect on hand hygiene.

Activity 7.1   Reflection

Consider the five moments for hand hygiene and reflect on an experience from clinical practice where you observed or participated in patient care. Were the five moments adopted by all those involved in the patient's care? If not, what opportunities for hand hygiene were commonly missed?

There are some possible answers to all activities at the end of the chapter, unless otherwise indicated.

The dermis

The dermis lies just below the epidermis and comprises the bulk of the skin. It provides the epidermis with nutrients, protects the body from mechanical injury, helps bind water, regulates heat loss and contains receptors for sensory stimuli. Blood vessels, nerve endings, hair follicles and sebaceous and sweat glands all reside in this layer. The dermis is the thickest and most robust layer of skin, around 1 to 4 mm thick.

The dermis and epidermis interact to form the dermal-epidermal junction and epidermal appendages. They also collaborate to repair and remodel the skin during wound healing (Kolarsick et al., 2011).

Cells of the dermis

Essentially, the dermis is an integrated system consisting of fibrous and filamentous connective tissue and numerous cells including macrophages, mast cells and fibroblasts.

Dermal macrophages

The dermis contains tissue-resident dermal macrophages (which are large phagocytic cells) and dermal dendritic cells, which play multiple roles in maintaining cutaneous homeostasis. Macrophages are involved in the regulation of inflammation and immunity. They are present during all three stages of wound repair, being essential participants in wound closure and full tissue regeneration (Yanez et al., 2017). Macrophages are also involved in hair follicle regeneration during catagen, helping to stimulate follicular stem cells to enter the active stage of hair growth (anagen).

Mast cells

Mast cells are specialised immune cells derived from bone marrow and distributed to connective tissues throughout the body. They are present in significant numbers in the dermis and help to regulate inflammation, host defence and innate immunity. Mast cells can undergo activation by antigens or allergens and are associated with the allergic response and the production of the inflammatory mediator, histamine, which dilates dermal blood vessels, resulting in skin redness.

Activity 7.2   Arm slapping!

Skin reactions can occur to minimal trauma such as mild physical stimulation like slapping the skin.

Slap your forearm gently a few times.

What happens?

Do you notice a change in the appearance of the skin?

Fibroblasts

The dermis is largely composed of a matrix containing a sturdy mesh of collagen and elastin fibres which give the skin its elasticity and resilience. Vital cells in the dermis are fibroblasts, which synthesise the collagen, elastin and other structural molecules of the dermis (which make up the extracellular matrix – ECM). Fibroblasts are actively dividing cells and are essential for wound healing and walling off infection.

Fibroblasts synthesise collagen fibres which form the major structural components of the dermis. These are strong, fat, white, wavy, cord-like bundles which cannot stretch. Collagen makes up over 70 per cent of the dermis (James et al., 2015). Collagen fibres are continually being degraded by proteolytic enzymes and replaced by new fibres. Collagen remodelling can go on for many years to ensure greater strength of the dermis is maintained. Elastic fibres maintain pliability and elasticity but do very little to resist deformation and tearing of the skin.

Structure of the dermis

The dermis is made up of loose connective tissue which is also called areolar tissue. In the dermis, collagen fibres are bundled relatively wide apart, while finer elastic fibres are interwoven around larger collagen bundles, together providing the tensile and elastic properties of the skin. As well as having loosely packed protein fibres, the space between them is filled with a matrix of loose consistency (like a cotton wool ball that has been pulled apart).

Layers of the dermis

The dermis is divided into two layers: the papillary layer and the reticular layer.

Papillary layer

This is the most superficial layer of the dermis. Here, hundreds of small extensions of the dermis protrude into the epidermis. These are known as dermal papillae: peg-like projections containing blood vessels that nourish the epidermis. The dermo-epidermal junction is characterised by an interdigitation of the dermal papillae of the dermis with reciprocal extensions of the epidermis known as the rete ridges. The impressions made by the papillary ridges of the thumbs and fingertips are also known as fingerprints.

These projections increase the surface area between the two layers, providing physical stability and nutrient exchange. If this layer is subject to shear forces, these can cause the separation of the ridges, causing fluid to collect and forming blisters (Growney et al., 2017). The papillary layer of the dermis is a matrix of loosely packed collagen fibres dispersed with nerves and capillaries throughout, providing nutrient exchange and sensory function to the epidermis.

Reticular layer

This is the deeper layer of the dermis which is made up of dense, irregular tissue. Most of the collagen fibres here run in bundles parallel to the surface, interwoven with elastin and matrix. This layer provides the physical strength of the skin; collagen prevents tearing of skin when stretched, and elastin allows it to return to its normal shape and size after stretching.

Sensory receptors

The skin represents our largest sensory organ, encompassing the entire body. Located in the dermis are sensory receptors which allow the body to receive stimulation from the outside environment and register a variety of sensations (including pain, heat, cold, itch and touch). Some of these are free (bare) nerve endings in the skin, and they extend into the middle of the epidermis. Free nerve endings are mainly sensitive to heat and painful stimuli. Several receptors play a role in communicating environmental information to the central nervous system. These receptors are named based on the nature of the stimuli they receive; for example, mechanoreceptors (touch), thermoreceptors (temperature), nociceptors (pain) and pruriceptors (itch).

The distribution of touch receptors in human skin is not consistent all over the body. Touch receptors are fewer in number in skin covered with any type of hair, which includes the arms, legs, torso and face. They are, however, denser in hairless (glabrous) skin, such as lips, palms, fingertips and the soles of the feet, and thus these areas are more sensitive than hairy skin.

Mechanoreceptors

The sensation of 'touch' involves more than one kind of stimulus and therefore has more than one type of receptor. Mechanoreceptors sense stimuli as they undergo a physical deformation of their plasma membranes. There are four primary tactile mechanoreceptors in human skin: Merkel discs, Meissner corpuscles, Ruffini endings and Pacinian corpuscles. A fifth type of mechanoreceptor, Krause end bulbs, detect cold and are found only in specialised regions in deeper parts of the dermis.

Merkel discs are found in the upper layers of skin near the base of the epidermis, both in hairy and hairless skin. They are, however, more densely distributed in the fingertips and lips and respond to gentle, but highly discriminative touch, for example edge detection, and are therefore useful for sensitive work like typing on a keyboard.

Meissner corpuscles, also known as tactile corpuscles, are located in the upper dermis, where they project within the dermal papillae into the epidermis (Zimmerman et al., 2014). They are found primarily in hairless skin, such as fingertips and eyelids, and can accurately perceive fine touch and pressure. Meissner corpuscles occur in greater abundance on the ventral sides of hands, highly concentrated in the fingertips.

Ruffini endings are located in deeper layers of the dermis and are highly branched nerve endings which respond to the displacement of connective tissue fibres and sense distension in the dermis. They are present in hairy and hairless skin, mainly for the detection of skin stretch, but can also detect warmth. Since these detectors are situated deeper in the skin than cold detectors, we tend to detect cold stimuli before we detect warm stimuli.

Pacinian corpuscles are located deep in the dermis of both hairy and hairless skin. They sense pressure and vibration by being compressed. There are fewer Pacinian corpuscles and Ruffini endings in the skin than there are Merkel discs and Meissner corpuscles. Pacinian corpuscles are also located deeper in the hypodermis.

Nociceptive receptors are located near the surface of the skin. They can detect pain and are critical to ensure the neural processing of potentially injurious stimuli that may cause tissue damage. Nociception starts at the sensory receptors, but pain itself is not perceived until it is communicated to the brain.

Pain, temperature and itch sensation are transmitted by free nerve endings also located around the base of hair follicles. Any thermal stimulus that is too intense can be perceived as pain because temperature sensations are conducted along the same pathways that carry pain sensations.

Skin capillaries

The dermis has a copious blood supply made up of intercommunicating networks of vessels (plexuses). Blood flow through the skin can be adjusted as part of the process of thermoregulation (Chapter 2).

Dermal capillaries are vulnerable to shear forces if the layers of the dermis separate, and also to external pressure. A pressure of 12 mmHg will occlude the venous capillaries, and a pressure of 32 mmHg will occlude the arterial capillaries, reducing the blood supply. This will initially cause skin redness of the pressurised area because venous drainage is interrupted and red blood cells cannot leave. If the pressure is allowed to continue, it will exceed the pressure in the arterial capillary (32 mmHg) and block the delivery of oxygen to the area. This may result in the development of ischaemic tissue and subsequent death of the dividing cells of the basal layer, leading to necrosis and the rapid formation of a pressure ulcer.

Pressure ulcers are most common in malnourished patients, those who are under or overweight, those who are incontinent and those who have limited mobility or significant cognitive impairment. Healthcare professionals should undertake a skin assessment within 6 hours of admission to hospital or a care home (NICE, 2015). The skin should be checked for:

- integrity;
- colour changes or discolouration;
- variations in heat, firmness and moisture;
- whether erythema or discolouration is blanchable.

Numerical scoring tools can be useful in identifying those at risk of pressure damage. These not only incorporate a skin assessment but also consider the patient's physical, nutritional and cognitive status. Among the most popular tool is that developed by Judy Waterlow in 1985 and revised in 2005. Patients scoring 10 or above are at high to very high risk of developing pressure ulcers. The correct interpretation of the results will identify the measures needed to reduce the risk of skin damage and pressure ulcers and will include interventions such as regular turning, managing incontinence and improving nutrition and use of pressure-relieving devices.

Lymphatic vessels

These are found throughout the dermis, in close association with the skin blood capillary networks, and have a major role in draining excess tissue fluid. Branches from the superficial lymphatic vessels extend into the dermal papillae and drain into the larger lymphatic vessels in the lower dermis.

The hypodermis

The dermis lies on a layer of subcutaneous tissue (panniculus). This layer, the hypodermis, is not considered true skin and predominantly consists of adipose tissue (small lobes of fat cells known as lipocytes) and a supply of nerves and blood vessels to the dermis. The hypodermis attaches the dermis to the bone and muscle, and since it sits above the tough connective tissue wrapping the skeletal muscles (fascia), it firmly, but loosely, anchors the skin to the underlying structures, and is therefore also known as the superficial fascia.

Remarkably, it holds about 60 per cent of the body's fat stores, and so roles of the hypodermis include insulation of the body to conserve heat, providing the body with buoyancy and functioning as a storehouse of energy. It also protects underlying structures from trauma by allowing fat to absorb the impact of physical shocks before they are transmitted deeper within the body.

Hormone conversion (testosterone) can also take place in the hypodermis and the fat cells (known as lipocytes) produce leptin, a satiety hormone that reduces food intake by binding to receptors in the hypothalamus.

The hypodermis varies in thickness depending on the skin site and on individual age, fat stores and gender. In the dorsogluteal site (buttocks), where certain intramuscular injections need to be administered, it can range from 1.2 to 14.4 cm thick. Extreme care is required here as administering drug preparations into fat rather than muscle can cause abnormal drug absorption, tissue damage, bruising and scarring.

Subcutaneous injections are administered when medication requires a slower absorption. Drugs commonly administered by this route include insulin and subcutaneous heparin. Only small volumes of medication (< 0.1 ml) can be given subcutaneously. Areas of the body commonly used for subcutaneous injections include the outer aspect of the upper arm, the anterior aspect of the thigh and the abdomen. Less commonly, the scapular areas of the back and the upper ventrogluteal and dorsogluteal regions may be used.

Patients who require repeated injections should rotate the sites to aid absorption, reduce tissue damage and minimise discomfort. Patients with diabetes need to be aware that insulin is absorbed at different rates in different sites, and the site of injection can affect their blood sugar. Insulin is absorbed most quickly when injected into the abdomen and most slowly when injected into the buttocks and thighs (Kozier et al., 2012).

Inflammation and wound healing

A wound can result from localised trauma, e.g. a tear or cut in the skin. This breach provides an immediate avenue for opportunistic microorganisms to enter the body, with the possibility and threat of an ensuing and potentially deadly infection. The body's response is naturally to prepare for and counteract such an eventuality and to attempt to close the breach as quickly and efficiently as possible. Thus (in healthy tissue) the most likely outcome of a wound will be a timely and ordered series of physiological events which should result in the restoration and functional integrity of the skin and underlying tissue.

A wound is termed acute if it resulted from a sudden, solitary insult such as a traumatic injury or a surgical intervention and if it can neatly and efficiently progress from one phase to the next. It has to be emphasised, though, that these three phases are not distinct, as each gradually rolls into the other as the wound heals. This sequence of events is termed 'wound healing' and is briefly summarised in Figure 7.4.

A wound progresses through three major phases on its way to complete healing. These are the phases of inflammation, proliferation and maturation (remodelling).

The inflammatory phase

This first phase is launched upon injury and serves to immediately protect the body from two undesirable consequences: blood loss and infection. To control any blood loss caused by the trauma, haemostatic mechanisms begin as soon as vascular tissue is injured. Haemostasis involves platelet coagulation and fibrin clot formation. After initial vasoconstriction at the wound site, there is an increase in vascular permeability, and some of the classic signs of inflammation (redness, warmth, swelling and pain) begin to manifest.

To deal with any lingering and potential pathogens, the inflammatory phase results in the active recruitment of leukocytes such as neutrophils (which become the predominant wound cell type within the first three days after injury). These phagocytic cells ingest and clear microorganisms, cellular debris and necrotic tissue, which may have resulted during the formation of the wound or the early progression of healing. This clearing-up process is termed debridement and is an essential prerequisite before the wound can progress into the next phase of healing.

Specialised leukocytes debride the wound at a microscopic level, producing a wide variety of vital substances such as immune mediators, growth factors and distinctive cytokines. At this point, the bacterial burden of the wound should diminish substantially, and the wound can progress into the next phase – proliferation.

The proliferative phase

The proliferative phase can begin two or three days post-trauma. Several physiological events occur during this phase, including granulation: the laying down of new foundation tissue in the wound base. Here, fibroblasts (described above) migrate inwards from the wound margins and begin to generate and assemble ECM, collagen and elastin to reform wound-connective tissue.

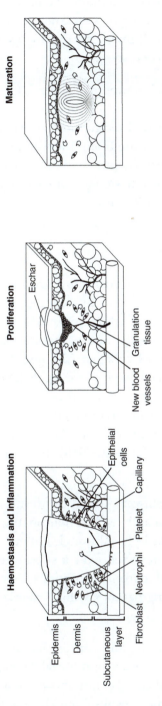

Figure 7.4 Stages of wound healing

Fibroblasts are stimulated by many chemical activators and messengers, mostly released by macrophages, which dominate towards the end of the inflammatory phase. Fibroblasts secrete a variety of cytokines (e.g. platelet-derived growth factor (PDGF), tissue growth factor beta (TGFβ) and keratinocyte growth factor), allowing other vital cells to proliferate and aid the healing process. Such cells include endothelial cells and angiocytes. Expansion of these cell numbers contributes to a process known as angiogenesis, the generation of new blood vessels.

These vessels begin as tiny buds but eventually form larger capillary loops, resembling 'granules' when examined macroscopically (hence the term granulation tissue). New blood vessels provide much-needed oxygen and nutrients, helping to facilitate the growth and proliferation of new tissue filling the wound. Towards the end of the proliferative phase, a process known as epithelialisation occurs. Epithelial cells migrate inwards from the wound edges, leapfrogging over each other to reach the centre of the wound. These will form the new epidermis.

The maturation phase

Fibroblasts are now induced to transform into myofibroblasts, which contain contractile fibres enabling the wound to shrink, leading to its eventual closure. Wound collagen is assembled into fibres, which are cross-linked and organised into bundles with increasing tensile strength. As the wound matures, collagen is remodelled into a more organised structure. Type III collagen (the initial, new collagen synthesised in the proliferative phase) is replaced by type I collagen. The body continues to heal the wound anywhere from six months to two to three years, depending on the patient's health. The collagen support structure is gradually strengthened until a plateau in tensile strength is achieved. This has been reported as never exceeding 80 per cent of the strength of the wound (Xue and Jackson, 2015), hence healed tissue will never be as strong as uninjured tissue.

In contrast to acute wounds, a chronic wound can result from a myriad of aetiologies such as pressure, venous, arterial and diabetic neuropathies and is not able to progress rapidly through the phases of healing. Although initiating as acute wounds, a wound becomes chronic if it has not resolved over a substantial period of time. Chronic wounds are often associated with chronic conditions such as cardiovascular disease or diabetes, diseases with underlying pathology that severely impacts on and impairs the ability of wounds to heal.

Leg ulcers typically occur below the knee on the leg or foot, which takes more than two weeks to heal. Venous leg ulcers account for 60–85 per cent of all leg ulcers. They usually develop on the inside of the leg, just above the ankle, and are caused by sustained venous hypertension, which results from chronic venous insufficiency and/or an impaired calf muscle pump but can also occur after a minor injury, where persistently high pressure in the veins of the legs has damaged the skin. Contributory factors include immobility, obesity, previous DVT or varicose veins.

The symptoms of a venous leg ulcer include pain, itching and swelling in the affected leg, and there may be an offensive discharge. The most effective treatment for venous leg ulcers is compression. Antibiotics may be required if a bacterial infection is present. Patients who have had a leg ulcer should be advised to wear compression stockings, lose weight if needed, take regular exercise, elevate legs when at rest and stop smoking to prevent a reoccurrence.

People with type I and type II diabetes are prone to ulcers on the lower leg and feet. Diabetes can cause peripheral diabetic neuropathy in which the nerves that transmit pain to the brain may not function as well as they should. Minor damage to the foot may go unnoticed, and an ulcer can develop. Impaired circulation will reduce blood supply to the feet and delay healing.

The risk of diabetic ulcers is increased by smoking, lack of exercise, obesity, high cholesterol and high blood pressure. Healing can be very slow, and compression must never be used. Good foot care is essential to prevent diabetic foot ulcers. People living with diabetes should be advised to take extreme care when walking barefoot, to wear comfortable, well-fitting shoes, to inspect their feet regularly and to have an annual consultation with a podiatrist.

Common skin disorders and diseases

The skin is the largest organ of the body and is vulnerable to trauma, ageing and disease. Skin and hair are central to perceptions of body image and managing patients with skin conditions is very important.

Eczema

Eczema or atopic dermatitis is probably the most common skin complaint. This is an irritating skin condition, particularly prevalent in babies and young children. Often it can affect any part of the body, causing itchy, dry, red and cracked skin, and can manifest as a long-term condition in older atopic individuals (those with a sensitivity to allergens such as pollen or food allergies). The treatment for eczema centres around providing relief of symptoms and daily use of emollients (topical skin moisturisers). During more troublesome flare-ups, application of topical steroids may be recommended.

Psoriasis

Psoriasis is a chronic skin disorder which affects about 2 per cent of the UK population. It varies in severity between individuals and results in an abnormal, rapid and increased production of skin cells. This build-up of cells produces red, flaky patches of skin covered in silvery, white scales (plaques). For many people, symptoms can get worse after a specific event or trigger, such as infection, stress or sunlight. It is believed that psoriasis is an autoimmune condition, and several different plaque patterns are recognised, which can cover large areas of the body.

Although many common skin disorders such as psoriasis and dermatitis are chronic, nurses frequently encounter infectious skin diseases which require careful management and advice to prevent spread among family members and communities. A common example is highlighted in Finley's case study.

Case study: Finley – impetigo

Finley is a 12-month-old boy who developed red sores and blisters around his mouth and nose. As they burst, these lesions left crusty, golden-brown patches. Finley had a four-year-old sister called Emily who developed similar symptoms around an area of eczema on her hand two days later. On investigation, it was found that several children in Finley's nursery had reported similar symptoms. The GP diagnosed impetigo and prescribed mupirocin (Bactroban), an antibiotic ointment, for both children, and the infection was treated successfully. Both children remained at home until they became non-infectious.

Impetigo is an extremely infectious skin infection usually caused by *Staphylococcus aureus* or *Streptococcus pyogenes*. It spreads rapidly, and outbreaks in schools and nurseries are common. It is spread by physical contact, and the infection can easily spread to other parts of the body or on to other people until it stops being contagious, which will occur 48 hours after the start of treatment or when the patches dry out and crust over if there is no treatment.

Now you have completed this chapter, test your acquired knowledge by attempting the short series of multiple-choice questions in Activity 7.3.

Activity 7.3   Multiple-choice questions

1. The outer layer of the epidermis is known as the

    a) Stratum basale
    b) Stratum spinosum
    c) Stratum granulosum
    d) Stratum corneum

2. How many scalp hairs are typically shed in one day?

    a) 10
    b) 100
    c) 1,000
    d) 10,000

3. Which of the following may cause hair loss?

    a) Penicillin allergy

    b) Sunburn

    c) Chemotherapy

    d) Dairy intolerance

4. Mechanoreceptors are most common in the

    a) Skin

    b) Lungs

    c) Intestines

    d) Spleen

5. What part of the body does not contain sebaceous glands?

    a) Face and scalp

    b) Palms of the hands and soles of the feet

    c) Genitalia

    d) Torso

6. What is the function of mechanoreceptors?

    a) Detection of light

    b) Detection of pressure

    c) Detection of hormones

    d) Detection of heat

7. Which of these is not a contributory factor for pressure ulcers?

    a) Being malnourished

    b) Obesity

    c) Having full mobility

    d) Significant cognitive impairment

8. Which of the following is not a stage in wound healing?

    a) Inflammation

    b) Destruction

    c) Proliferation

    d) Elimination

(Continued)

(Continued)

9.   What percentage of leg ulcers are venous in origin?

   a)   10–15 per cent

   b)   20–25 per cent

   c)   50–80 per cent

   d)   100 per cent

10.   Which of the following is not a function of the skin?

   a)   Thermoregulation

   b)   Storage and synthesis

   c)   Blood cell maturation

   d)   Protection

Chapter summary

The skin is a malleable, tough structure covering and protecting the body from microbe invasion and the external environment. Structurally, it is made up of the epidermis, dermis and hypodermis.

The epidermis contains an uppermost layer of dead, keratinised cells, which along with skin melanocytes offer a unique protective layer. The dermis forms the majority of skin tissue, containing important nerve endings that can detect and act upon environmental fluctuations, and blood vessels which serve to feed the germinal layers of skin cells. The hypodermis lies beneath the dermis, attaching it to bone and muscle.

In addition to protection, the skin and its accessory structures such as sweat glands, hair and nails perform a variety of functions including thermoregulation, storage and cutaneous sensation. Skin trauma can often lead to a wound which will hopefully heal. Wound healing takes place in three distinct phases – inflammation, proliferation and maturation.

Activities: Brief outline answers

Activity 7.1: Reflection (page 184)

My five moments for hand hygiene (WHO, 2009) are:

* before touching a patient;
* before clean/aseptic procedures;
* after body fluid exposure/risk;
* after touching a patient;
* after touching patient surroundings.

Activity 7.2: Arm slapping! (page 185)

Your skin may turn red where you have slapped it.

Mast cells here locally release the inflammatory mediator histamine, dilating blood capillaries near the skin's surface so that the skin appears red.

Activity 7.3: Multiple-choice questions (pages 194–6)

1) d, 2) b, 3) c, 4) a, 5) b, 6) b, 7) c, 8) d, 9) c, 10) c

Further reading

Nigam Y and Knight J (2017) Anatomy and physiology of ageing 11: The skin. *Nursing Times*, 113(12): 51–5.

A short summary of how the skin ages.

Tortora G and Derrickson B (2017) *Tortora's Principles of Anatomy and Physiology* (15th edition). New York: John Wiley & Sons.

In-depth coverage of human anatomy and physiology.

Useful websites

www.nice.org.uk/about/nice-communities/social-care/quick-guides/helping-to-prevent-pressure-ulcers

A review of risk factors, assessment and care planning for pressure ulcers.

www.nursinginpractice.com/wound-care/effective-wound-care

An expert-authored article on effective wound care.

www.nursingtimes.net/clinical-archive/tissue-viability/pressure-ulcer-education-3-skin-assessment-and-care-18-11-2019

An article detailing education of pressure ulcers with a focus on skin assessment and care.

Chapter 8   The musculoskeletal system

Chapter aims

After reading this chapter, you will be able to:

- provide an overview of the axial and appendicular skeletons;
- describe the nature of long and flat bones;
- explain how bones develop and grow;
- highlight how bone density is maintained and regulated;
- describe the nature of fixed and articular joints;
- describe the nature of skeletal, cardiac and smooth muscle;
- describe the physiology of muscle contraction.

Introduction

Case study: Nikki – bone fracture

Yesterday evening, Nikki, an eight-year-old girl, was playing outside with her friends when she fell and landed heavily when her skateboard skidded on some loose gravel. Initially, her parents thought she had just suffered some bruising but gradually the area around her elbow began to become swollen and tender, so her mother took her to the local accident and emergency department.

After an examination and an X-ray, it was revealed that Nikki had suffered an oblique distal fracture to her left humerus. The bone fracture was correctly realigned, a plaster cast was fitted and Nikki was discharged with some ibuprofen for pain relief.

The adult musculoskeletal system consists of the 206 bones which form the skeleton, together with the associated skeletal muscles that allow coordinated physical movement. Although bones are incredibly strong, even young bones are susceptible to fracture when exposed to physical trauma, as we have just seen in Nikki's case study.

We will begin this chapter by exploring the structure and function of the human skeleton, highlighting the nature of long and flat bones. Since nurses routinely encounter broken bones in clinical practice, the common types of fracture and their physical characteristics will be highlighted. Once you have a sound knowledge of bone structure and function, we will examine how bones form, grow and are maintained and highlight the role played by the two major types of bone marrow. Where two or more bones come together, they form a joint. We will describe the structure and function of both fixed and articular (movable) joints and explain how joint pathologies such as arthritis can affect joint mobility. Finally, we will turn our attention to muscle, initially examining the three muscle types and their locations before exploring the physiology of skeletal muscle contraction.

The skeleton

The skeleton has two major divisions (Figure 8.1). The axial skeleton consists of the bones which form the central axis of the body; its major components are the skull, the vertebral column and the ribcage. The axial skeleton is predominantly composed

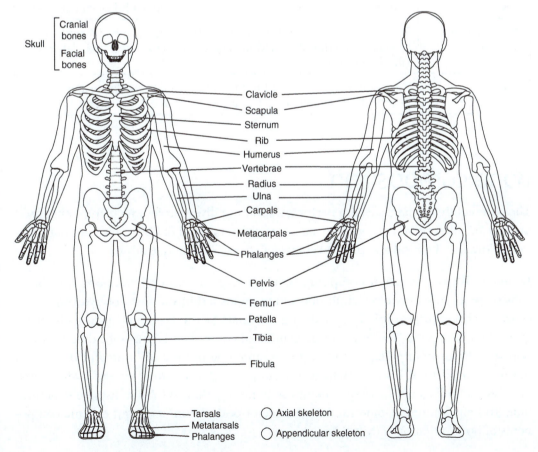

Figure 8.1 The axial and appendicular skeletons

of flat bones that cover and protect our major internal organs and provide points of attachment for the limbs. The appendicular skeleton consists of the bones which form the arms and legs (appendages), together with the shoulder and pelvic (hip) bones.

The appendicular skeleton is largely composed of long bones which function as levers to allow physical movement of the body and objects in the environment. The vast majority of bone fractures that nurses encounter are long-bone fractures, although with age, as bones lose their density, fractures to the flat bones of the axial skeleton (particularly the ribs) become more common.

Table 8.1   Major functions of bone

Function	Example
Support	The skeleton forms a rigid framework to support the soft tissues of the body
Protection	Bones cover vulnerable delicate regions of the body, e.g. the skull surrounds and protects the brain; the ribcage surrounds and protects the heart, lungs and other thoracic organs
Movement	Articular joints facilitate movement via contraction of skeletal muscles
Production of blood cells	Red bone marrow produces the formed elements of blood including red blood cells (erythrocytes), white blood cells (leukocytes) and platelets (thrombocytes)
Storage	The skeleton is a reservoir for minerals, particularly calcium and phosphate. The long bones also act as a region of fat storage

Bone composition

The bones of the human skeleton perform a variety of diverse roles which are summarised in Table 8.1. Before we examine the nature of different types of bone, it is important that we explore the chemical and physical characteristics of this complex tissue.

Bone consists of two major components. The inorganic mineral component of bone consists predominantly of calcium phosphate deposited in the form of hydroxyapatite crystals. This is responsible for imparting hardness to the bone; unfortunately, as we grow older, bones may lose some of their mineral content and density, leading to osteoporosis. The protein collagen forms the organic component of bone and this is laid down in the form of fibres which form a supporting framework for the hydroxyapatite crystals. Collagen also serves to knit the bone together to form a discrete structural unit. To help you understand the importance of both the mineral and organic components of bone, attempt Activity 8.1.

Activity 8.1   Practical experiment

Take two long chicken bones (a cooked leftover from a meal would be perfect), place one of these in a jar of vinegar (an empty jar of pickled onions with remaining vinegar would be suitable), and leave it for three days. With the second bone, heat the end over a naked flame (e.g. a gas hob) for around a minute and allow to cool for another two minutes (ideally use an oven glove or kitchen tongs to avoid burning your fingers).

Try bending both bones.

What do you notice about the first bone when you remove it from the vinegar?

What do you notice about the second bone that was heated over the gas hob?

There are some possible answers to all activities at the end of the chapter, unless otherwise indicated.

Once you have completed Activity 8.1 and reviewed the answer at the end of this chapter, you will be aware how changing the collagen or calcium phosphate composition of a bone can dramatically affect its physical properties. We will now explore the importance of these building blocks of bone further.

Changes in bone composition

Bones are incredibly strong; indeed, weight for weight, bone is stronger than both steel and concrete. However, bones only reach such strengths if the collagen and calcium phosphate are present in the correct amounts. Many diseases, including osteoporosis, rickets and brittle bone disease, affect bone strength.

Case study: Indra – osteogenesis imperfecta

Indra is 19 years old and has just started studying pharmacology at university. She was diagnosed with brittle bone disease shortly after birth and has become very knowledgeable about the condition and its consequences. It came as no surprise to Indra's parents that she was born with this disease since several other family members, including her mother, are also sufferers. Indra quickly learnt that the medical term for

(Continued)

(Continued)

brittle bone disease is osteogenesis imperfecta (OI) and that it is a genetic disorder affecting around 1 in 20,000 people caused by problems associated with the production of collagen.

Since collagen provides the structural framework which holds bones together, issues with collagen production within bone result in bones losing their structural strength and becoming fragile and susceptible to fracture, even when exposed to minor stresses. Over the years, Indra has suffered multiple fractures to her limbs, meaning she has not grown to her expected height. To help protect her skeleton from unnecessary stress, Indra spends a lot of time in her specially adapted wheelchair; fortunately, her university has excellent wheelchair access throughout and Indra is progressing well in her studies.

Diet and bone health

To maintain bone density, it is essential that our diets are rich in calcium and phosphate. Animal-derived products, particularly dairy products, form the major source of calcium and phosphate in the UK diet, although many types of seeds and nuts are excellent vegetarian alternatives. To help maintain bone health, many vegetarians and vegans choose to boost their intake of calcium and phosphate through the use of commercially available supplements which are frequently sold combined with vitamin D.

Vitamin D is essential for the absorption of both calcium and phosphate in the digestive tract. Even if intakes of calcium and phosphate are optimal, if the patient is deficient in vitamin D these minerals will not be absorbed into the blood, and the levels of calcium and phosphate in bone will fall, and bones may lose their hardness and become deformable. Vitamin D is a fat-soluble vitamin found at high concentrations in dairy products, fatty cuts of meat and oily fish. In association with the kidneys, the skin can synthesise vitamin D when exposed to direct sunlight; however, because of the risk of skin cancer, many people avoid direct sun exposure or wear sunblock when going out on sunny days.

A lack of vitamin D commonly occurs through a combination of dietary deficiency and lack of sun exposure and can lead to rickets in childhood or the adult form of rickets, which is called osteomalacia. Contrary to popular belief, rickets and osteomalacia are not confined to developing countries and are routinely encountered by nurses in the UK. It is worth noting that cases of both of these diseases increase when we have a poor summer and in particular when we have a run of poor summers.

Nurses should also be aware that patients with eating disorders such as anorexia nervosa and bulimia are likely to be deficient in calcium, phosphate and vitamin D, and as a result they may be at a significantly increased risk of bone fractures because of a decrease in bone density.

Long and flat bones

Now that we have examined the nature of bone tissue, we will explore the structure of long and flat bones. It is essential that nurses are familiar with the terminology used when describing the anatomy of bones since these terms are encountered when dealing with bone fractures.

Long bones

Long bones are found predominantly in the appendicular skeleton where they function as levers. A typical long bone (Figure 8.2) consists of a diaphysis, which is the anatomical term for the shaft of the bone, and two epiphyses, which correspond to the rounded bulbous ends of the bone. The proximal epiphysis of the long bone corresponds to the portion in closest proximity to the trunk of the body (the point where the limb attaches), and the distal epiphysis corresponds to the portion furthest away from the trunk.

Nurses need to familiarise themselves with these terms since they are used to identify the location of bone fractures, e.g. a distal fracture of the humerus (as in Nikki's case study) would be close to the distal epiphysis of the bone (towards the elbow), while a proximal fracture of the humerus would be close to the proximal epiphysis (towards the shoulder).

Running longitudinally through the diaphysis is a hollow chamber called the medullary cavity. In children, this is filled with red bone marrow which produces red and white

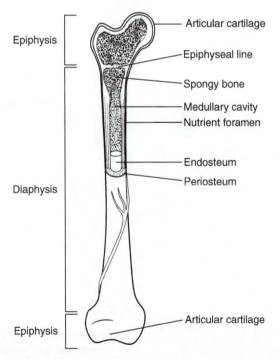

Figure 8.2 Structure of a long bone

blood cells (see below). In adult bones, the red bone marrow is gradually replaced with yellow bone marrow, which is predominantly composed of adipose tissue (fat). The exact role of yellow bone marrow is unclear, although as an adipose tissue it can function as an energy storage area and is also a region where toxins that cannot be metabolised by the liver can be locked away relatively safely. During severe infections and fever or during significant blood loss, yellow bone marrow can revert back to red bone marrow to release red and white blood cells.

Since the forces exerted on a long bone are directed through the diaphysis, it is incredibly strong, with the bone surrounding the medullary cavity being composed of dense, compact bone. This contrasts with the epiphyses, which are composed of a much softer bone with a honeycombed spongy appearance (Figure 8.3). This softer, spongy bone,

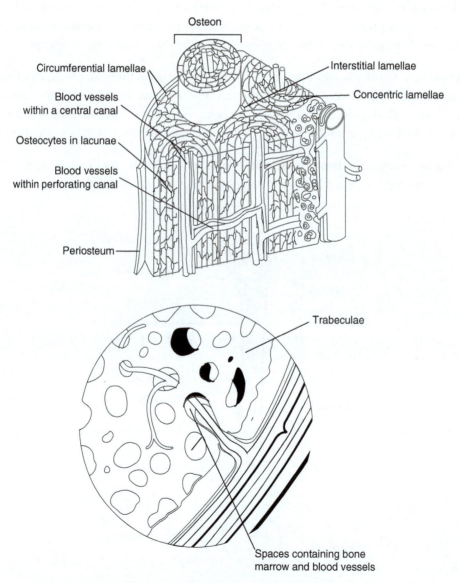

Figure 8.3 Nature of compact and cancellous bone

which is also known as cancellous bone, is slightly deformable, allowing the epiphyses of a long bone to be very efficient at absorbing impacts.

Additionally, the epiphyses of a long bone are usually covered by a layer of articular cartilage which further serves to absorb any mechanical stresses. The spongy bone of epiphyses usually contains small amounts of red bone marrow, which contributes to the production of red and white blood cells; however, the vast majority of red bone marrow is located within the central portions of the flat bones of the axial skeleton. All bones are surrounded by a thin sheath termed the periosteum, which is largely composed of collagen and contains blood vessels which permeate into the bone.

Long-bone fractures

In their daily role, functioning as levers, the long bones of the body are exposed to significant loading forces. As we will see below, this is a good thing since when stressed, bones become denser and stronger. However, when bones are exposed to unusual and excessive forces, e.g. a sudden sharp impact as a result of falling over, a bone fracture may occur. There are various types of fracture that may be observed. Broadly speaking, fractures are divided into simple fractures where only the bone itself is broken, and compound fractures where the bone is broken and it penetrates into the surrounding structures and usually out through the skin.

Simple fractures

Simple fractures come in many varieties. Since young children have relatively soft bones, fractures in children may be incomplete, with the bone breaking in a similar manner to a soft twig; indeed, the term 'greenstick fracture' is frequently used to describe these types of incomplete fracture. Transverse fractures occur perpendicular to the diaphysis of the bone, while oblique fractures (as the name implies) occur at a diagonal angle to the diaphysis.

When bones are twisted, spiral fractures are frequently observed, with the fracture spiralling along the length of the diaphysis in a corkscrew-like manner. If bones are exposed to sudden powerful impacts, e.g. following a car accident, then the bone may literally explode into multiple bone fragments. This type of fracture is called a comminuted fracture and can be particularly dangerous since the bone fragments can penetrate into soft tissues and blood vessels, causing significant bleeding and sometimes bone emboli (fragments of bone circulating in the blood).

Compound fractures

Compound fractures are also known as open fractures since the fractured bone usually breaks through the skin. These types of fracture are always regarded as serious since the broken bone is exposed to bacteria and other infectious agents on the skin and in the environment. Bacteria such as *Staphylococcus aureus* (a common skin microbe) will readily grow in bone tissue, leading to bone infections and inflammation (osteomyelitis), which can be incredibly painful and difficult to treat. There is always the risk that infections in bone can become more widespread if they enter the blood and potentially may even lead to sepsis and septic shock.

Flat bones

The vast majority of flat bones are located in the axial skeleton and overlay and protect vulnerable vital organs, e.g. the skull protects the brain while the ribs protect thoracic organs such as the heart and lungs. Flat bones have a simple sandwich-like structure consisting of outer layers of compact bone (the bread) and an inner layer of spongy, cancellous bone (the filling). This arrangement of bone tissue is very effective at absorbing physical impacts since the inner spongy portion of the bone is slightly deformable and able to absorb and dissipate forces of impact.

Like the spongy bone present in the epiphyses of long bones, the spongy bone in the centre of flat bones is populated by red bone marrow which acts as the major haemopoietic tissue in humans, producing the formed elements of blood including erythrocytes (red blood cells), leukocytes (white blood cells) and platelets (Chapter 9).

Flat-bone fractures

While flat bones are excellent at absorbing most types of physical impact, when exposed to excessive forces, they can fracture. Flat-bone fractures become more common with age, and in particular the ribs are vulnerable to fracturing in the elderly following falls. When flat bones do fracture, they frequently fracture in an irregular and unpredictable manner; this can cause significant issues in skull fractures where there is the potential for irregular bone fragments to penetrate into the meninges (membranes surrounding the brain) and the brain itself.

Flat bones, again particularly bones of the skull, may also show depression fractures where directed forces (e.g. a blow to the head) can cause the bone structure to collapse inwards. This is commonly associated with significant bleeding beneath (subdural haematoma) which may press on the brain, reducing blood flow, which can lead to permanent brain damage. Compound fractures of flat bones are rarer than in long bones and occur most frequently with longer flat bones such as the ribs, e.g. during crushing chest trauma.

Bone formation

The process of bone formation is called ossification (also known as osteogenesis) and begins in early foetal development. Initially, the primitive embryonic skeleton is composed entirely of soft cartilage and is referred to as the skeletal template. At around eight weeks into prenatal development, the skeletal template is invaded by bone-forming cells called osteoblasts. These progressively begin to replace the cartilage by depositing calcified bone in the central region of the diaphysis; this process is termed primary ossification (Figure 8.4).

Gradually the diaphysis is ossified and osteoblasts move into the epiphyses of the bone, creating areas of secondary ossification. At the time of delivery, the regions of primary and secondary ossification have usually extended until only two bands of the cartilaginous tissue which initially formed the skeletal template remain at the epiphyses of the bone. These two thin bands of cartilage are called the epiphyseal growth plates and allow the bones to grow in length throughout prenatal development, childhood and adolescence.

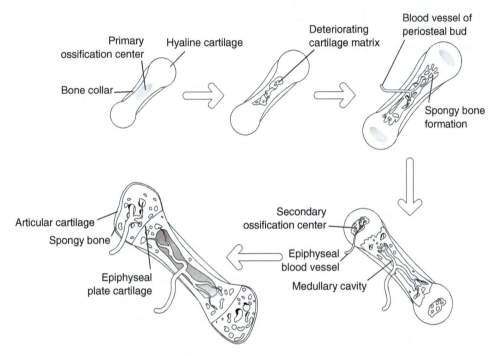

Figure 8.4 Bone formation: ossification

Bone growth

The growth of bones is predominantly under the control of the anterior pituitary gland, which secretes somatotropin (growth hormone). Somatotropin promotes cell division of the cartilage-producing cells (chondrocytes), which causes the epiphyseal growth plates to widen. As both growth plates expand, the bone increases in length and the portion of cartilage in closest proximity to the diaphysis becomes ossified at the same rate, ensuring that the growth plates remain at around the same width.

At around the age of 22, the maximal adult height is usually achieved, and the growth plates become entirely ossified. Today, the growth of children is usually closely monitored, and if growth is not proceeding at the anticipated rate, interventions are available, including the prescription of synthetic growth hormone.

Maintaining bone density

To ensure that a healthy bone density is retained, it is essential that adequate nutrition and levels of exercise are maintained throughout our lifespan. Earlier in the chapter, we discussed the importance of dietary calcium, phosphate and vitamin D intake to ensure the inorganic mineral components of bone are retained. It is also essential that protein intake is sufficient to allow the collagen components of bone to be synthesised and maintained.

Bone is a dynamic tissue that is perpetually in a state of flux and is continually being broken down and rebuilt. This is a gradual process, with an estimated 5–10 per cent of adult bone replaced each year (Walsh, 2015).

The bone-forming cells called osteoblasts that were responsible for initially building our bones remain active, laying down new bone throughout our lifespan. The activity of these cells is offset by the action of a second population of cells called osteoclasts, which are continually breaking down bone and releasing calcium into the blood. When we are active and mobile, the osteoblasts and osteoclasts work at roughly the same rate, ensuring that bone density is kept relatively constant.

During periods of immobility, e.g. extended time in a hospital bed, the bone-forming osteoblasts become less active and lay down less new bone. However, the bone-digesting osteoclasts retain their level of activity and during the period of immobility bone density is gradually lost. This explains why an elderly patient admitted to hospital with a bout of pneumonia may suffer a fracture on returning home that requires hospital readmission.

Today it is well understood that to retain their activity, osteoblasts require the weight of the body to be directed through the skeleton (skeletal loading). For this reason, anyone with a history of osteoporosis or with a recorded low bone density should be encouraged to get up on their feet and engage in exercise as much as is safely possible.

The activity of the osteoclast and osteoblast populations is tightly regulated via the hormones calcitonin and parathyroid hormone. These antagonistic hormones help maintain bone density while ensuring a stable concentration of calcium in the blood (Chapter 5).

Osteoporosis

The term osteoporosis refers to a group of diseases where the rate of bone breakdown (resorption) is greater than the rate of bone deposition. This leads to reduced bone density and increased pore spaces within the bone, which can increase the risk of fracture. It has been estimated that one in three women and one in five men will experience a fracture as a result of osteoporosis in their lifetime (Sözen et al., 2017). There are two broad categories of the disease recognised.

Type I osteoporosis is the most common and is usually associated with a decline in male and female sex hormones at the time of the andropause and menopause. Women are at greatest risk of type I osteoporosis as they go through the menopause and there is a sudden drop in the levels of oestrogen. Oestrogen stimulates osteoblast activity, and so reduction at the time of the menopause is usually associated with a decrease in the rate of bone deposition. The effects of osteoporosis are often insidious and may not be noted until 10–15 years post-menopause (typically the mid-60s or later).

Like oestrogen, the male sex hormone testosterone also stimulates osteoblast activity, and so as men age and levels of testosterone fall, there is a tendency for bones to progressively lose density. However, unlike in women, the reduction in testosterone levels is more gradual, and even men in their 80s and beyond usually still retain significant testosterone levels in their blood which help maintain osteoblast activity and bone density.

In both men and women, hormone replacement therapy (HRT) is available to help offset the decline in sex hormones. Although oestrogen and testosterone supplementation may help maintain a healthy bone density, HRT has well-established risks, including increasing the risk of clots and breast cancer in women and testicular shrinkage and increased risk of heart disease in men.

Type II osteoporosis is frequently referred to as senile osteoporosis since it is usually seen in elderly people of both sexes. It is usually associated with age-related reductions in the numbers of osteoblasts and calcium deficiency, either as a result of reduced calcium intake or a lack of vitamin D which, as we have seen, is essential for calcium and phosphate absorption in the gut.

Secondary osteoporosis

As the name implies, secondary osteoporosis occurs secondary to another pathology or medication which skews the healthy balance in bone turnover in favour of bone demineralisation. It is essential that nurses are aware that there are multiple causes of secondary osteoporosis, all of which can significantly increase the risk of fractures.

Common causes include liver disease, blood disorders such as thalassaemias and leukaemias, scurvy (vitamin C deficiency) and medications such as steroids, methotrexate, anticonvulsants and heparin. Occasionally secondary osteoporosis may be linked to overactivity of the parathyroid glands, with increased parathyroid hormone (PTH) secretion reducing osteoblast activity, resulting in a progressive loss of bone density.

Joint structure and function

Where two or more bones meet, a joint is formed. Joints can be broadly divided into synarthroses and synovial joints: synarthroses are fixed, non-articular joints such as the sutures of the skull and pelvis. As the bones here are usually knitted together with collagen fibres, these joints are also called fibrous joints. Joints that are capable of articulation (movement) are termed synovial joints and have a characteristic internal structure (Figure 8.5). Synovial joints that are freely movable are referred to as diarthroses and include major articular joints such as the elbow and shoulder.

In a typical synovial joint, the epiphyses of each bone are covered by a layer of incredibly smooth articular cartilage. The smoothness of the cartilage surfaces ensures that resistance is minimal during movement, while the soft rubbery nature of the cartilage acts as a cushion and an effective shock absorber should the joint be exposed to stresses, e.g. a sudden impact. The whole of the articular joint is held together by the outer joint capsule, which is composed predominantly of elastic ligaments that allow free joint movement while simultaneously retaining the integrity of the joint and helping to prevent dislocation.

A membrane called the synovium or synovial membrane lines the inner portion of the joint capsule. It has a serous component that produces a watery synovial fluid which fills the internal joint capsule. Synovial fluid is slippery and acts as an effective lubricant, ensuring the articular cartilages can move freely during joint articulation.

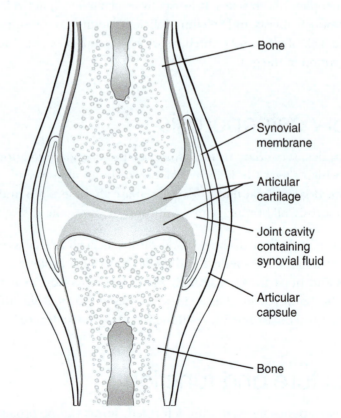

Figure 8.5 Synovial joint structure

Diarthrotic joints may be further subdivided according to the planes of movement they allow; for example, the knee joint is a typical hinge joint allowing movement in one plane analogous to the hinges of a door, while the hip joint is a ball-and-socket joint allowing multidirectional movement. Some of the articular synovial and cartilaginous joints such as those in the spine only allow minimal movement. Such joints are referred to as amphiarthroses.

It is important to realise that while each amphiarthrotic joint in the vertebral column is only capable of small limited movement, cumulatively the collective movements of all the individual bones give the spine its inherent flexibility.

Arthritis

The term arthritis literally means inflammation of the joints; in most cases, arthritis is associated with significant pain and swelling, which can significantly reduce joint mobility and function. There are many causes of arthritis including age-related general wear and tear, which can lead to osteoarthritis, joint infections, which can lead to septic arthritis, and autoimmune reactions, which can lead to debilitating rheumatoid arthritis.

Rheumatoid arthritis

Like most autoimmune diseases, rheumatoid arthritis (RA) disproportionally affects women, with a 3:1 ratio of females to males diagnosed (Intriago et al., 2019). In addition to gender, there are many risk factors associated with RA, including inheriting specific genes associated with autoimmunity such as HLA DR4, smoking and infection from certain viruses such as Epstein Barr virus (EBV).

Rheumatoid arthritis can usually be differentiated from osteoarthritis as it is a symmetrical disorder generally affecting both sides of the body equally. Rheumatoid arthritis usually begins in either the phalangeal joints of the fingers or toes, while some patients may show a prolonged insidious onset that is frequently associated with general lethargy and progressive joint stiffness without any initial pain.

Patients with rheumatoid arthritis usually have detectable autoantibodies (antibodies that bind to the body's own tissues) that react with the collagen that holds together the articular cartilage in synovial joints. Progressively, the patient's immune system will attack this cartilage, which is gradually replaced by an abnormal inflammatory tissue termed pannus. As pannus tissue accumulates in the joints of the fingers and toes, the joint becomes deformed as the phalangeal bones of the fingers and toes are pushed out of alignment. A key diagnostic feature of RA is that the fingers start pointing towards the ulna bone of the forearm (ulnar deviation).

As RA progresses, autoimmune reactions can begin to affect larger joints such as the wrists, hips, elbows and knees. In some patients, other organs and tissues may be affected by autoimmune reactions, including the skin (rheumatoid nodules), eyes (scleritis), blood vessels (vasculitis) and lungs (rheumatic lung disease).

To further your understanding of arthritis, read through Edward's case study.

Case study: Edward – septic arthritis

Edward is a 54-year-old man who was recently working in his garden shed when he was bitten on his right elbow by a spider. He thought little of the incident until his wife noticed a large red patch of skin which appeared to be spreading up his right arm. On ringing NHS 111, Edward was asked to draw a line around the margins of the redness with a pen and immediately arrange to either see his GP or visit the local A&E department.

Edward's GP agreed to see him immediately, and by the time he arrived at his doctor's surgery, his right elbow had become incredibly painful and felt as if it had been struck by a hammer. His GP noted that the redness had extended another 2 cm outside the margins of the pen circle that Edward had drawn around two hours previously. Edward was diagnosed with cellulitis and septic arthritis in his right elbow joint. He was prescribed a broad-spectrum antibiotic and told to immediately go to A&E should he start to develop a fever or feel unwell. Within two days, the redness around the elbow began to subside, and within a week, his elbow was pain-free.

Activity 8.2   Evidence-based practice and research

Edward's septic arthritis and cellulitis were clearly precipitated by the spider bite in his shed.

Ultimately, what was the likely cause of the cellulitis and elbow pain?

Why did the symptoms respond so well to the broad-spectrum antibiotic?

Why did the GP insist that Edward immediately go to his local A&E should he develop a fever or begin to feel unwell, or if the nature of the skin around the bite changed?

Edward's case study highlights the importance of identifying the cause of joint pain to be able to offer the best form of treatment. Now that you have a good understanding of bone structure and function, we will explore the nature of muscle tissue.

Types of muscle

There are three major types of muscle tissue present within the human body: cardiac muscle, smooth muscle and skeletal muscle. The first two types are referred to as involuntary since they cannot, under most circumstances, be consciously controlled. Skeletal muscle differs in that it is under direct conscious control.

Cardiac muscle

Cardiac muscle is restricted to the myocardium (muscle layer) of the heart and consists of individual muscle cells separated from each other by specialised tight junctions termed intercalated discs. Cardiac muscle has a branching structure which makes it incredibly durable and resistant to tearing, and has an inbuilt ability to contract at a regular rate (intrinsic rhythm) which is essential to its role within the heart (Chapter 3).

Smooth muscle

Smooth muscle consists of individual diamond-shaped cells usually organised into layers or sheets. It is found in multiple locations throughout the body including in the airway, blood vessels, uterus and gastrointestinal tract. Smooth muscle is controlled by the autonomic nervous system or via locally acting hormones (autacoids) such as prostaglandins.

Skeletal muscle

Skeletal muscle is also known as striated muscle since under the microscope it has a striped (striated) appearance. It is essential that skeletal muscle is under conscious control since this allows us to perform the highly coordinated physical movements necessary to carry out our day-to-day activities. As implied by the name, most skeletal muscle is found attached to bone (Figure 8.6); some skeletal muscles such as the external anal and urinary sphincters are not associated with bone but are still under conscious control to facilitate the processes of micturition (urination) and defaecation.

Skeletal muscle is usually attached to bone by a non-elastic collagen-rich tissue that forms tendons. It is essential that tendons are non-elastic since the force generated by muscular contraction needs to be exerted directly and efficiently on the bone to facilitate bodily movement.

Each skeletal muscle is surrounded by a thin elastic membrane called the epimysium, which functions as an outer sheath to protect the inner muscular components. Skeletal muscles have a complex Russian doll-like structure with structures found within structures.

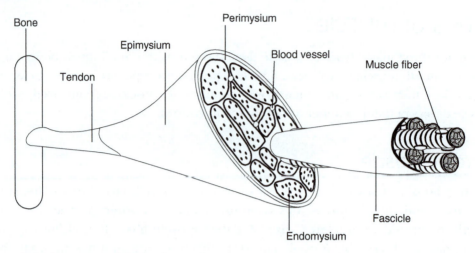

Figure 8.6   Structure of skeletal muscle

Within the epimysium are located parallel running tubular bundles of muscular tissue called fascicles. Each fascicle has its own elastic protective sheath around it called the perimysium which surrounds bundles of parallel running muscle fibres.

Unlike cardiac and smooth muscle, there are no recognisable individual muscle cells in skeletal muscle, but tubular muscle fibres with nuclei distributed along their outer peripheries. Each individual muscle fibre has its own protective sheath called the endomysium, within which are found parallel running myofibrils.

Each myofibril is surrounded by a specialised area of endoplasmic reticulum called the sarcoplasmic reticulum (unique to muscle) which concentrates and stores calcium ions (Ca^{++}). Myofibrils are the actual contractile structures within a skeletal muscle and are composed predominantly of two proteins called actin and myosin.

The sliding filament mechanism

The proteins actin and myosin are present within myofibrils in the form of filaments. The myosin filaments are relatively thick, while the actin filaments are comparatively thinner. Skeletal muscles contract by the thick myosin filaments physically sliding over the thinner actin filaments. The process of muscle contraction requires energy that is provided in the form of adenosine triphosphate (ATP).

For this reason, skeletal muscle usually has densely arranged populations of mitochondria. Although the proposed mechanics of the sliding filament mechanism are thought to be largely accurate, the mechanism is yet to be fully proven, and so this mechanism is still frequently referred to as the sliding filament hypothesis or theory.

To help you understand the physical mechanism of muscle contraction, now attempt Activity 8.3.

Activity 8.3   Practical analogy

A simple way of visualising the sliding filament mechanism is to open the fingers of your right and left hands and slide your fingers in between each other. The fingers of your left hand are representing the myosin (thick) filaments, and the fingers of your right hand are representing the actin (thin) filaments.

Now that you have a working understanding of the physical events that occur within a muscle as it contracts, we will explore how muscular contraction is initiated.

Control of muscular contraction

Contraction of the skeletal muscle groups is controlled by the somatic motor cortex within the frontal lobes of the brain (Chapter 6).

The neuromuscular junction

The action potentials that initiate muscular contraction arrive at muscles through motor neurones, which form specialised synapses termed neuromuscular junctions at the muscle site. Motor neurones release the neurotransmitter acetylcholine into the synaptic cleft of the neuromuscular junction, which rapidly binds to cholinergic receptors present on the surface of the muscle fibres. The binding of acetylcholine to its receptors initiates the release of Ca^{++} ions which have been concentrated within the sarcoplasmic reticulum, and it is this release of intramuscular calcium stores that initiates the sliding filament mechanism that leads to muscular contraction.

Muscle relaxants

It is essential that nurses have a good understanding of the neuromuscular junction since an important group of drugs termed muscle relaxants exert their effects at this site. Muscle relaxants are most frequently used during surgery that requires cutting into muscle tissue, e.g. opening up the abdominal cavity. These drugs typically work by blocking the cholinergic receptors, preventing acetylcholine from binding and triggering the release of calcium that would normally initiate muscle contraction.

Muscle relaxants ensure that muscles are relaxed during surgery to prevent muscle spasms and fasciculation that would otherwise occur. Use of muscle relaxants during surgery usually requires that the patient is intubated and mechanically ventilated during the surgical procedure, since these drugs also paralyse the major breathing muscles.

Muscle groups and injection sites

Nurses are frequently involved in administering intramuscular injections and so need to learn early on in their training the location of some of the major muscle groups used as injection sites. Intramuscular injections allow for faster absorption and distribution of pharmaceutical agents compared to subcutaneous routes, since muscle is very vascular and can also absorb a higher volume of injected material which is then progressively released into the blood. The deltoid muscle of the shoulder (Figure 8.7) is the most common site for intramuscular injection because of its prominence, excellent blood supply and easy accessibility.

Many drug injections and virtually all needle vaccinations are given at this site, although its anatomical position makes it less suitable for patients to self-inject. The dorsogluteal muscles of the buttocks used to be a common injection site, although this site is used less frequently today because of the recognised risk of sciatic nerve damage. Other common injection sites include the ventrogluteal muscles at the side of the hip, which are away from major blood vessels and nerves, and the vastus lateralis muscles of the thigh, which is particularly useful as a site for patients to self-inject since it is readily accessible for the patient without uncomfortable contortion of the body.

Now that you have completed this chapter, attempt the multiple-choice questions in Activity 8.4 to test your understanding of the subject material.

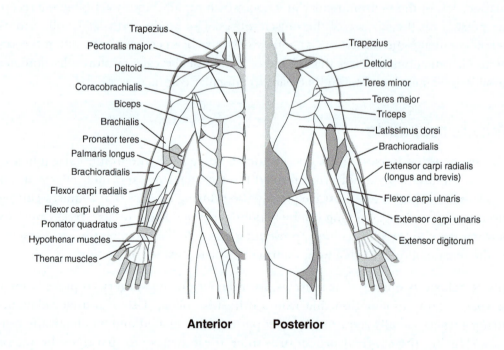

Anterior **Posterior**

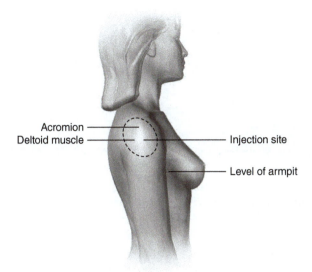

Correct place to give shot
in the deltoid muscle

Figure 8.7   Major muscle groups

Source of second image: BruceBlaus. Available at: https://commons.wikimedia.org/wiki/File:Injection_
Sites_Intramuscular_Rear-End_%26_Deltoid.png

Activity 8.4   Multiple-choice questions

1.   Which of the following bones is part of the appendicular skeleton?

   a)   The mandible

   b)   The sternum

   c)   The radius

   d)   The sacrum

2.   Which of the following forms the mineral component of bone?

   a)   Calcium carbonate

   b)   Calcium phosphate

   c)   Calcium silicate

   d)   Calcium citrate

(Continued)

(Continued)

3. In adults, the medullary cavity found running through the diaphysis of a long bone is usually filled with

    a) Yellow bone marrow

    b) Red bone marrow

    c) White bone marrow

    d) Serous fluid

4. Osteomyelitis is frequently seen following

    a) Simple fractures

    b) Joint dislocations

    c) Osteoarthritis

    d) Compound fractures

5. Which of the following is not a flat bone?

    a) The sternum

    b) The vertebrae

    c) The ulna

    d) The frontal bone of the skull

6. Which of the following types of bone fracture is also known as a greenstick fracture?

    a) A spiral fracture

    b) An oblique fracture

    c) An incomplete fracture

    d) A compound fracture

7. Which of the following statements concerning osteoblasts is true?

    a) Osteoblasts break down bone, releasing calcium into the blood

    b) Osteoblasts are only found in flat bones

    c) Osteoblasts deposit new cartilage

    d) Osteoblasts deposit bone

8. Which of the following components of a joint are found in the outer joint capsule?

    a) Articular cartilage

    b) Ligaments

    c)   Synovial membrane

    d)   All of the above

9.   Which of the following statements concerning muscle tissues is true?

    a)   Skeletal muscle fibres are not composed of individual cells

    b)   Cardiac muscle cells are separated by intercalated discs

    c)   Smooth muscle is not under conscious control

    d)   All are true

10. In skeletal (striated) muscle, actin forms the

    a)   Epimysium

    b)   Thin filaments

    c)   Thick filaments

    d)   Perimysium

Chapter summary

The musculoskeletal system consists of the 206 bones of the adult skeleton and the associated joints and skeletal muscles that facilitate movement. The skeleton consists of two divisions: the axial skeleton consists of the skull, vertebral column and ribcage, while the appendicular skeleton consists of the bones of the arms, legs and pelvis. Bone is a dynamic tissue predominantly composed of collagen and calcium phosphate, which is continually being deposited by bone-forming cells called osteoblasts and broken down by bone-digesting cells called osteoclasts.

To maintain a healthy bone density, an adequate intake of calcium and vitamin D is required, together with regular loading of the skeleton with the weight of the body, which is best achieved through regular exercise. Three major types of muscle tissue are recognised: cardiac muscle is restricted to the myocardium of the heart, smooth muscle is found in multiple locations throughout the body, including blood vessels, the gut wall and the walls of hollow organs such as the uterus and bladder, and skeletal muscle is also known as striated muscle.

(Continued)

(Continued)

Both cardiac and smooth muscle types are involuntary and cannot be controlled consciously. Conversely, skeletal muscle is voluntary, and most skeletal muscle groups can be consciously controlled to facilitate movement. Muscle contraction occurs when action potentials arrive at neuromuscular junctions, initiating the sliding filament mechanism which is powered by ATP. Since skeletal muscles have a good blood supply, they are used as injection sites, with the deltoid muscle of the shoulder used most frequently by nurses for both drug administration and needle vaccination.

Activities: Brief outline answers

Activity 8.1: Practical experiment (page 201)

The bone placed in vinegar for three days will have lost most of its mineral components (calcium phosphate) which will have dissolved in the vinegar. This will leave predominantly soft collagen. The bone should be soft and pliable like a piece of rubber.

The bone that has been heated over a naked gas flame will have had its collagen fibres denatured, leaving the calcium phosphate. This bone will be very fragile and break easily when a bending force is applied.

This simple experiment highlights that both the mineral and collagen components are essential for bone to retain its strength.

Activity 8.2: Evidence-based practice and research (page 212)

The ultimate cause of Edward's cellulitis and septic arthritis is bacteria introduced into the skin following the spider bite. These bacteria could be common skin microbiota such as *Staphylococcus aureus* or a streptococcal species, or a more exotic species associated with the spider. As bacteria began to replicate in the favourable environment of the dermis, the body's immune system has attempted to limit the spread of infection by initiating an inflammatory response; the area has become swollen and painful. The pain in the joint indicates that the bacteria have gained access to the joint capsule and began to replicate rapidly within the synovial fluid (septic arthritis).

A broad-spectrum antibiotic has started to kill bacteria at the wound site; gradually, as bacterial numbers fall, the inflammatory response and painful swelling resolve.

The GP suggested that Edward visit A&E if he developed a fever, felt unwell or noticed skin changes around the site of the bite because he was concerned that this could indicate: either the infection has spread into the blood (septicaemia) which increases the risk of sepsis or septic shock, or more rapid bacterial growth may be occurring in the deeper layers of the skin, potentially leading to necrotising fasciitis.

Activity 8.4: Multiple-choice questions (pages 217–19)

1) c, 2) b, 3) a, 4) d, 5) c, 6) c, 7) a, 8) b, 9) d, 10) b

Further reading

Boore J et al. (2016) Chapter 15: The musculoskeletal system – Support and movement, in *Essentials of Anatomy and Physiology for Nursing Practice*. London: SAGE Publications Ltd.

A textbook to develop your knowledge of human anatomy and physiology that is aimed specifically at nurses.

Tortora G and Derrickson B (2017) *Tortora's Principles of Anatomy and Physiology* (15th edition). New York: John Wiley & Sons.

In-depth coverage of human anatomy and physiology.

Useful websites

www.medicalnewstoday.com/articles/173312.php

What is a fracture? A clear, informative overview of different fracture types.

www.youtube.com/watch?v=Ktv-CaOt6UQ

Muscles, Part 1 – Muscle Cells: Crash Course. A simple overview of skeletal muscle structure together with a good description of the sliding filament mechanism.

Chapter 9

Blood, immunity and the lymphatic system

Chapter aims

After reading this chapter, you will be able to:

- list the components of blood, including plasma and plasma proteins;
- describe the structure and function of erythrocytes;
- explain the ABO and Rhesus blood grouping systems;
- describe the process of blood clotting (haemostasis), including the structure and function of platelets;
- highlight the roles of the different types of leukocyte and describe the immune responses of the body;
- explain the role of the lymphatic system in immune responses.

Introduction

Case study: Erika – secondary anaemia

Erika is a 53-year-old woman who consulted her GP after several months of experiencing progressive tiredness. She was pale and felt short of breath after even slight exertion and occasionally suffered from palpitations. Her haemoglobin (Hb) was found to be 10.7 gram/100 ml. Erika had previously experienced heavy, frequent vaginal bleeding for approximately six months. She assumed this was due to the menopause, but on investigation the bleeding was found to be due to uterine fibroids. Erika's anaemia was secondary to the bleeding.

Anaemia is the most common blood disorder and has a variety of courses ranging from dietary deficiencies to secondary anaemia precipitated by blood loss, as seen in Erika's case study. Nurses encounter a variety of blood diseases in clinical practice and quickly learn to understand the use of blood samples in screening for a variety of disorders and homeostatic imbalances. This chapter will begin with an overview of the nature of blood, examining both the fluid plasma and formed elements of blood. We will review the structure and function of erythrocytes and the importance of blood groups in blood transfusions. We will discuss the physiological processes of haemostasis, and the role of platelets in blood clotting. We will also cover the different types of leukocytes together with an overview of their immune function, and conclude this chapter by examining the lymphatic system.

Overview of blood, lymphatics and immunity

The blood is a fluid connective tissue composed of four main constituents: plasma, red blood cells (erythrocytes), white blood cells (leukocytes) and platelets, which are also known as thrombocytes. Leukocytes are sentinel cells which form a key element of an effective immune system to guard and defend the body against pathogens. The lymphatic system is aligned to this immune system, although it does play its own role and has other functions in the body.

Together, these systems transport substances including vital gases (oxygen, O_2) and carbon dioxide (CO_2), and regulate the body's fluid and electrolyte balance and body temperature. They also protect the body from loss of blood by the action of clotting. The lymphatic system additionally cleanses the cellular environment and returns proteins and tissue fluids to the blood (drainage).

Blood

As the only fluid tissue in the body, blood forms the perfect medium for the delivery of oxygen to all cells of the body and transport of the major metabolic waste carbon dioxide to the lungs for elimination. Blood performs many other key roles, including distribution of body heat, hormones, wastes and the products of digestion. Average adult males have approximately 5–6 litres of blood, whereas average females tend to have less at between 4 and 5 litres.

The four major constituents of blood are summarised in Table 9.1. Blood cells are generated in the red bone marrow by a process called haematopoiesis. In children, haematopoiesis occurs in marrow cavities of the axial skeleton and all long bones. In adults, it only occurs in the vertebrae, sternum, ribs, upper ends of the humerus, femur and pelvic girdle.

Table 9.1 Summary of blood constituents

Constituent	% in whole blood	Blood count	Descriptive features	Size (average diameter)	Main functional role
Plasma	55%	–	Pale yellow liquid	–	1) Fluid to carry blood cells around body 2) Transport of proteins, ions, nutrients, hormones and waste
Erythrocytes (RBCs)	44%	$4\text{--}6 \times 10^9$ cells/ml	Red, anucleate biconcave discs	7–8 micrometres	1) Transport of O_2 2) Transport of CO_2
Leukocytes (WBCs)	<1%	$4 \times 11 \times 10^6$ cells/ml	Large, nucleated cells	10 micrometres	1) Protect the body against pathogens such as bacteria and viruses 2) Clear old, dead and diseased cells
Platelets	<1%	$200\text{--}400 \times 10^6$ cells/ml	Cellular fragments	2–4 micrometres	Blood clotting

Blood constituents

Plasma

Plasma consists mainly of water (90 per cent) and is the medium in which the three cellular constituents of blood are carried. The temperature, pH and chemical composition of plasma are tightly regulated by negative feedback mechanisms to maintain homeostatic balance (Chapter 2). The aqueous medium of plasma contains a variety of other molecules, including plasma proteins which make up around 8 per cent of the total plasma volume.

Plasma proteins

The main groups of plasma proteins are albumins, globulins and the clotting proteins. Nearly all plasma proteins are made in the liver, so patients with liver failure may have low concentrations of albumins and clotting proteins. Plasma protein concentrations may also be decreased in patients with malnutrition, malabsorption and renal dysfunction.

Functions of the plasma proteins

Transport

Several plasma proteins act as 'carrier' proteins, which bind other substances such as ferritin (iron), hormones (see Chapter 5) and bilirubin for transport around the body. The protein-bound molecules act as transport and storage reservoirs and only the unbound molecules are biologically active.

Clotting

The clotting proteins fibrinogen, prothrombin and other clotting factors circulate in the plasma. Higher concentrations of certain plasma proteins, e.g. fibrinogen, increase the risks of stroke and cardiovascular disease. It has been shown that smokers and individuals exposed to high concentrations of dust and tobacco smoke have greatly increased concentrations of fibrinogen and other clotting factors in their plasma (Muddathir et al., 2018). Furthermore, studies also indicate that smoking cessation (one year of abstaining) has little effect on plasma fibrinogen levels (King et al., 2017).

Viscosity and osmotic pressure

Plasma proteins contribute to the viscosity (thickness) and density of blood and can affect blood pressure and blood flow. Because of their large size and negative charge, plasma proteins are unable to leave the capillaries. This creates an osmotic pressure gradient, pulling fluid back into the capillaries. This is essential for effective capillary exchange at tissues (a vital role of the lymphatic system). Loss of plasma proteins can cause problems with the regulation of capillary exchange and may lead to fluid accumulation and oedema (see Chapter 3).

Immunity

Some proteins, the globulins (gamma-globulins or immunoglobulins), are involved in immunity and defending the body against pathogens (see below). Additionally, a cascade of plasma enzymes, termed the complement system, is present in the plasma and can be activated to defend the body against bacterial infection.

Other plasma components

Organic substances make up 1.1 per cent of plasma weight. These include nutrient amino acids, glucose and also waste materials such as urea and creatinine. Inorganic substances make up 0.9 per cent of plasma weight. These are the electrolytes such as sodium (Na^+), potassium (K^+), calcium (Ca^{++}), chloride (Cl^-) and bicarbonate ions (HCO^{3-}).

Serum is the term often given to plasma, but strictly serum is plasma that has had blood clotting factors removed. Proteins such as albumin and globulins are often referred to as serum proteins.

The formed elements of blood: blood cells

Erythrocytes

Red blood cells (RBCs) (Figure 9.1a) are known as erythrocytes and their primary role is in the transport of oxygen and carbon dioxide. There are around 5 million RBCs in each µl of blood. The structure and function of erythrocytes and their role in the transport of respiratory gases were discussed in detail in Chapter 4.

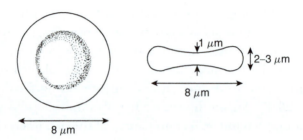

Figure 9.1a   Red blood cell

Formation of red blood cells (erythropoiesis) and the role of erythropoietin

The formation of erythrocytes is regulated by the hormone erythropoietin (EPO) which is synthesised and released from the kidneys. Release of EPO is stimulated by hypoxia, which may be a result of lung disease, smoking, heart failure, high altitudes or high concentrations of corticosteroid or thyroid hormones.

In kidney failure, the production of EPO may decline dramatically, causing a profound and disabling anaemia, which is largely managed by injections of synthetic EPO.

EPO is also reportedly used illicitly by elite athletes and sports competitors to increase their red cell numbers, thereby increasing their oxygen-carrying capacity and tissue oxygenation. However, if erythropoietin concentration is excessive for any reason, the number of circulating red cells increases. An increase in circulating RBCs is known as polycythaemia (see below). This condition causes an increase in the viscosity (thickness and stickiness) of blood, and therefore a raised blood pressure. Polycythaemia can also make the blood flow sluggish, which increases the risk of blood clot formation.

Erythrocytes are manufactured in the red bone marrow at a phenomenal rate of 2.5 million per second. Erythrocyte formation usually takes about seven days. If not enough new red blood cells are produced, the oxygen needs of the body's cells will not be met. Formation of red cells requires three major dietary nutrients: iron, folic acid (vitamin B9) and vitamin B12.

Red blood cells are also affected when DNA formation is hindered by a lack of folic acid or vitamin B12. Without adequate DNA, red cells become enlarged (macrocytosis), misshapen and fragile and the rate of red cell breakdown is increased. Macrocytic anaemia occurs when haemoglobin concentration is very low and RBCs are enlarged. The size of red cells is measured as mean corpuscular volume (MCV), but a raised MCV is a relatively late sign of deficiency, and measurements of serum concentrations of folate and B12 are more sensitive. Adequate intake of folic acid and B12 is essential and may be compromised by poor diet or malabsorption syndromes. Folate and B12 deficiencies also cause nervous system disturbances and have been linked to dementia (Blundo et al., 2015).

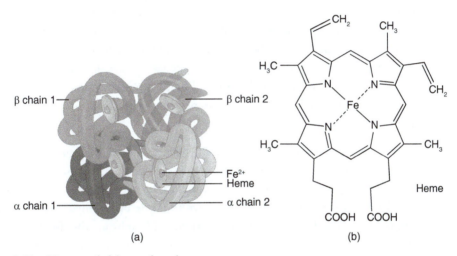

Figure 9.1b   Haemoglobin molecule

Dietary iron deficiency is also relatively common and iron intake is vital for the formation of haem, which involves a complex synthesis process in the bone marrow and liver, where enzymes incorporate ferrous iron into a ring-like molecule known as a porphyrin.

Anaemia

If the number of red blood cells becomes insufficient, a condition called anaemia can develop and oxygen delivery to the tissues becomes suboptimal. Normally a person's haemoglobin (Figure 9.1b) is measured in grams per litre of blood. For adult males, normal haemoglobin concentrations range from 130–180 g/100 ml; for females, 115–165 g/100 ml. A low haemoglobin concentration (i.e. below 130 g/100 ml in males and below 115 g/100 ml in females) is referred to as 'anaemia'. If haemoglobin levels fall below 8 g/100 ml (11 g/100 ml in the elderly), there is insufficient oxygen delivered to the tissues, and symptoms of inadequate tissue oxygenation will ensue. These may include fatigue, weakness, dizziness, insomnia, indigestion, angina, paraesthesia (pins and needles), palpitations and poor healing.

In severe anaemia, cardiac insufficiency develops, causing shortness of breath on exercise. Anaemia also causes thinning of mucous membranes, resulting in soreness of the mouth and tongue, malabsorption and vaginal atrophy in post-menopausal women. There are many causes of anaemia, including under-nutrition, chronic inflammation, blood loss and excessive destruction of red cells.

To help you understand the importance of adequate iron intake, read through Alan's case study.

> ## Case study: Alan – iron-deficiency anaemia
>
> Alan is a 32-year-old male who is concerned over the way in which animals bred for food are treated. Recently, he has been reading about the impact increased meat consumption has on greenhouse gases. As a consequence, he has decided to become a vegan. Unfortunately, over a period of several months, Alan has started to develop symptoms of anaemia similar to those experienced by Erika in our first case study in this chapter.
>
> A vegan diet is sometimes deficient in iron and Alan's GP referred him to a dietitian who advised him on a suitable diet, and recommended that he increase his intake of dark-green leafy vegetables like watercress and curly kale, pulses, cereals and bread fortified with extra iron, and to avoid foods with high levels of phytic acid, such as wholegrain cereals, which can inhibit the absorption of iron from other foods.

Polycythaemia

Primary polycythaemia (polycythaemia vera) is usually due to a gene defect in the erythrocyte stem-cell line (haemocytoblasts), from which all erythrocytes are derived. Red cell production is unable to stop even when too many cells are already present. Venesection (blood-letting) is sometimes used to reduce the numbers of erythrocytes.

Polycythaemia can be associated with dehydration and other causes of decreased plasma volume. Secondary polycythaemia may result from an increase in plasma erythropoietin due to hypoxic conditions. This can be apparent in people living at high altitudes, patients with cardiac failure, smokers or patients with chronic bronchitis and emphysema.

Haematocrit

When a blood sample is centrifuged in a tube the erythrocytes collect at the bottom since they have the greatest density; above the erythrocytes is a thin layer of leukocytes called the buffy coat, with the remainder of the sample consisting of the straw-coloured plasma. The haematocrit is the percentage of whole blood occupied by erythrocytes and is often referred to as the packed red cell volume. Haematocrit scores are routinely used in clinical practice to assess the patient's current red cell volume, with normal values around 47±7 per cent for men and 42±5 per cent for women and children. However, haematocrit may fall to very low levels in severe chronic anaemia, or rise as high as 65–70 per cent in polycythaemia.

Destruction of red blood cells (haemolysis)

Old and worn-out red blood cells are removed by phagocytic macrophages in the spleen and liver. The haem and globin portions of haemoglobin are split apart. Globin is broken down into its constituent amino acids, which can be utilised in the synthesis of new protein. Iron is removed from the haem, transported and reused to make new haemoglobin, or stored as ferritin so that very little is lost from the body.

The non-iron part of haem, the ring-shaped porphyrin, is converted into the green pigment biliverdin, and then into a yellow-orange pigment, bilirubin. Bilirubin, the more toxic pigment, is conjugated to glucuronic acid in the liver to form a less toxic compound. Any liver problems may lead to build-up and subsequent backflow of bilirubin into the blood. This can be detected as a raised serum bilirubin concentration but is also visible as a yellowing of the skin or sclera of the eyes and is known as jaundice.

Case study: Martha – cirrhosis of the liver

Martha is 59 years old, divorced and unemployed. Martha has always been a heavy drinker, but since losing her job, her alcohol intake has increased significantly and she now drinks at least a bottle of vodka a day. Martha was admitted to hospital following a fall. Her injuries were minor but she was also noted to have a grossly distended abdomen, swollen ankles and jaundice, including yellowing skin and sclera, itching, dark urine and pale fatty stools. It was also noted that she smelt of alcohol and was irritable, anxious and sweating. She had a tachycardia and slight tremor, all of which are signs of alcohol withdrawal. A provisional diagnosis of cirrhosis of the liver was made.

Blood groups

Blood transfusions are common procedures necessary for a variety of medical conditions, and also under critical conditions when there is a need to replace important missing blood components. Transfusions involve transferring whole blood or components (e.g. erythrocytes, plasma) from one individual (donor) into another (recipient) intravenously. Most blood transfusions involve the transfer of donor RBCs (in saline dextrose) to a recipient. However, if blood groups are incorrectly or incompletely matched, the makeup of the donor's erythrocyte membranes may trigger damaging transfusion reactions in the recipient.

Antigens

All cells and cell fragments, living or dead, possess molecules known as antigens on their surface membranes. Many different types of antigens exist; those present on our own cells are known as self-antigens. If a cell enters the body, and carries surface antigens that are not recognised as self (non-self-antigens), the body will react to these foreign antigens by making antibodies. These antibodies are created and directed against a specific antigen, to which they will bind and cause agglutination, clumping and subsequent destruction of the invading cell.

This defence strategy is important and useful if the foreign cells are pathogens, but in certain circumstances (e.g. organ transplants or blood transfusions), antibodies against non-self, foreign cells can cause unwanted damage. There are several different types of antigens on the surface of erythrocytes (and most other cells). Blood groups are named according to the absence or presence of erythrocyte antigens. About 33 different human blood grouping systems are recognised (Mitra et al., 2014) including ABO, Lewis (Le), Duffy (Fy) and Rhesus (Rh) systems.

However, two blood grouping systems that are of greatest clinical significance are the ABO and Rhesus systems.

ABO blood grouping

This blood grouping system is dependent on the existence of two surface erythrocyte antigens, A and B. All humans can be split into four groups on the basis of the ABO blood system.

An individual whose erythrocytes possess:

1. antigen A is blood type/group A;
2. antigen B is blood group B;
3. both antigens A and B is blood group AB;
4. neither antigen A nor antigen B is blood group O.

Thus, four distinct ABO blood groups exist, depending on the presence or absence of one or both of these two antigens, A and B. The frequency of occurrence of each of the four ABO blood groups varies within different populations.

Problems may occur if a person belonging to a particular blood group donates or receives blood from a person of a different blood group. This is because antibodies to antigen A and/or antigen B are found pre-formed in virtually everyone who lacks the corresponding antigens. These antibodies are present in the plasma soon after birth. Thus, for example, an individual of blood type A has antigen A on the surface of his/her erythrocytes, but also has antibody to antigen B in his/her plasma. If this individual receives blood donated from a person of blood type B (with antigen B on the erythrocytes), agglutination (clumping) of the donor erythrocytes occurs in the body of the recipient (Table 9.2a).

The size and spread of the erythrocyte clumps would depend on the strength of the recipient's antibody response to antigen B. Clumping leads to intravascular haemolysis (bursting of erythrocytes) and can happen whenever incompatible erythrocytes are transfused.

Table 9.2a ABO blood groups and corresponding antibodies

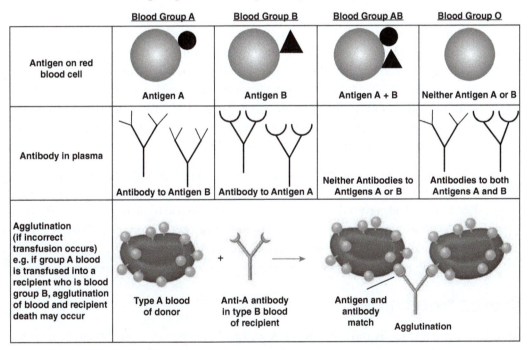

Close observation, BP monitoring and questioning of patients receiving transfusions are needed to recognise and minimise potential problems. Many symptoms of incorrect blood transfusions become apparent early on, often within the first 30 minutes of transfusion. Acute haemolytic reactions (caused by the clumping of erythrocytes) are characterised by hypotension, fever and chills, and chest or flank pain. Table 9.2b summarises the ability of various blood types to donate and receive blood.

Table 9.2b Ability of persons with different blood types to donate and receive blood

	Blood Group A	Blood Group B	Blood Group AB	Blood Group O
Can donate blood to:	Group A Group AB	Group B Group AB	Group AB	Group O Group A Group B Group AB
Can receive blood from:	Group A Group O	Group B Group O	Group A Group B Group AB Group O	Group O

Case study: Michael – transfusion reaction

Michael is a 45-year-old male who was admitted to his local A&E following a fall at a building site where he was employed as a labourer. Significant blood loss ensued which required surgery and a blood transfusion. Michael was cross-matched for five units of packed red blood cells. Three units of blood were transfused without incident. However, 25 minutes after the fourth unit of blood was commenced, Michael's blood pressure fell to 90/45 and his temperature was recorded as 38.2°C. The transfusion was stopped immediately because of a suspected haemolytic transfusion reaction. Michael was commenced on intravenous fluids for the hypotension and diuretics to promote urine output and improve renal blood flow.

The blood bank was contacted and pre-transfusion samples, post-transfusion samples and a segment from the fourth unit transfused were tested. It was subsequently discovered that an error had occurred and the fourth unit of blood had been incorrectly labelled as type A, when in fact it was type AB. The fact that nurses were monitoring Michael closely meant that the reaction was identified early and there were no long-term consequences.

Rhesus blood group

About 85 per cent of us have the Rhesus antigen (D) present on the surface of our erythrocytes. Those that do are termed Rhesus positive (Rh+ve). Approximately 15 per cent of us do not have this antigen and we are Rhesus negative (Rh-ve). Even though there are no pre-formed antibodies to Rhesus antigens (unlike antibodies to the ABO blood group antigens), the Rhesus system is of great clinical significance. This is because individuals without Rhesus antigen (D) can readily form antibodies once exposed to it. Formation of Rhesus antibodies to antigen D (Anti-D) will happen if Rh-positive blood is transfused to a Rh-negative person in about 90 per cent of cases.

However, the most important clinical situation can arise if a Rh-negative woman is pregnant with a Rh-positive foetus. The pregnancy of the first child is without incident, but at the birth, when maternal and foetal bloods mix, the baby's Rhesus D antigen on its red blood cells will be detected by the mother post-birth, who will rapidly begin to form antibodies to it within 3–7 days. Months or years later during any subsequent pregnancies, Rhesus antibodies (Anti-D) from the maternal circulation are capable of crossing the placenta, causing clumping and destruction of foetal red blood cells carrying the D antigen.

This haemolytic activity can give rise to severe jaundice, anaemia, hypoxia and oedema in the foetus (haemolytic disease of the newborn). To combat this, maternal blood is taken for grouping early in the first pregnancy, so that at the birth of the first child, Rhesus-negative women can receive intramuscular injections (anti-D). Administration of this antibody will destroy any rogue baby RBCs and prevent the detection of the baby's Rhesus antigens by the mother's immune system. This will prevent antibody formation in the mother and ensure the normal development and survival of any future foetuses.

White blood cells

These cells form < 1 per cent of whole blood (Table 9.1), and will be discussed below under immunity.

Platelets

Platelets play a hugely important role in blood clotting (coagulation) and help to prevent blood loss by the body. When blood vessels are damaged, clotting mechanisms are activated with the aim of sealing off the vessel to limit blood loss. Platelets (thrombocytes) are cellular fragments produced in the bone marrow under the influence of the hormone thrombopoietin. Large cells, megakaryocytes, undergo fragmentation and each cell is capable of budding off up to 4,000 cell-membrane-bound thrombocytes. Platelets live for about 7–10 days in the circulation (Drelich and Bray, 2015). In adults the platelet count is usually between 150 and 450×10^9/L, which means there are 150,000 to 450,000 platelets per microlitre of blood (Table 9.1).

Platelet count

A low platelet count (less than 150×10^9/l) is known as thrombocytopenia. It may lead to bruising (purpura), petechiae (small purple markings) or spontaneous bleeding. There may be many reasons for thrombocytopenia, including leukaemia or other conditions affecting the bone marrow, liver disease, some infections, folate or B12 deficiency, clotting disorders such as idiopathic thrombocytopenic purpura (an autoimmune disease) and cytotoxic therapy. A high platelet count (more than 450×10^9/l) is known as thrombocytosis. It is usually associated with certain cancers or chronic inflammation. This condition increases the risk of spontaneous clotting and blood vessel occlusion.

Blood clotting

Initially, upon injury, the damaged blood vessel immediately constricts. Then, as blood begins to leak out of it, mechanisms to initiate blood coagulation begin. First, a temporary plug of platelets forms. This is then converted into a permanent and more robust clot, as the soluble plasma protein fibrinogen is converted into insoluble fibrin.

Formation of the platelet plug

Normally, platelets are not attracted to each other, or to the lining of healthy vessels. When blood vessels are damaged, however, the epithelial lining is torn and the collagen(s) in underlying connective tissue are exposed. These collagen fibres become coated with a protein, Von Willebrand factor, which is secreted by cells lining the blood vessels. Von Willebrand factor attracts platelets, which now stick to the exposed collagen. As platelets stick, they degranulate, releasing three main chemicals, which contribute to clotting:

1. Serotonin. This stimulates and maintains vasoconstriction of vascular smooth muscle, decreasing blood flow to the injured vessel, thereby preventing further blood loss. Serotonin has complex effects on the microcirculation: it dilates arterioles and constricts venules. Serotonin also causes platelets to aggregate.

2. Adenosine diphosphate (ADP). This changes the platelet surface membrane so that the platelet becomes a more spherical, fatter structure. Membrane extensions (pseudopodia) form, which cause platelets to become 'sticky'.

3. Thromboxane A2 (TxA2). This prostaglandin is a very powerful inducer of vasoconstriction and platelet aggregation. The common household drug aspirin irreversibly inhibits platelet enzymes responsible for synthesis of TxA2, thereby reducing clot formation. In patients at risk of or those who have suffered a prior stroke or heart attack, low doses of aspirin may be effective in prevention of further cardiac incidences. Since the effects of aspirin last as long as the platelets survive (about 7 days), the full ability of the blood to clot is not restored for a week after aspirin is discontinued, so aspirin is avoided before planned operations and in late pregnancy.

ADP and thromboxanes attract more platelets to the site of injury. These adhere to platelets already stuck to the collagen. Platelets in this second layer then degranulate, releasing the three main platelet-derived factors above, thus attracting even more platelets. The resulting positive feedback ensures that layer upon layer of platelets aggregate, leading to the rapid formation of the platelet plug (Figure 9.2). This plug can be quite fragile and may be washed away if blood flow in the injured vessel is too vigorous, so this now needs to be stabilised.

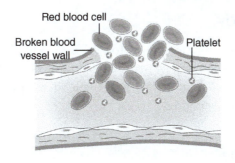

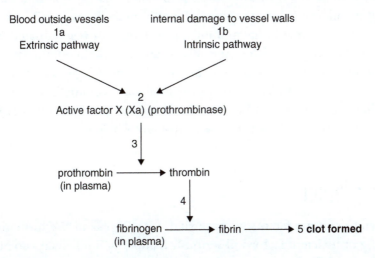

Figure 9.2   Blood vessel with platelet plug

Formation of the fibrin clot

To reinforce the platelet plug and stop blood loss, a more robust clot is formed. This relies on the synthesis of a tough, fibrous, rope-like protein called fibrin. Fibrin forms a meshwork around the platelet plug, sealing an injured vessel and trapping blood cells.

Fibrin is formed from the plasma protein fibrinogen in a complex series of reactions involving several blood clotting factors (I–XIII), which can proceed via one of two pathways, the extrinsic and/or intrinsic pathways. Initially, the extrinsic pathway normally predominates. A simplified clotting cascade is shown in Figure 9.3a.

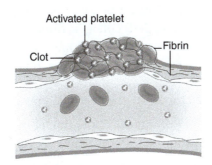

Figure 9.3a   Simplified clotting cascade (steps 1–5)

The extrinsic pathway

When blood leaves the vessels, clotting factor VII interacts with tissue factor. This is a large protein found on the surface of many cells and on the cells lining the blood vessels when they are damaged. The complex of tissue factor plus factor VII triggers the clotting mechanisms within seconds.

The intrinsic pathway

The intrinsic pathway refers to clotting factors that are present within (intrinsic to) blood. When vessel walls are damaged, collagen fibres are exposed. Contact with collagen fibres activates a protein known as Hageman factor (factor XII). Over several minutes, a sequence of reactions unfolds, whereby each factor activates the next:

1. Both pathways activate factor X, an enzyme called prothrombinase.
2. Factor X forms a complex with other factors (including factor V), which converts the plasma protein prothrombin into the active enzyme thrombin.
3. Thrombin converts fibrinogen into fibrin, which forms a permanent clot. Thrombin also activates a fibrin stabilising factor (factor XIII), which strengthens the fibrin strands into a tough clot.
4. Thrombin also intensifies the actions of the clotting factors, thereby accelerating and reinforcing the process.

Blood coagulation is necessary to combat blood vessel injury and blood loss. However, some 10 days after an operation, the concentration of clotting factors and platelets is at its maximum, so patients post-op must be kept as mobile as possible and provided with support stockings, high fluid intake and prophylactic anticoagulant (e.g. heparin), if necessary.

Clot formation is restricted by anti-clotting mechanisms. Normally, a balance exists between clotting and anti-clotting forces. If clotting mechanisms fail, excessive bleeding may occur, for example in haemophilia, liver failure or disseminated intravascular coagulation. If anti-clotting mechanisms fail, or are overwhelmed, thrombi (clots) may form. Fragments of clots (emboli) may break away and lodge in distant vessels, particularly the lungs or brain. Thrombi and emboli can occlude/block any part of the circulation, but the coronary and cerebral arteries and the deep veins of the calf and pelvis are the most frequently affected (see thrombosis below).

Haemophilia

Since the various clotting factors all have vital roles to play in the formation of fibrin clots, a missing or deficient factor will seriously hamper an individual's ability to control blood loss. Haemophilia is the most common inherited clotting disorder. There are two types, both caused by deficiency in a factor from the intrinsic pathway: type A, deficiency of factor VIII; and type B, deficiency of factor IX (a milder condition). Haemophilia can be managed by intravenous administration of concentrates of the missing factor.

Thrombosis

Thrombosis is the formation of unwanted clots in blood vessels. These can narrow or block a vessel and restrict blood supply to the tissues being fed by that particular vessel. This can have serious, even fatal outcomes such as strokes or heart attacks.

In 1856, Rudolf Virchow proposed three causes of thrombosis, known as 'Virchow's Triad'. This stated that the composition of blood, the lining of blood vessels and the rate and state of blood flow are all closely interlinked, for example: endothelial injury can be initiated by abnormal blood flow and any endothelial injury is likely to promote the coagulability of the blood, and dehydration can affect both blood flow and coagulability.

Factors preventing thrombosis

There are some key proteins in the body that contribute to adjust the rate of blood clot formation; in particular, two anticoagulant proteins, protein C and protein S, help. When a blood vessel is injured, the body initiates the clotting cascade and platelets are activated, as are clotting factors, and this results in the formation of a stable blood clot, preventing further blood loss and protecting the injury as it heals.

Thrombin is a clotting factor that can accelerate or decelerate blood clot formation by promoting or inhibiting its own activation (intrinsic pathway). It forms a feedback loop that uses protein C and protein S to slow down the clotting cascade process. Thrombin first combines with a protein called thrombomodulin, then activates protein C. This activated protein C (APC) then combines with protein S (a co-factor) and together they work to degrade coagulation factors VIIIa and Va which are required to produce thrombin. This has the net effect of slowing down the generation of new thrombin and inhibiting further clotting. If there is not enough protein C or protein S, however, then thrombin generation goes on unchecked. This can lead to excessive or inappropriate clotting that may block the flow of blood in the veins.

Oestrogens inhibit the actions of activated protein C, which may account for the increased risks of venous thrombosis associated with pregnancy, or the combined oral contraceptive pill and hormone replacement therapy (Devis and Knuttinen, 2017).

Septicaemia

Septicaemia can occur if an infection is caused by large amounts of bacteria in the blood. Usually in association with septicaemia is a serious condition known as disseminated intravascular coagulation or DIC. This is often visible as a non-dispersing 'rash' under the skin. It arises if cells lining blood vessels trigger the clotting cascade but once all the clotting factors have been expended, bleeding can be uncontrollable.

Sepsis

Sepsis is a life-threatening condition which results following an infection. This is not necessarily a blood-borne infection. Sepsis is characterised by a raised serum lactate and falling blood pressure (often needing urgent administration of vasoconstrictors). It usually overwhelms the body and can lead to multi-organ failure and death.

Anticoagulants

Most of the proteins involved in haemostasis are synthesised by liver cells. Patients with liver failure may therefore bleed excessively because of the failure to produce enough clotting factors. Heparin is a common anticoagulant given intravenously, usually by injection. It is most likely to be used as a prophylactic anticoagulant, and works by inhibiting the formation of thrombin.

Vitamin K is essential for synthesis of some vital clotting factors (prothrombin, VII, IX and X). Dietary sources of this vitamin are not abundant, and the majority of our Vitamin K is acquired from resident colonies of commensal bacteria (*E.coli*) harboured in the large intestine. These bacteria produce vitamin K, which is fat-soluble, and easily absorbed through the lining of the colon into the blood and passed to the liver.

In the first few weeks of life, until their colons are colonised by *E.coli*, neonates have low levels of vitamin K. This is therefore administered to most neonates shortly after birth to facilitate clotting in the event of any bleed or haemorrhage.

Warfarin inhibits activation of vitamin K, and therefore reduces the production of some clotting factors. It is prescribed as an anticoagulant to inhibit the formation of new clots for patients who may be at risk from thromboses, heart attack or stroke.

Dissolution of the fibrin clot

Once a clot has served its purpose to stop the loss of blood from a damaged vessel, scar tissue is formed and the clot is ready to be dissolved by the fibrinolytic system.

Fibrinolysis is very important. If clots were left in place, they could dislodge, travel (as emboli) in the circulation and get stuck in important blood vessels, impeding blood flow. The fibrinolytic system is constantly in operation, removing unnecessary clots. The key enzyme in this cascade of reactions is plasmin (Figure 9.3b).

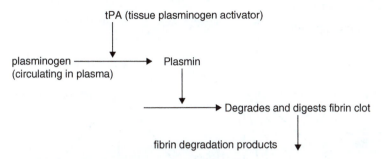

Figure 9.3b Dissolution of the fibrin clot: simplified diagram of the fibrinolytic system

1. Tissue plasminogen activator (tPA) is released from cells lining blood vessels. It is normally regulated by several inhibitors.

2. tPA converts an inactive plasma protein, plasminogen (produced by the liver), into a potent enzyme, plasmin.

3. Plasmin splits fibrin and fibrinogen into fragments known as fibrin degradation products or 'D dimers', thereby dissolving the clot. (The D-dimer blood test is often used to determine if a patient has recently formed any blood clots.)

4. The remains of the clot are removed by scavenger white blood cells – the macrophages.

Immunity

White blood cells (leukocytes)

Like all blood cells, leukocytes are produced in the red bone marrow from stem cells during haematopoiesis (Figure 9.4). Leukocytes are the principal components of the immune system and form less than 1 per cent of whole blood. Most leukocytes undergo daily fluctuations exhibiting a diurnal variation such that the highest levels usually occur late in the day or in the middle of the night (Druzd et al., 2017).

The five main types of white blood cells are divided into two groups: granulocytes and agranulocytes (Table 9.3). Neutrophils, eosinophils and basophils are granulocytes, named because of the presence of an intense number of cytoplasmic granules. Monocytes and lymphocytes are agranulocytes. The normal total white blood cell counts in adults ranges from $4.0–11.0 \times 10^9$ cells/l. An increased number of white cells in the circulation may be associated with exercise, stress, disease, infection or leukaemia.

A low white blood cell count may indicate bone marrow disorders (sometimes secondary to anti-cancer therapy), nutritional deficiency or an immunocompromised state. Changes in white cell numbers can occur in hypersensitivity or allergic responses. Each of the five types of leukocytes has its own function, but all are involved in, and form an integral part of, the body's immune system.

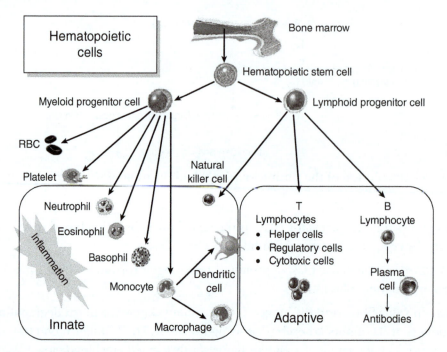

Figure 9.4 Formation of immune cells in bone marrow

© Wayne W. LaMorte and Boston University School of Public Health. Reprinted with permission.

Table 9.3 Differential white blood cell count

Type	Percentage (%)	Number of cells/ml blood
Neutrophils	50–60%	3000–7000
Eosinophils	1–4%	50–400
Basophils	0.5–2%	25–100
Lymphocytes	20–40%	1000–4000
Monocytes	2–9%	100–600
Total Count	100%	4100–10900

The immune system

The survival of the human body depends on its ability to protect itself against environmental dangers, foreign and harmful substances and persistent attack from a hostile array of pathogenic microorganisms. The body defends itself using three interdependent immune systems:

1. A range of non-specific physical barriers and reflexes which include the skin, and provide protective defences, internal and externalised secretions, such as mucus and lysozyme (an enzyme which can lyse bacteria).

2. A whole army of innate immune defences, comprising non-specific (four out of the five) leukocytes, peptides and chemical mediators (called chemokines and cytokines), bolstered by the inflammatory response, which increases the flow of blood to damaged areas, and encourages phagocytic leukocytes to move into injured tissues to engulf potential pathogens, limiting their proliferation and spread.

3. The specific, adaptive immune system whose responses develop more gradually, yet more definitively, specifically targeting individual pathogens and ridding the body of malignant cells. The leukocyte involved here is the lymphocyte.

Unbroken physical barriers and innate immune defences provide the initial immediate and effective response to most pathogens (Table 9.4). Such barriers and defences are scattered at many entry portals throughout the body (Figure 9.5). The more sophisticated and expansive adaptive immune system is called upon as a second line of defence and comes into play usually several days after the innate response has been initiated.

Table 9.4 Mechanical and chemical defences of the body

DEFENCE	DESCRIPTION
Coughing/sneezing	These reflex actions help to prevent entry and expel foreign material from the respiratory tract
Ciliary escalator	The wavy motion of cilia on cells lining the respiratory tract pushes mucus and trapped microorganisms upwards towards the mouth and nose, away from the lungs (see Chapter 4)
Skin and mucous membranes	These prevent organisms from entering and spreading within the body. Protective mechanisms include: • keratin in epidermal cells. This is resistant to microbial enzymes; • desquamation. The regular removal of skin cells and transient microorganisms; • low pH. Slight acidity and fatty acids keep several pathogens at bay; • resident microflora act as commensals and reduce the spread of potential pathogens; • skin secretions containing antibodies (mainly IgA) and lysozyme (see below)
Gastric juice	Stomach hydrochloric acid. Most bacteria exposed to this will die in about 60 seconds
Drainage	If urine is allowed to stagnate, infection is likely If a patient remains in a supine position for a protracted period, the decreased drainage of mucus leads to chest infections
Secretions: mucus, lysozyme, antibodies (IgA)	These provide a physical barrier and a medium for antimicrobial substances, such as lysozyme Lysozyme occurs in tears, saliva and nasal, respiratory and GI secretions. Kills and digests (hydrolyses) many bacteria

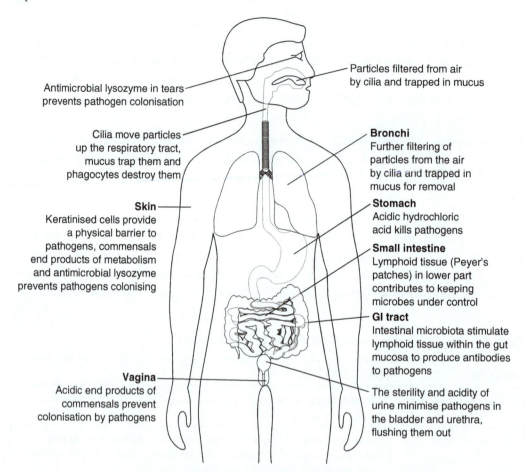

Antimicrobial lysozyme in tears prevents pathogen colonisation

Cilia move particles up the respiratory tract, mucus trap them and phagocytes destroy them

Skin
Keratinised cells provide a physical barrier to pathogens, commensals end products of metabolism and antimicrobial lysozyme prevents pathogens colonising

Vagina
Acidic end products of commensals prevent colonisation by pathogens

Particles filtered from air by cilia and trapped in mucus

Bronchi
Further filtering of particles from the air by cilia and trapped in mucus for removal

Stomach
Acidic hydrochloric acid kills pathogens

Small intestine
Lymphoid tissue (Peyer's patches) in lower part contributes to keeping microbes under control

GI tract
Intestinal microbiota stimulate lymphoid tissue within the gut mucosa to produce antibodies to pathogens

The sterility and acidity of urine minimise pathogens in the bladder and urethra, flushing them out

Figure 9.5   Physical and chemical barriers to infection

The innate immune system

The innate defence system relies on secreted molecules including antimicrobial factors such as defensins, which can pierce pathogen membranes, thereby impeding infection through the body. Our innate defence also depends heavily on cellular components such as the phagocytes – neutrophils, monocytes and macrophages. In addition, dendritic cells, mast cells, eosinophils and natural killer cells all play a key role in innate clearing. Other chemicals and substances of the innate immune defence system include the plasma-based 'staircase' of the complement cascade of proteins and enzymes.

Complement proteins help to promote inflammation, enhance antibody action and 'coat' (opsonise) unwanted microbes, highlighting them for destruction. Complement further activates phagocytic cells to help mediate clearance of pathogens, resulting in an amplification of the immune response to attack pathogen membranes and kill invading cells. Additional humoral components include C-reactive protein (CRP) which is produced by the liver. By binding specifically to certain molecules and cells such as phagocytes, this can quickly raise cytokine production and levels of other mediators, increasing the inflammatory response to help rapidly destroy invading organisms.

Immune cells

Haemopoietic stem cells are found in the red bone marrow. These stem cells are triggered and directed to form the various immune cells, either of the myeloid or lymphoid lineage (Figure 9.4). There are four white blood cells which form part of the innate immune system which are highlighted below and are split into two populations called granulocytes and agranulocytes, based on the appearance of their cytoplasm.

Granulocytes

As implied by their name, these cells have a cytoplasm with multiple granular inclusions, most of which are essential to their function such as digestive enzymes or inflammatory mediators. There are three major granulocyte populations:

Neutrophils

Neutrophils are the most abundant leukocytes (Table 9.3), forming part of the general attack system. They are attracted to sites of injury and infection in the tissues where they constitute the primary immune defence against rapidly proliferating bacteria, yeast and fungal infections.

The immune system is regulated by soluble local hormones called cytokines, produced by leukocytes. Cytokines act as chemical messengers, communicating between leukocytes, orchestrating the control and movement of cells, and protecting the body from foreign invaders. Following localised injury, trauma or stimulation by an infectious agent, certain cytokines are produced which control and direct the migration of immune cells, particularly neutrophils. This process of chemical attraction or chemotaxis is essential for the accumulation of phagocytes around traumatised or infected tissue.

To exit blood vessels and reach infected or damaged tissue, neutrophils adhere to vessel walls. Then, by 'cell walking', or diapedesis, neutrophils squeeze through pores in the vessel endothelial wall, migrating into tissue and secreting an enzyme, collagenase, which breaks down collagen as they move through tissues. Neutrophils then engulf foreign material and invading pathogens, in a process known as phagocytosis. These phagocytes are capable of deploying antimicrobial mechanisms such as the generation of reactive oxygen (superoxide burst) and nitrogen species to destroy pathogens. Following microbial stimulation, they can also kill extracellularly through the extrusions of NETs (neutrophil extracellular traps) – their own DNA thrust out into the extracellular environment to trap foreign cells. Neutrophils often die after this process.

The body's neutrophils are present within the bone marrow (90 per cent), tissues (7–8 per cent) and circulation (2–3 per cent). Some of these sit in the margins of blood vessels and are mobilised when needed, redistributing in response to stress. Adrenaline mobilises marginated neutrophils into the circulation during conditions such as exercise,

243

anger, fear or anxiety. Corticosteroids mobilise both marginated neutrophils and those in the bone marrow following tissue damage such as a myocardial infarction (Hellebrekers et al., 2018).

Basophils

Basophils contain large, prominent cytoplasmic granules, distributed throughout the whole cell. These granules contain several compounds including heparin and histamine. Heparin is one of the body's natural anticoagulants, and histamine is a potent mediator of inflammation. Basophils are associated with the immediate immune response to foreign antigens and are involved in allergic conditions such as asthma, hay fever and anaphylaxis. Mast cells are granular cells believed to have similar origins to basophils but are located in solid organs and tissues. Mast cells increase in numbers in tissue following allergic reactions or chronic irritation or injury. Both basophils and mast cells are activated by Ig-E antibodies (see below).

Case study: Hongyi – anaphylaxis

Hongyi, a 26-year-old, was celebrating her birthday by visiting a seafood restaurant where she ate crab salad. Approximately 10 minutes after eating, Hongyi felt her throat beginning to swell, and she felt dizzy and weak. Her husband rang 999 and the paramedics arrived 8 minutes later. On examination, her airway was partially obstructed, her respiratory rate was 20 and regular but shallow, and there was an audible wheeze present. Hongyi's heart rate was 100 and regular and capillary refill was normal. Her blood pressure was 90/55. Her skin was flushed. Hongyi was given 100 per cent oxygen and 0.5 ml of 1:1000 adrenaline IM. She was commenced on salbutamol 5 mg/2.5 ml nebuliser and given a second 0.5 ml dose of 1:1000 adrenaline IM, administered with good effect. Symptoms began to resolve quickly but Hongyi was taken to hospital where she remained under observation for six hours before being discharged home.

Shellfish allergy is one of the few allergies that can present for the first time in adulthood and can be caused by food that one has enjoyed before with no ill effects.

Eosinophils

The two main functions of eosinophils include combatting invasive parasitic infestations and reduction of inflammation caused by histamine. Eosinophils are highly granular cells able to release their potent chemicals onto parasitic worms such as tapeworms to damage and destroy the worm. Eosinophils are able to reduce inflammation through the release of histaminase, an enzyme which neutralises histamine. They can also inactivate other chemicals involved in anaphylaxis. Increased numbers of eosinophils may be seen in some individuals with chronic allergic conditions such as asthma.

Agranular leukocytes

These leukocyte populations have significantly fewer visible granules within their cytoplasm. In addition to the monocytes discussed below as part of the innate immune system, the agranular population also include the lymphocytes which form the cornerstone of the specific adaptive immune system.

Monocytes and macrophages

These are leukocytes which also belong to the reticuloendothelial system (RES), a network of cells dispersed throughout the organs of the body and the lymph nodes. Precursor cells in bone marrow develop into monocytes, which are released into the bloodstream. Monocytes are highly mobile white blood cells making up between 5 and 10 per cent of the circulating leukocyte pool (Table 9.3). Following a short period of circulation of about 8 days, monocytes leave the blood and enter the tissues, where they can differentiate into larger cells, the macrophages. These large cells are phagocytes too, able to engulf microbes and other foreign material. Unlike the smaller neutrophils, they are able to survive this process.

Macrophages can engulf most foreign material, such as bacteria, viruses, dust particles and other foreign substances. They also ingest and clear away worn-out, dead or abnormal body cells, including dead neutrophils (or pus). In this way, they act as a general 'rubbish collection and disposal' system. While macrophages can digest most organic matter, they cannot digest some particles, such as coal dust and foreign bodies. These particles therefore remain in the tissues and can cause problems such as chronic inflammation.

Macrophages act as antigen-presenting cells to lymphocytes. This means that they process foreign cells (such as bacteria) and, as a result, display antigens on their own cell surface. The trapping, processing and presentation of material by macrophages typically take place within the lymph nodes and spleen.

Monocytes and macrophages both recognise pathogens through specific cell-surface receptors. These bind to molecules shared by pathogens, triggering the induction of a vast range of important chemicals – cytokines and chemokines, inflammatory mediators which encourage the recruitment of other phagocytes. Thus, monocytes and macrophages are central to the initiation and propagation of the inflammatory process.

Inflammation

The inflammatory response is an important part of both innate and specific immunity and serves to isolate and protect the body from further injury or the spread of invading pathogens. The signs and symptoms of inflammation are associated with the mobilisation of the body's defences towards the site of tissue trauma or damage so that the area of injury can be isolated, pathogens destroyed, and tissue repair and healing can proceed. Minutes after cell injury, numerous powerful, chemical substances are released from the injured tissue.

Histamine release (see below) increases blood flow to the injured site and prostaglandins allow white blood cells and plasma to migrate out of the capillaries. The cascade of complement proteins in the plasma can help this physiological process, resulting in vasodilation, chemotaxis, neutrophil migration and increased vascular permeability, which in turn lead to the classically unpleasant symptoms of inflammation – redness, heat, swelling and pain. Despite this, inflammation is a very important and beneficial phenomenon designed to protect the body and limit and reduce the spread of infection.

Many different chemicals are involved in inflammation and the immune response.

These include:

Histamine: This is released by basophils, mast cells and platelets. It causes local vascular dilation and an immediate increase in vascular permeability, swelling and itching. It is released following tissue damage or irritation, e.g. contact with stinging nettles or allergens. The problems caused by histamine can be ameliorated by antihistamine creams or tablets.

Prostaglandins: These are lipid mediators synthesised by many cell types, and have many roles to play in localised inflammation, including increase in vascular permeability, platelet aggregation and interacting with nerve endings to cause pain.

Leukotrienes: Like prostaglandins, leukotrienes are lipid mediators; their major role, particularly that of leukotriene B4, is mediating chemotaxis of neutrophils to sites of inflammation. Their production is decreased by corticosteroids.

Cytokines: These regulate the growth and activation of immune cells and mediate immune and inflammatory responses.

Kinins: Kinins are peptides which act directly on local smooth muscle, causing vasodilation and increasing vascular permeability. Some kinins, e.g. bradykinin, are responsible for the pain and sometimes itching associated with inflammation.

Interleukins: Over 50 interleukins have been identified; these small peptides are produced by a variety of leukocytes. Interleukin 1 (IL-1) is responsible for some of the classic signs and symptoms of infection such as pyrexia, malaise and anorexia and interleukin 11 (IL-11) is responsible for release of acute phase proteins.

Acute phase proteins: These are released by the liver during acute inflammation, atherosclerosis and infection. They include clotting factors, complement and C-reactive protein (CRP). Elevated CRP concentrations are associated with high blood pressure, alcohol, ageing and smoking and may indicate a link between inflammatory process and coronary artery disease. Monitoring CRP is useful for identifying the presence of general inflammation or inflammatory diseases in the body.

Lymphocytes

Lymphocytes are small cells arising from the lymphoid lineage in the bone marrow (Figure 9.4). After neutrophils, lymphocytes are the most numerous leukocytes in circulation (Table 9.3). They are capable of recognising and responding to specific foreign antigens which occur on microorganisms, e.g. bacteria, parasites, cells infected with viruses, tumour cells and another person's cells or transplanted organs.

Lymphocytes are of three main types: natural killer (NK) cells, T-cells and B-cells.

Natural killer cells

Natural killer cells (NKCs) are large, non-specific, cytotoxic white blood cells (lymphocytes) involved in early defence. Known as the 'pitbulls' of the defence system, they recognise and eliminate a variety of virus-infected cells and some malignant cells by detecting general abnormalities within them. They make up approximately 10–15 per cent of all circulating lymphocytes and kill by direct contact with cells, through azurophilic granules filled with potent chemicals. Stress, such as bereavement, may decrease the number of NKCs. People who are bereaved may be more vulnerable to viral infections, such as shingles.

Well-preserved NKC cytotoxicity is seen in healthy, physical fit, elderly individuals, whereas low NKC activity is associated with the development of medical disorders and a higher incidence of infections such as respiratory tract infections.

Although primarily cytotoxic in nature, NKCs also provide a rich early source of chemical mediators and cytokines which help amplify the innate immune response and the early phases of the adaptive immune response.

The other two types of lymphocytes, the T- and B-cells, are involved in the adaptive immune response.

The adaptive immune system

The adaptive immune system is a highly evolved complex of cellular and humoral responses and is gifted with immunological memory. Small molecules called antigens invoke the adaptive immune system. Antigens, found on the surface of pathogenic cells, foreign proteins and self-cell debris, are mostly processed by dendritic cells of the innate system and then displayed to stimulate adaptive immune responses.

Our own cells possess a set of self-antigens called major histocompatibility complex (MHC) proteins which the adaptive immune response recognises as 'self'. Invading pathogens and foreign substances, however, lack the self-MHC marker set and are identified as 'non-self', becoming targets for immune attack and destruction. While this detection system is exceptionally refined and elegant, abnormalities can exist which result from several aberrations within this system. These abnormalities include the development of autoimmune disease (see later) and conditions such as allergies and anaphylactic shock.

The two main weapons of the adaptive (acquired) immune system are the T- and B-lymphocytes. Both these cell types work to create and 'acquire' immunity to specific antigens (rather than relying on innate immunity present from birth). Since the adaptive immune response is antigen specific, it needs priming by initial exposure to specific foreign antigen. This priming takes a while to initially develop, and thus the adaptive immune response usually kicks in a few days after the innate response. The ability of the adaptive immune system to recognise pathogens is outstanding and its recall (second encounter) with the same pathogen usually results in extremely rapid and complete pathogen elimination. The adaptive immune system also functions to prevent cancers, through a complicated surveillance network.

T-lymphocytes

T-lymphocytes, commonly referred to as T-cells, the 'T' denoting their maturation and release from the thymus gland, make up about 65–85 per cent of blood lymphocytes, and circulate through lymph, blood and back to lymph nodes once a day (Druzd et al., 2017), increasing their encounters with a large variety of antigens. The activation of T-cells depends absolutely on interaction with antigen-presenting cells, which 'show' them the foreign antigen. The cells then proliferate and migrate to the site of inflammation. Antigen-presenting cells include dendritic cells which are found at the body's frontiers such as skin and resident macrophages within the lymph nodes.

Dendritic cells

Dendritic cells are a vital link between the innate immune system and the adaptive immune system. So-called because their surface membrane looks similar to the tree-like dendrites of neurones, dendritic cells are key in activating T-lymphocytes, by presenting microbial antigen to them. These wispy extensions make them efficient antigen catchers. They phagocytose antigen and present this to the T-lymphocytes. This process is very important to ensure that lymphocytes encounter invading antigen, and dendritic cells are known to be the most effective antigen-presenting cell, playing a pivotal role in the onset and regulation of the adaptive immune response.

Differentiation of T-cells

T-cells mature under the influence of cytokines in the thymus gland (see lymphatics section below). On their surface, T-cells display thousands of identical T-cell receptors

(TCRs) which interact with antigens and protein molecules brought to them by macrophages or other APCs. A series of events occurs to activate T-lymphocytes:

1. foreign cells (tumour, transplant or virus-infected cells) are engulfed by macrophages;

2. protein from these phagocytosed cells is broken down into peptide fragments within macrophages;

3. macrophages now present the antigen fragments on their cell surface together with the MHC proteins;

4. antigen fragments, presented by macrophages, in association with an MHC molecule, can interact with a T-lymphocyte which has the specific, matching T-cell receptor (TCR) on its surface.

Once they have bound with an antigen, T-cells are activated and stimulated to proliferate. Activated T-cells can differentiate into different sub-types: cytotoxic T-cells (CD8+), which mediate the direct cellular killing of target cells through the release of potent molecules such as lymphotoxin; Helper T-cells (CD4+), central cells which 'help' all other immune cells do their job (particularly B-cells with their production of antibody and CD8+ cells with their cytotoxicity); T-suppressor cells; and T-memory cells.

TC (cytotoxic T-cells)

CD8 cytotoxic T-cells destroy the cells to which they attach (via their T-cell receptors). Such cells may be foreign (transplant) cells, tumour cells or even host cells which may have become infected with viruses. Cytotoxic T-cells adhere to target cells and release lethal granules at the point of attachment. These granules include a group of proteins termed perforins which attack and rupture the cell membrane of target cells, initiating lysis and cell death.

TH (helper T-cells)

Helper T-cells are key cells in the immune response. These cells enhance the effects of other cells of the immune system. By the release of various cytokines, they attract inflammation-promoting cells such as monocytes and macrophages, and also play a role in helping B-cells produce antibodies (see below). Additionally, helper T-cells make sure that immune cells can proliferate to increase in number when needed (clonal expansion). They help phagocytes with their functions and direct other innate cells to sites of infection.

T-cells may also differentiate into regulatory T-cells (T-suppressor cells) which try and dampen any excessive immune response, and T-memory cells (which will remain dormant, but will reactivate upon subsequent re-exposure to the same antigen).

Ts (suppressor cells)

This group of CD8 T-cells act as monitors of other immune cells to keep a check on T-cell activity. The number of regulatory T-suppressor cells increases during pregnancy, suppressing the mother's immune responses and decreasing the chance of foetal attack and spontaneous abortion (Jørgensen et al., 2019).

T-cells can direct and attract other important immune cells by the secretion of their own cytokines and chemokines. Some of these, for example interleukin-6, are pro-inflammatory and attract neutrophils to infection sites. Other cytokines are produced by T-cells with multiple roles, e.g. transforming growth factor-beta, TGFβ, works to prevent tissue damage by negating inflammation. Interferon allows a degree of antiviral protection. Interferons are proteins produced by virally infected cells which alert healthy neighbouring cells of the infection, allowing them to produce factors which will block their own infection. Synthetic forms of interferon can be prescribed to combat serious viral infection.

B-lymphocytes (B-cells)

B-lymphocytes originate in the bone marrow. The exact location of B-cell maturation is not confirmed in humans although the intestines, the liver and bone marrow are all proposed sites (Bilder, 2016). B-cells are responsible for humoral immunity, a type of immunity to infection conferred by proteins termed antibodies. The process of antibody production begins with receptors for antigens on the surface of B-cells which interact with foreign antigens found on microorganisms. This interaction triggers the B-cell to divide and develop into a clone of cells. This mechanism is termed clonal selection. Aided by T-helper cells, antigen-stimulated B-cells subsequently develop into larger cells called plasma cells which begin to synthesise and secrete large amounts of specific antibody.

Antibodies are soluble within the plasma and are also frequently referred to as immunoglobulins. Antibodies help deal with infection via several mechanisms which are summarised below:

Agglutination: Bacteria, viruses and other cells are located by antibodies which have been created to bind to their antigens. The resulting 'bridge' that forms between antibodies and foreign cells causes the agglutination or clumping of the foreign invaders. Agglutinated pathogens are then readily phagocytosed by neutrophils, monocytes and macrophages.

Neutralisation: Toxins and other harmful chemicals released by bacteria are neutralised when a specific antibody binds to them. This prevents the toxins causing further damage to the host.

Opsonisation: This is the 'coating' of foreign cells by the specific region of antibody molecules and makes the foreign cell more attractive to circulating phagocytes such as neutrophils. Opsonisation effectively marks out and labels pathogens for destruction. Phagocytes then rapidly engulf the opsonised cells and particles.

Complement activation: Antibodies, when bound to their corresponding antigens, are capable of activating a system of potent serum enzymes termed complement. This group of 20 or so proteins, once activated, forms a protein conglomerate termed a membrane attack complex (MAC) which attacks and ruptures the membranes of pathogens, leading to cell lysis and death. The complement system can be activated by antigen-antibody complexes or by recognition of bacteria.

There are five structurally different types of antibody described to date. Table 9.5 lists the currently understood functions of these.

Table 9.5   Types and functions of immunoglobulins

Class of immunoglobulin (I$_g$)	Type of heavy chain	Properties and function	Clinical implication
I$_g$G	• Gamma heavy chains • (4 subclasses)	• most versatile immunoglobulin • major I$_g$ in serum (75%) • can cross placenta • fixes complement • good opsonin • binds to cells	Increases in: • infection of all types • liver disease • severe malnutrition • rheumatoid arthritis Decreases in: • chronic lymphoblastic leukaemia
I$_g$M	• Mu heavy chains	• 3rd most common serum • 1st I$_g$ to be made by foetus • 1st I$_g$ made by B cells upon antigenic stimulation • fixes complement • efficient in leading to lysis of microorganisms	Increases in: • certain parasitic infections such as malaria • infectious mononucleosis (glandular fever) • SLE/DLE • rheumatoid arthritis Decreases in: • Lymphoproliferative disorders
I$_g$A	• Alpha heavy chains • 2 subclasses	• 2nd most common serum I$_g$ • major I$_g$ in secretions, e.g. tears, saliva, colostrum, mucus • can bind to some cells • does not normally fix complement	Increases in: • liver cirrhosis • certain autoimmune disorders • some chronic infections Decreases in: • immunological deficiency status • malabsorption syndromes

(Continued)

Table 9.5   (Continued)

Class of immunoglobulin (I$_g$)	Type of heavy chain	Properties and function	Clinical implication
I$_g$D	• Delta heavy chains	• found in low levels in serum • found on B-cell surfaces where it functions as a receptor for antigens	Increases in: • chronic infections
I$_g$E	• Epsilon heavy chains	• least common serum I$_g$ • binds tightly to basophils and mast cells • involved in allergic reactions • plays a role in killing parasitic helminths • does not fix complement	Increases in: • atopic skin disease, e.g. eczema • hay fever • asthma • anaphylactic shock

Memory B-cells

Some B-cells can become memory B-cells, capable of 'remembering' their specific antigen which triggered antibody production. Each specific antigen for a specific disease (e.g. rubella) causes the body to produce matching, specific antibodies. Once produced, 'the blueprint' for each antibody is remembered by memory B-cells. A recall antigen will induce a much more avid and extremely rapid response, with large quantities of antibodies being generated to ensure swift elimination of a repeating offensive microbe and usually offering lifelong protection against previously encountered microbes. Vaccination to protect against pathogens is one mechanism which exploits this principle, since administering an inactive or killed pathogen or pathogen fragment in a small dose elicits antibody generation and the creation of immunological memory. B- and T-memory cells are on continuous patrol in the circulation and will be rapidly activated if a previously encountered antigen is reintroduced into the body.

During the primary exposure to a pathogen, the individual may succumb to the disease. The antibody response is too little and too late. However, the next time the disease is encountered, the antibody response is rapid and large enough to overwhelm the pathogen, and the individual does not succumb. Therefore, an individual usually only suffers the infectious illness once. Vaccines act as the primary exposure, so that antibodies can be produced rapidly as soon as the pathogen is encountered. The lifespan of lymphocytes can range from several days to a lifetime. It is, however, possible that memory cells will only last a lifetime if they are re-stimulated by contact with their specific antigen. Authorities remain uncertain on this point, but it is recognised that some vaccinations may only offer temporary protection, e.g. yellow fever vaccination is usually recommended for renewal after 10 years, typhoid vaccine after 3 years, diphtheria, tetanus and polio immunisation after 10 years and hepatitis B (for healthcare workers) once only after 5 years (Public Health England and Department of Health, 2013).

To help you understand the process of vaccination in a real-world scenario, attempt Activity 9.1.

Activity 9.1   Decision making

While on a clinical placement with a district nurse, you visited a 65-year-old gentleman, Mr Jones, who was living with chronic obstructive pulmonary disease (COPD). The visit was to administer the flu vaccine to Mr Jones. He lived with his extended family including his wife, daughter and two grandchildren aged 9 months and 4 years. The family didn't know much about the vaccine and asked about whether they should be vaccinated too. Where could Mr Jones and his family access advice?

There are some possible answers to all activities at the end of the chapter, unless otherwise indicated.

Now that we have explored the components of the immune system and the nature of vaccination, we will examine the roles of the lymphatic system and its overlap with immunity.

The lymphatic system

The lymphatic system consists of two major components; firstly, a fluid called lymph, which flows around the body within a system of lymphatic capillaries and vessels, and secondly, various glands and organs distributed around the body which contain lymphatic tissue and whose cells are capable of mounting an immune response to pathogens or abnormal cells.

Lymph and the lymphatic vessels

Lymph is a milky fluid formed from excess fluid which surrounds the bodies' tissues (interstitial fluid). Lymph drains into special thin tubes, the lymphatic vessels, which permeate virtually every major organ and tissue (Figure 9.6).

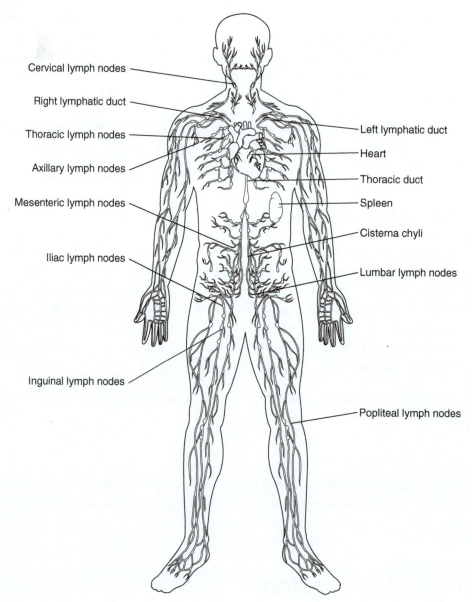

Figure 9.6 The components of the lymphatic system and major lymph nodes

The lymphoid glands and organs

These include the spleen, thymus and clusters of lymph nodes (Figure 9.7). They have many roles, most notably removal of damaged red blood cells (the spleen), maturation of immune cells (thymus) and trapping of foreign material (lymph nodes and spleen).

The lymphatic system has three major functions: tissue drainage, fat transport and trapping of antigen. For this chapter, only the latter function will be discussed since it forms an integral part of our immune defence system.

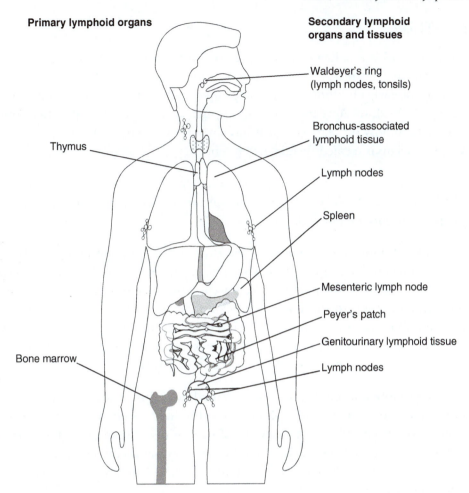

Figure 9.7 The lymphoid organs

Immune function of the lymphatic system

Since lymphatic capillaries are present in virtually all organs and tissues and are continually draining interstitial fluid, infections that occur anywhere in the body eventually end up circulating within the lymph. The human lymphatic system has evolved to take advantage of this phenomenon and strategically located throughout the body are areas highly effective at trapping pathogenic material. These are the lymph nodes.

Primary lymphatic organs

The bone marrow and the thymus are considered to be primary lymphoid organs because it is here that the majority of immune cells originate.

The thymus

The thymus gland is a bi-lobed pinkish-grey organ located just above the heart in the mediastinum where it rests just below the sternum (Figure 9.7). It is a large and very active organ in early childhood, regressing rapidly thereafter at a constant rate until middle age. Indeed, by 20 years of age the thymus is 50 per cent smaller than the size it was at birth and by 60 years of age it has shrunk to a sixth of its original birth size (Bilder, 2016). This is termed thymic involution.

The thymus matures T-cells. Maturing T-cells that have not yet been exposed to antigen are called naïve cells. Naïve T-cells are calm, quiescent cells that will only become active when exposed to foreign antigen.

One of the most important functions of the thymus is in programming T-cells to recognise 'self' antigens through a process termed 'thymic education'. Thymic education allows mature T-cells to distinguish foreign (potentially pathogenic material) from antigens which belong to the body. Several studies have shown an immune system derangement following thymectomy and it has been strongly hypothesised that removal of the thymus (thymectomy) may lead to an increase in autoimmune diseases as the ability to recognise self is diminished (Panarese et al., 2014).

Each of the two lobes of the thymus is surrounded by a capsule within which are found numerous micro-lobules, typically 2–3 mm in width, held together by loose connective tissue. Each lobule consists of a framework of thymosin-secreting epithelial cells and a population of T-lymphocytes. Each lobule has two distinct areas: a dense outer cortex that is rich in actively dividing T-cells and an inner medulla that is much paler in colour and functions as an area of T-cell maturation.

The role of the thymus in T-cell maturation

T-lymphocytes originate as immature stem cells (haemocytoblasts) from the red bone marrow of most flat bones. A population of these haemocytoblasts infiltrate the thymus and undergo further divisions within the cortical regions of the thymic micro-lobules. This immature population of T-cells then migrate into the medullary regions where they mature into active T-lymphocytes.

Secondary lymphatic organs

The lymph nodes and spleen are peripheral lymphoid organs playing a role in filtering out and destroying unwanted pathogens and maintaining the population of mature naïve lymphocytes to enable commencement of the adaptive immune response. At these organs, foreign antigens initiate lymphocyte activation and subsequent clonal expansion and maturation. Mature lymphocytes can then leave the secondary organs to enter the circulation to target the foreign antigen.

Lymph nodes

Lymph nodes vary in size and shape; they are typically bean-shaped structures found clustered at specific locations throughout the body (Figure 9.6). The central portions of the lymph node are essential to its function. Here are large numbers of fixed macrophages which phagocytose foreign material such as bacteria on contact. In addition to macrophages, lymph nodes also contain populations of B- and T-lymphocytes. Lymph nodes are crucial to most antibody-mediated immune responses; pathogenic material is trapped by the central phagocytic macrophages and presented to lymphocytes so that antibodies can be generated. Each lymph node is supplied by one or more afferent lymphatic vessels which deliver crude, unmodified lymph direct from the neighbouring tissues.

A healthy, fully functioning node will remove the majority of pathogens (e.g. bacteria) from the lymph before they pass out of the node via one or more efferent lymphatic vessels. In addition to its lymphatic supply, each lymph node is supplied with blood via a small artery. These arteries deliver a variety of leukocytes which populate the inner regions of the node. When infection is present, the nodes become increasingly metabolically active and their oxygen requirements increase. A small vein carries deoxygenated blood away from each node and returns it to the major veins. In times of infection, this venous blood may carry a variety of chemical messengers (cytokines) which are produced by the resident leukocytes within the nodes. These cytokines act as general warning signals, alerting the body to the potential threat as well as ramping up a variety of specific immune reactions.

Although the size of the lymph nodes varies, each node has a characteristic internal structure (Figure 9.8).

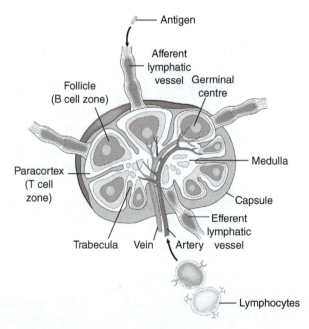

Figure 9.8   Internal structure of a lymph node

Structure of a lymph node

The structure of a lymph node is not unlike that of the spleen (see below). Each lymph node is divided into several regions.

- **Fibrous capsule:** The capsule forms a protective outer sheath and has processes (trabeculae) that extend periodically into the node, subdividing it into small compartments.
- **Outer cortex (nodular cortex):** This region (just inside the capsular margin) consists of numerous follicles rich in B-lymphocytes. When pathogens are present, these follicles expand and prominent germinal centres containing actively dividing, antibody-secreting B-lymphocytes become visible.
- **Inner cortex (paracortex):** This area is found just below the outer cortex and is particularly rich in T-lymphocytes which also continually circulate throughout most other regions of the node.
- **Medulla:** The central inner portion of the node contains large numbers of fixed phagocytic macrophages. These are continually monitoring the lymph (immuno-surveillance) for potentially pathogenic foreign material which they phagocytose on contact.

Lymph node swelling

As the antibody-producing B-lymphocytes begin to proliferate within the germinal centres, the affected lymph nodes begin to enlarge, and may become palpable and tender. Depending on the site of location in the body, swollen lymph nodes may be indicative of different conditions (Table 9.6). Some of the cytokines released are pyrogenic (i.e. they cause fever) and act directly on the thermoregulatory centre (within the

Table 9.6 Major groups of lymph nodes and indication of swelling

Name	Location	Swelling commonly indicative of:
Cervical lymph nodes/tonsils	Neck/pharynx	Upper respiratory tract infections
Axial lymph nodes	Armpits	Lower respiratory tract infections, carcinoma of lung/breast
Mammary plexus	Circular clusters around the areolae	Mastitis, carcinoma of the breast
Gut-associated lymphoid tissues (GALT), also known as Peyer's patches	Throughout the inner layer (mucosa) of the gastrointestinal tract	Gastrointestinal disturbances, infections and malignancies
Inguinal lymph nodes	Groin	Infections/malignancies of the reproductive system, urinary system and colon

hypothalamus) to increase body temperature. Since the majority of human pathogens divide quickly and optimally at around 37°C, this measurable increase in body temperature serves to slow down bacterial replication. This allows the infection to be dealt with more efficiently by the patient's immune system. In fact, both swollen lymph nodes and a fever are sure signs that the patient is mounting an effective immune response against the offending pathogen.

Swollen lymph nodes are readily detected by palpation and provide valuable clues as to the location of infection. To help you understand the value of examining lymph nodes in clinical practice, read through Dylan's case study.

Case study: Dylan – swollen cervical lymph nodes

Dylan is a 16-month-old child who is normally healthy. One evening he developed a slight cough which initially didn't worry him too much. However, overnight, Dylan's cough became worse and by morning he seemed generally unwell and had a temperature of 38°C. His mother gave him some paracetamol which reduced his temperature but his cough persisted. By that afternoon, Dylan's mother could feel two pea-sized lumps beneath his jaw. Having read that lumps in the neck could be a sign of cancer, Dylan's mother made an emergency appointment with the GP where fortunately she was reassured that Dylan's lumps were the result of swollen lymph nodes in response to a bacterial chest infection. Dylan was prescribed amoxycillin 250 mgs three times a day.

Now that you have an understanding of the role played by lymph nodes in trapping foreign material, we will examine the role of the spleen which is often regarded as a giant version of a lymph node.

The spleen

The spleen is considered the largest lymphoid organ. Situated in the left hypochondriac region of the abdominal cavity between the diaphragm and the stomach (Figure 9.7), this dark-purplish organ is approximately 12 cm long, oval in shape, highly vascular and enclosed in a dense, fibro-elastic capsule.

The spleen primarily functions as a filter for the blood, bringing it into close contact with scavenging phagocytes and lymphocytes. It is made up of two regions: the stroma and parenchyma. The stroma consists of the outer capsule with its trabeculae, some fibres and fibroblasts (cells that secrete connective tissue collagen). The parenchyma of the spleen is composed of two types of intermingling tissue called white pulp and red pulp (Figure 9.9). The white pulp consists mainly of lymphocytes and macrophages arranged as lymphatic nodules around branches of the splenic artery. Blood flows into the spleen via this splenic artery, entering smaller, central arteries of the white pulp, eventually reaching the red pulp.

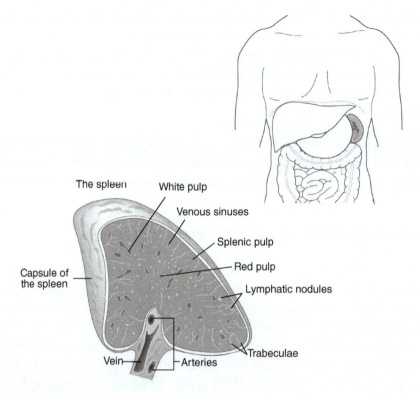

Figure 9.9 Internal structure of the spleen

The red pulp of the spleen consists of blood-filled venous sinuses and splenic cords. Splenic cords are made up of red and white blood cells and plasma cells (antibody-producing B-lymphocytes). It is in the red pulp that most of the filtration occurs.

Function of the spleen

The main immunological function of the spleen serves to remove microorganisms from the circulation. Lymphocytes (B- and T-cells) and macrophages are arranged as sleeves around the blood vessels, bringing blood into the spleen. Within the white pulp are nodules, called Malpighian corpuscles, which are rich in B-lymphocytes, and thus this portion of lymphoid tissue is quick to respond to foreign antigenic stimulation by producing antibodies.

The walls of the meshwork of sinuses in the red pulp contain phagocytes that engulf foreign particles and cell debris, effectively filtering and removing them from the circulation. The main function of red pulp is the removal of aged and damaged erythrocytes and the phagocytosis of opsonised bacteria. The red pulp is also a storage site for platelets and can act as a reservoir for blood.

Other lymphatic components

A few other types of lymphatic tissue also exist. Mucosa-associated lymphoid tissue (MALT) includes gut-associated lymphoid tissue (GALT – see Table 9.6), bronchus-associated lymphoid tissue (BALT) and the tonsils. MALT is positioned to protect the respiratory and gastrointestinal tracts from invasion by microbes. The tonsils are aggregates of lymphatic tissue strategically located in the pharynx (palatine), oral cavity (lingual) and nasal cavity (pharyngeal, or adenoids), to prevent foreign material and pathogens from entering the body. The tonsils themselves are therefore under high risk of infection and inflammation, a common condition called tonsillitis.

The lymphatic system and the metastatic spread of malignancy

We have seen previously that virtually all areas of the body are infiltrated by lymphatic vessels. Unfortunately because of this, tumours undergoing metastatic fragmentation can readily spread to other regions of the body via the lymphatic system. It is common for a primary tumour to quickly establish secondary spread in the neighbouring lymph nodes, e.g. carcinoma of the breast is often followed by secondary involvement of the axial lymph nodes. Malignant involvement of the lymph nodes often leads to obstruction to lymphatic flow and sometimes complete occlusion of the lymphatic vessels. This can cause a 'backing up' of lymph and swelling of the elastic lymphatic vessels – lymphoedema.

To help consolidate your understanding of how metastatic spread of cancer can lead to lymphatic obstruction, attempt Activity 9.2.

Activity 9.2   Evidence-based practice and research

Alison is a 52-year-old lady who has recently undergone a left mastectomy and removal of lymph nodes for stage 3 breast cancer. Although her immediate post-operative recovery from surgery was uneventful, she is aware of the risk of lymphoedema and has asked you what she can do to prevent it. Using online resources, identify what Alison can do to reduce the risk of lymphoedema.

Lymphomas

Lymphomas are cancers that originate in the lymphocytes when normal lymphoid tissue is replaced by abnormal, rapidly dividing cells of lymphoid origin. This results in the formation of solid tumours of the lymph nodes. The tumours appear firm, immovable and painless, in contrast to lymph node enlargement caused by infection, which often presents as a movable, tender lump. Most lymphomas are classified as either Hodgkin's or non-Hodgkin's.

Autoimmunity

Autoimmunity results when the body mistakenly begins to attack its own self-antigens and healthy cells, often leading to painful and inflammatory conditions which can affect either specific organs or the whole body. Usually, this results in the creation of auto-antibodies. Autoimmune diseases, which are usually more typical in women than in men, include type I diabetes, rheumatoid arthritis and systemic lupus erythematosus.

Oedema

Any disruption in the collection or passage of lymph from organs and tissues into the lymphatic vessels, or leakage of fluid from blood vessels, may result in an accumulation of fluid. This is known as oedema and causes swelling of the surrounding tissue. Since oedema is subject to gravity, it becomes more apparent in dependent parts of the body such as ankles and wrists. Most oedema is 'pitted' – pressing the area will cause a 'pit' to form as the fluid is pushed away. After several seconds, this pit slowly disappears as fluid returns.

Common causes of oedema include immobility such as sitting or standing for long periods which causes an increase in fluid pressure as a result of venous stasis. Cardiac failure (venous insufficiency), where increased capillary blood pressure may result from heart failure and an increased back pressure in the venous system, can cause oedema (see Chapter 3). This is typically visible as ankle swelling and/or pulmonary oedema, due to increased pulmonary capillary pressure and therefore greater movement of fluid into the interstitial spaces around the lungs.

Now that you have completed the chapter, attempt the multiple-choice questions in Activity 9.3 to assess your understanding.

Activity 9.3   Multiple-choice questions

1. The process of synthesis of blood cells is called

   a) Haemoptysis
   b) Haematemesis
   c) Haematopoiesis
   d) Haemolysis

2. Haem is formed of four ring-shaped molecules called

   a) Pyrroles
   b) Pyuria

c)   Pyaemia

d)   Pyorrhoea

3.   An acute haemolytic reaction is *not* characterised by

  a)   Hypotension, fever, chills, chest and abdominal pain

  b)   Hypertension, fever, chills, chest and flank pain

  c)   Hypotension, fever, chills, abdominal and flank pain

  d)   Hypotension, fever, chills, chest and flank pain

4.   Which of these statements about vitamin K is *untrue?*

  a)   Vitamin K is plentiful in a balanced diet

  b)   Neonates have low levels of vitamin K for the first few weeks of life

  c)   *E.coli* produce vitamin K in the colon

  d)   Vitamin K is essential for the synthesis of prothrombin, factor VII, factor IX and factor X

5.   In what clinical circumstances would IgA decrease?

  a)   Liver cirrhosis

  b)   Certain auto-immune disorders

  c)   Diabetes insipidus

  d)   Diabetes mellitus

6.   Which site has been suggested as the location of B-cell maturation?

  a)   Heart

  b)   Spleen

  c)   Bone marrow

  d)   Lungs

7.   Thymic involution is

  a)   The shrinkage of the thymus gland with age

  b)   The growth of the thymus gland with age

  c)   The size of the thymus gland in relation to body mass

  d)   The growth of the thymus gland in response to disease

(Continued)

(Continued)

8. Waldeyer's ring is a ring of lymphatic tissue formed by the

    a) Cervical lymph nodes
    b) Spleen
    c) Axillary lymph nodes
    d) Tonsils

9. Blood flows into the spleen via the

    a) Renal artery
    b) Hepatic artery
    c) Splenic artery
    d) Coronary artery

10. Haemophilia is most commonly caused by a deficiency of which clotting factor?

    a) VII
    b) VIII
    c) X
    d) XI

Chapter summary

Blood is a circulating fluid composed of fluid, plasma and cells. The cellular components of blood are erythrocytes (red blood cells), leukocytes (white blood cells) and platelets (thrombocytes). Oxygen, carbon dioxide and glucose are among the most vital molecules transported in blood. Blood cells are essential for normal metabolic and immune system functions. Red blood cells contain haemoglobin molecules which bind to oxygen so it can be transported to tissues. Red blood cells have surface-expressed proteins that act as antigens, which are molecules that can elicit an immune system response, and belong to different groups on the basis of the type of antigen they express.

Blood type ABO and Rhesus are two of the clinically most important blood groups. Blood matching determines compatibility for receiving blood transfusions from other people. White blood cells are the main functional component of the body's immune system. They help the body fight infection and other diseases. The different types of white blood cells are neutrophils, eosinophils, basophils, monocytes and lymphocytes (T-cells and B-cells).

Immune cells destroy and remove old or aberrant cells and cellular debris, as well as attacking pathogens. Immune responses are innate (non-specific) or acquired (adaptive). The adaptive immune response includes the ability to recognise and remember specific pathogens to generate immunity, and mount stronger attacks each time the pathogen is encountered. Platelets are sticky fragments of cells which accumulate at the site of damaged blood vessels to form a clot, due in part to the release of clotting factors that occurs during endothelial injury to blood vessels. This process is called haemostasis and involves the formation of a platelet plug and a fibrin clot.

The lymphatic system is a linear network of lymphatic vessels and secondary lymphoid organs. It is the site of many immune system functions as well as its own functions. The thymus and bone marrow constitute the primary lymphoid tissues that are the sites of lymphocyte generation and maturation. The secondary lymphoid tissues consist of lymph nodes, tonsils, Peyer's patches, spleen and mucosa-associated lymphoid tissue (MALT).

Activities: Brief outline answers

Activity 9.1: Decision making (page 253)

If Mr Jones and his family have access to the Internet, there are several very informative and user-friendly sites that they can easily access, including the following:

www.nhs.uk/conditions/vaccinations/who-should-have-flu-vaccine

www.nhs.uk/conditions/vaccinations/child-flu-vaccine

www.boots.com/health-pharmacy-advice/vaccinations/flujab

Advice is also available from GPs and other healthcare professionals including local pharmacies.

However, as you and the district nurse are already visiting Mr Jones, now would be a good opportunity for a discussion with him and his family. All nursing students should be aware of the current guidance on vaccination and should set a good example by getting vaccinated themselves.

Activity 9.2: Evidence-based practice and research (page 261)

According to Cancer Research UK (2019a), the following advice should be followed to reduce the risk of lymphoedema:

Infection in a cut or graze can increase fluid collection in your arm and increase your risk of lymphoedema.

There are things you can do to help:

- wearing gloves when gardening or doing housework
- using nail clippers rather than scissors
- using an electric razor if you shave under your arms
- take care when playing with pets

If you get a cut or graze, wash it well and cover it up with a plaster or dressing until it's healed.

Go to your GP straightaway if it looks red or swollen. You might need antibiotics.

Severe heat sunburn can increase your risk of lymphoedema. You can:

- wear factor 50 sunscreen
- avoid very hot baths and showers
- use a non-scented moisturiser every day to keep your skin moist

Putting too much strain on your arm after surgery can increase your risk of lymphoedema. Don't use your arm for anything heavy until your team say you can. You should carry on the arm and shoulder exercises you started after surgery.

Activity 9.3: Multiple-choice questions (pages 262–4)

1) c, 2) a, 3) b, 4) a, 5) b, 6) b, 7) a, 8) d, 9) c, 10) b

Further reading

www.bbc.co.uk/news/health-51065430

Interesting article about male blood donation.

www.msdmanuals.com/home/blood-disorders/symptoms-and-diagnosis-of-blood-disorders/overview-of-blood-disorders

A comprehensive overview of blood disorders.

https://courses.lumenlearning.com/boundless-ap/chapter/overview-of-blood

A clear summary chapter on blood.

Useful websites

www.nhs.uk/conditions/blood-clots

Summary NHS guide to blood clots.

www.nhs.uk/conditions/embolism

Summary NHS guide to an embolism.

www.bmj.com/content/351/bmj.h5832

NICE guidelines on blood transfusion.

Chapter 10 The digestive system

Introduction

Case study: Janet – acute cholecystitis

Janet is a 47-year-old lady who presented to her local Emergency Department at 9.30pm with a three-hour history of severe right-upper quadrant pain radiating to her back and shoulder. She was also showing signs of mild jaundice. An ultrasound scan revealed gallstones in the gall bladder and common bile duct. Stones travelling down the common bile duct are the most likely cause of Janet's pain. These are preventing bile from being released from the gall bladder into the gut and causing yellow bile pigments such as bilirubin to accumulate in the blood, leading to jaundice. Janet was added to the waiting list for a laparoscopic cholecystectomy.

The gastrointestinal (GI) tract is essential to allow the digestion of food and absorption of nutrients which can then be distributed and utilised throughout the body. However, this organ system is vulnerable to a vast variety of common diseases ranging from mild heartburn (acid reflux) and the agonising painful gallstones experienced by Janet in our opening case study, through to life-threatening malignancies such as pancreatic and bowel cancer.

This chapter will examine the anatomy and physiology of the digestive system sequentially from mouth to anus. We will explore the physiological processes that allow ingestion, digestion, absorption of nutrients and the egestion of indigestible waste. We will also explore the nature of some of the key disorders and pathologies that nurses may routinely encounter in clinical practice.

Overview of the digestive system

A digestive system is necessary to break down food we eat from large, complex molecules into simple molecules which can be absorbed and used by the body. Several organs make up this system, each playing a distinct role in the process of digesting and/or absorbing digested molecules. In addition to the organs within the GI tract are the accessory organs (the liver and pancreas), which help in this process. The GI tract also harbours a diverse variety of microorganisms (predominantly bacteria) which are essential to our health and well-being. These are known as the microbiome, a unique and balanced ecosystem of billions of bacteria and other microbes that live on or in us.

Why do we need a digestive system?

The body needs to intake seven classes of nutrients to function, grow and repair. These are:

1. Carbohydrates
2. Proteins
3. Fats
4. Vitamins
5. Minerals
6. Fibre
7. Water

Most carbohydrates, proteins and fats that we eat are large, complex molecules that require digestion (the mechanical and chemical breakdown of food particles into smaller molecules) before they can be assimilated and used by the body. Digestive enzymes (proteins produced by the body that act like chemical scissors to 'snip' bonds linking large ingested molecules) are very important in the creation of simple molecules that can be absorbed easily across the gut wall into the body.

Digestion of carbohydrates, proteins and fat

In the body, digestion occurs via two means:

1. Mechanical, e.g. chewing (mastication) or churning by the GI tract wall.
2. Chemical, e.g. enzymes.

Carbohydrates

There are three types of carbohydrates. The basic sub-unit of a carbohydrate is a saccharide molecule. The three types of carbohydrate are named depending on the number of saccharide units present in the carbohydrate (Figure 10.1a):

- one saccharide unit = monosaccharide (e.g. glucose);
- two saccharide units = disaccharide (e.g. maltose);
- more than two units = polysaccharide (e.g. starch).

The body absorbs the simplest type of carbohydrate (monosaccharides), so ingested carbohydrates need to be broken down into monosaccharides. The enzymes that are able to do this are carbohydrases, e.g. amylase. Carbohydrases are located in strategic positions in the gut and secreted to help break up saccharide units (Table 10.1).

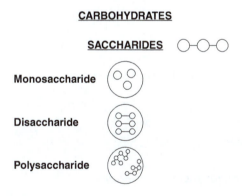

Figure 10.1a Carbohydrates

Proteins

Proteins are large, complex molecules with a primary, secondary and tertiary structure. Before they can be absorbed, all ingested proteins must be broken down into amino acids (Figure 10.1b). This is achieved by the action of enzyme proteases such as pepsin and trypsin (Table 10.1), which break chemical bonds between chains of amino acids to release individual small amino acids.

There are approximately 22 naturally occurring amino acids. Eight of these are essential (cannot be synthesised by the body and thus must be included in the diet); the rest are non-essential (can be synthesised by the body). This involves a complex process in the liver, called transamination.

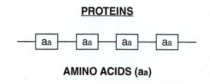

PROTEINS

AMINO ACIDS (aa)

Figure 10.1b Proteins

Fats

Fats or lipids are large, complex molecules. The most important and abundant lipids in the body are triglycerides. (Excess carbohydrates, proteins, fats and oils are converted into triglycerides and deposited in adipose tissue.) Triglycerides are made up of three molecules of fatty acid and one molecule of glycerol (Figure 10.1c).

Fats are emulsified in the gastrointestinal tract by the action of bile (see liver) and digested enzymatically (e.g. by lipases) (Table 10.1).

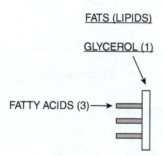

FATS (LIPIDS)

GLYCEROL (1)

FATTY ACIDS (3) →

Figure 10.1c Fats (lipids)

Table 10.1 Location of major digestive enzymes

Enzyme	Location
Carbohydrases – act to break down carbohydrate	
Salivary amylase	Mouth – salivary glands
Pancreatic amylase	Pancreas (acinar cells)
Maltase	Small intestine
Sucrase	Small intestine
Lactase	Small intestine

Proteases – act to break down protein	
Pepsin	Stomach (chief cells)
Trypsin	Pancreas (acinar cells)
Chymotrypsin	Pancreas (acinar cells)
Peptidases	Small intestine
Lipases – act to break down fats	
Lingual lipase	Serous glands of tongue
Gastric lipase	Stomach (chief cells)
Pancreatic lipase	Pancreas (acinar cells)
Colipase (assists pancreatic lipase)	Pancreas (acinar cells)

Water and other simple molecules such as vitamins and minerals can usually be absorbed as they are. Dietary fibre cannot be absorbed.

Anatomy of the digestive tract (GI tract)

The digestion of food needs time and space. The latter is provided by the GI tract (Figure 10.2). This is a long, muscular tube in which food is digested into small molecules. Nutrient molecules are then absorbed and the remaining matter (fibre and waste) is egested from the body as faeces. The GI tract consists of:

- mouth;
- pharynx;
- oesophagus;
- stomach;
- small intestine: duodenum, jejunum and ileum;
- large intestine: caecum, appendix, colon and rectum.

Also two major accessory organs, the pancreas and liver, play a vital role in digestion.

The mouth

Food is ingested using the teeth, lips and tongue. Lips are important; they grasp food, aid in sipping drinks and prevent dehydration of the mouth. They also form a muscular passageway into the GI tract. Once food has been placed in the mouth, the lips close the entrance to the GI tract so that chewing can be undertaken without loss of food particles. Teeth are a vital starting point in the digestive process since they mechanically grind food into smaller particles (chewing/mastication).

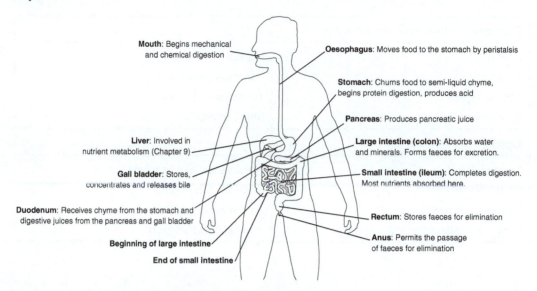

Figure 10.2 Components of the digestive system

The tongue helps to keep food moving around in the mouth during mastication and also mixes the food with saliva, a chemical mix of water, mucus, bicarbonate ions and enzymes. Saliva is secreted from three sets of salivary glands which open into the mouth: the parotid, submandibular and sublingual glands (Figure 10.3).

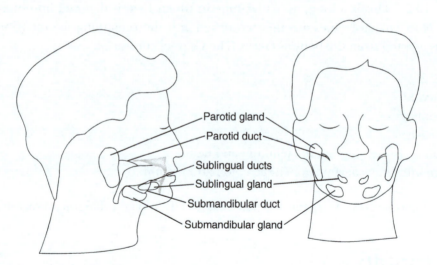

Figure 10.3 Salivary glands

Saliva has many functions: it provides lubrication for food in the mouth and later for food entering the pharynx and oesophagus; it also has an antimicrobial, defence role. Saliva contains immunoglobulin A (IgA) which is also known as secretory antibody, and lysozyme. Lysozyme is an enzyme which attacks and breaks bacterial cells. Any bacteria ingested in or with food is first dealt with by lysozyme in the mouth, before being later and more harshly handled by the stomach acid.

Saliva also protects the teeth from erosion. The bicarbonate ions present in saliva act to neutralise any acid formed by bacteria acting on refined and sugary foods in the mouth, and thus chewing gum after meals is believed to protect teeth as it encourages saliva production which reduces acidity in the mouth. Saliva also initiates digestion.

With a pH approaching 7.0, saliva contains an enzyme, salivary amylase (which acts on ingested starch), and a tiny proportion of a lipase (lingual lipase), secreted by serous cells which lie under certain papillae on the surface of the tongue. A neutral pH in the mouth favours the action of amylase but salivary lipase functions best at a lower pH of around 3–4, so this enzyme only becomes fully active and begins fat digestion properly in the acidic environment of the stomach.

Control of salivation

Stimulation by the parasympathetic branch of the autonomic nervous system promotes the continuous, moderate secretion of saliva. Parasympathetic fibres of specific cranial nerves (VII and IX; see Chapter 6) are responsible for this. However, the secretion of saliva is also is activated by a number of factors including the smell and sight of food, swallowing of irritating foods and when feeling nauseous. The touch and taste of food activate receptors that convey impulses to two salivary nuclei in the brain.

Daily, the body can produce up to 1.5 litres of saliva. Basal saliva secretion acts to keep the mucous membranes of the mouth moist and this need is met mainly by the submandibular glands. The parotid glands are mainly responsible for induced saliva secretion in the presence of food and the sublingual glands contribute only with small volumes of saliva (around 5 per cent). The volume of saliva produced can vary according to the nature of the food that is currently being chewed.

Taste is important in ensuring adequate nutrition. Food that tastes pleasant is more likely to be tolerated by patients. Furthermore, as we have seen above, saliva protects the teeth and initiates digestion. As we age, we produce less saliva. This can be compounded by other factors including smoking, poor fluid intake, alcohol consumption, high salt intake and some medication which can cause a dry mouth, known as xerostomia. Activity 10.1 asks you to consider this aspect of care.

Activity 10.1   Reflection

Consider a patient you have cared for over a period of time on clinical placement. Reflect on the oral care you provided and how that care would have affected the well-being of your patient.

As this activity is based on your own reflections, there is no exact model answer, but some general points are provided at the end of the chapter.

Having considered the importance of good oral care and the role taste plays in encouraging patients to eat in Activity 10.1, we can now consider the mechanics of chewing and swallowing.

After being chewed and mixed in the mouth, the tongue and roof of the mouth collect and manipulate the food to form a torpedo-shaped ball: a bolus. This is then pushed to the back of the mouth and into the oropharynx (anterior portion of the throat) to prepare for swallowing. Mucus present within saliva coats the bolus and provides a slippery outer surface to make swallowing and subsequent passage of the bolus easier. As the bolus gets to the back of the throat (posterior pharyngeal wall), the swallowing reflex is initiated. Swallowing (deglutition) involves several structures which work with precision and coordination to funnel the bolus down the correct tube.

To prevent food and fluids from entering the nasal cavity, the uvula (Figure 10.4) closes the entrance to the nasal cavity at the nasopharynx. Likewise, the epiglottis (a cartilage flap covering the glottis – the opening to the larynx) (Figure 10.5) is raised to protect

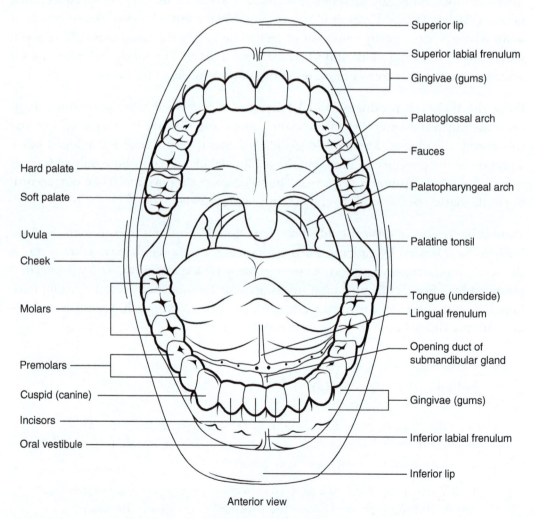

Anterior view

Figure 10.4 Structure of the mouth

the respiratory system from unwanted particles of food and drink. The bolus of food is therefore directed down through an upper oesophageal sphincter (Figure 10.5) into a muscular tube (lying posterior to the trachea), the oesophagus, which connects the throat to the stomach. Swallowing, or deglutition, occurs in three phases: voluntary, pharyngeal and oesophageal.

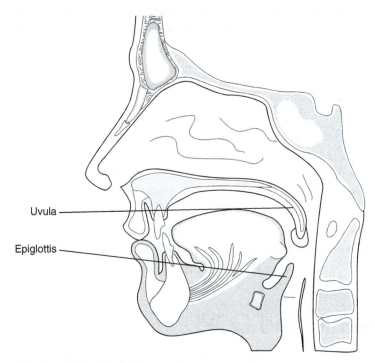

Figure 10.5   The uvula and epiglottis

Control of swallowing

Swallowing, like coughing, sneezing and vomiting, is a reflex response under the control of the medulla oblongata region of the brain. The voluntary movement of a bolus of food towards the pharynx triggers impulses in several cranial nerves, which starts a wave of involuntary contraction in the pharyngeal muscles, pushing food into the oesophagus. Following each mouthful swallowed, the upper oesophageal sphincter closes firmly to prevent any food from regurgitating back into the mouth. Stretching of the oesophageal wall here initiates peristalsis – rhythmic muscular contractions which enable transport of food along the length of the oesophagus. Watery drinks take 1–2 seconds and food can take 6–15 seconds to reach the stomach (Maurer, 2015).

Some patients may experience difficulty in swallowing or dysphagia. Dysphagia may be commonly caused by a dry mouth, stroke, head and neck cancer, neurological conditions such as Parkinson's disease, multiple sclerosis and motor neuron disease, but other less common causes have been identified. The consequences of dysphagia include food spillage, the inability to chew effectively, dry mouth, pooling of food in the mouth, choking, aspiration pneumonia, malnutrition and dehydration. To manage dysphagia, the underlying condition must be treated where possible. Where the underlying condition cannot be successfully treated or cured, thickened fluids that are easier to swallow may be advised.

A speech and language therapist may be able to help patients develop techniques to help them swallow more effectively and teach them exercises to strengthen the muscles needed for swallowing. If these measures are unsuccessful, then tube feeding may be necessary or surgery may be considered to release an overly tight muscle, remove strictures or place a stent to maintain the patency of the oesophagus.

The oesophagus

Food travels slowly down the oesophagus, aided by large amounts of lubricating mucus secreted by its walls. The oesophagus is about 25 cm long and, in order to reach the stomach, it pierces the diaphragm through an opening known as the oesophageal hiatus. The oesophagus is guarded both at its beginning and end by sphincters. The lower oesophageal sphincter controls the entry of food into the stomach, and needs to relax and dilate to allow this to happen. It is important that the lower oesophageal sphincter can close rapidly as soon as food hits the upper portion of the stomach to ensure that none of the extremely acidic gastric contents can regurgitate back into the oesophagus.

Hiatus hernia and GORD

A hiatus hernia occurs when a portion of the stomach protrudes through the hiatus into the chest. This may be a sliding hiatus hernia whereby the join between the oesophagus and stomach slides up into the chest, followed by the top part of the stomach, or a rolling hiatus hernia in which part of the stomach passes up into the chest to lie alongside the oesophagus.

Hiatus hernias are relatively common in the over-50s but do not necessarily cause symptoms, in which case treatment is unnecessary. However, a sliding hiatus hernia can cause gastro-oesophageal reflux disease (GORD) in which gastric acid rises back up into the oesophagus. Symptoms include a burning pain in the chest especially on bending or lying, acid reflux, belching, coughing – especially at night –and difficulty in swallowing.

Medical treatment is aimed at managing symptoms and comprises antacids, alginates, proton pump inhibitors and H2 receptor antagonists. In severe cases an operation known as a fundoplication may be necessary.

The micro-anatomy of the oesophageal and GI tract wall is illustrated in Figure 10.6. This basic layered structure is consistent through the whole length of the GI tube, expanding periodically into sacs, e.g. stomach and rectum.

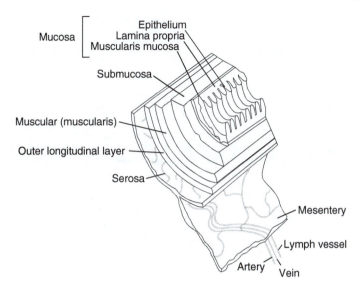

Figure 10.6   Tubular structure of the digestive tract

The stomach

The stomach lies in the upper-left quadrant of the abdomen (Figure 10.7a). Its connection with the oesophagus terminates at the lower oesophageal sphincter (also known as the cardiac opening because of its proximity to the heart).

Food will usually stay in the stomach for 3–6 hours, although this depends on its composition; a meal rich in carbohydrates will usually leave quicker than protein or fat-rich meals.

Because of its thick lining of mucus, very few substances can be absorbed by the stomach. Those that are include water, alcohol, lipid-soluble compounds and drugs such as aspirin and other non-steroidal anti-inflammatory drugs (NSAIDS).

In the stomach, food is converted into chyme, and there is some enzymatic digestion. Anatomically, the stomach is divided into three regions (Figure 10.7a), i.e. the fundus, body and antrum. (These regions are flanked within two curves: the greater curvature and the lesser curvature.) The mucosa and submucosa of the stomach are arranged in pleats, called rugae, which are distinct and visible when the stomach is contracted and empty, but disappear when the stomach is full and distended with food.

The point at which the stomach meets the next major portion of the GI tract, the small intestine (duodenum), is known as the pylorus. The pyloric sphincter controls the entry of stomach contents into the duodenum.

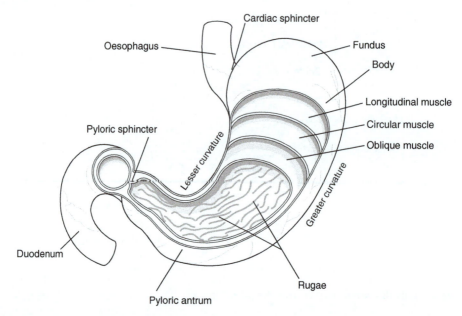

Figure 10.7a Parts of the stomach

Secretions of the stomach

The stomach daily secretes 2–3 litres of gastric juice, which is made up of three major constituents.

1. Hydrochloric acid (HCl) creates an acidity of approximately pH 2.0 (pH range 1.0–3.5) in the stomach; it is responsible for killing unwanted microbes that may enter the stomach with ingested food and water. Stomach enzymes involved in protein digestion also function optimally in an acidic environment. In addition, HCl causes the denaturing of complex protein structures, e.g. collagen fibres in meat, which helps with protein digestion.

2. Pepsinogen is a protein-digesting enzyme, secreted in an inactive form. With the aid of HCl, it is converted into a potent protease, pepsin, which can break up protein into smaller fragments called peptides. Peptides will later be acted upon by enzymes of the small intestine to become single and free amino acids.

3. Mucus is secreted to protect the stomach lining (mucosa), which could easily become irritated and damaged by HCl, or even auto-digested by pepsin. Luckily, in healthy individuals, released mucus forms a thick gel layer which coats and protects the delicate mucosa. Intake of certain substances, e.g. aspirin, NSAIDs, alcohol and vinegar, can disrupt this mucosal barrier.

Although the acidic environment of the stomach is inhospitable to most pathogens, some can survive here and are associated with a variety of pathologies. You are invited to explore the most famous microbial inhabitant of the stomach in Activity 10.2.

Activity 10.2   Evidence-based practice and research

Research the link between *H. pylori* and gastric ulcers.

There are some possible answers to all activities at the end of the chapter, unless otherwise indicated.

In Activity 10.2 you examined one of the most common gastric pathologies. We can now return and continue to examine the role of the stomach in the process of digestion.

Regulation of gastric juice production

The secretion of gastric juice begins when food is in the mouth and continues after chewing has ceased. This is due to both nervous and hormonal mechanisms. The secretion of gastric juice occurs in three phases.

1. A cephalic phase, which occurs as a result of the sight or smell of food, well before food has entered the stomach.
2. A gastric phase, which begins once food has entered the stomach.
3. An intestinal phase, which continues briefly while food is in the duodenum.

The cephalic phase is triggered by nervous mechanisms; the next phases occur because of the presence of food in the stomach, which triggers the release of the hormone gastrin. Gastrin controls the secretion of gastric juice. Mastication signals the onset of gastrin secretion by cells in the stomach lining. Gastrin production is also increased by the presence of foods such as proteins, coffee and alcohol in the gastric lumen.

The stomach wall is made up of the same four layers as the rest of the GI tract (Figure 10.6). However, adaptations here include an extra layer of smooth muscle in the muscularis, which allows the stomach to undergo robust churning, thereby enabling vigorous mechanical digestion into smaller food particles. In addition, the mucosal epithelial lining of the stomach is indented, and these hollow depressions are known as gastric pits (Figure 10.7b). Each gastric pit marks the position of a gastric gland from which the various constituents of gastric juice are secreted. There are reported to be almost 35 million gastric glands in the epithelial lining of the stomach, which enable production of around 2–3 litres of gastric juice a day.

Mucus cells produce the protective mucus. These cells are distributed throughout the stomach but are found in greatest abundance at the neck and surface of gastric pits. Parietal cells mainly secrete HCl and are mostly concentrated in the gastric pits found

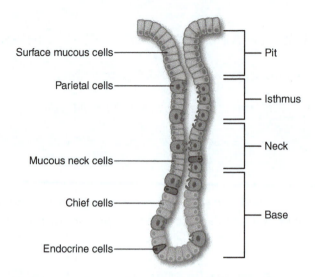

Figure 10.7b Four major types of secretory epithelial cells extend down into these gastric pits and glands

in the body of the stomach, but almost absent from those in the pyloric region. Parietal cells secrete intrinsic factor, a factor necessary for the absorption of vitamin B12, a vital vitamin involved in many body functions including the production of red blood cells. Chief cells secrete pepsinogen. They also secrete small quantities of gastric lipase (Kiela and Ghishan, 2016).

G-cells (endocrine cells) are mainly distributed in gastric pits from the mucosa of the antrum and secrete the hormone gastrin. Food is churned, mixed and ground with gastric juice into a white blend known as chyme. Periodically, about every 20 seconds, small portions of semi-liquid chyme are squirted through the pyloric sphincter into the duodenum. This is so the duodenum does not become overwhelmed with a vast volume of gastric contents. Gastric emptying is controlled by the stomach and duodenum; chyme in the duodenum activates receptors that inhibit gastric emptying.

When all the stomach contents have entered the duodenum, mild contractions begin in the stomach. These may persist and increase in intensity. If no food is received, these waves of hunger contractions can become quite painful.

Hunger and satiety

Hunger is under complex hormonal and neural control. A series of specialised contractions, termed the migrating motor complex (MMC), cause the rumblings that signify hunger and hunger pangs. These are under the control of a hormone, motilin. Additionally, another hormone, ghrelin, is released when the stomach is empty, and signals the brain to inform us of hunger. Ghrelin stimulates the production and secretion of gastric juice in anticipation of receiving food; if food is not provided, the stomach acid may begin to attack the lining, causing the pain sometimes associated with severe hunger.

Cortisol, a hormone produced by the adrenal glands, is released in certain situations including acute stress. Like adrenalin, it prepares us for a flight-or-fight response by flooding the body with glucose, making it available for rapid cell metabolism and energy production. It therefore temporarily causes a 'shut down' of processes that are required for immediate survival, like the digestive system. Subsequently, these cells become starved of energy, and to regulate this, they send hunger signals to the brain (Aronson, 2009). Cortisol may also directly influence appetite and cravings for high-calorie foods as well as indirectly influencing appetite by modulating other hormones and stress-responsive factors known to stimulate appetite (Table 10.2).

Table 10.2   Major appetite-controlling hormones

Hormone	Produced by	Function
Ghrelin	Stomach (in response to fasting)	Increases appetite
Peptide tyrosine tyrosine (PYY)	Ileum and colon (in response to food intake)	Suppresses appetite
Cholecystokinin (CCK)	Small intestine (in response to presence of fat and protein)	Suppresses appetite
Insulin	Pancreas (in response to high blood glucose)	Suppresses appetite
Leptin	Adipose tissue (secretion linked to BMI)	Inhibits hunger

The small intestine

The small intestine comprises the duodenum (25 cm long), the jejunum (2.5 m long) and the ileum (3.5 m long) (Figure 10.8). Most of this is held suspended from the body wall by a structure called the mesentery, an extension of the peritoneum. Chyme, with a pH of approximately 2.0, arrives here immediately after gastric emptying. The majority of enzymatic digestion occurs in the small intestine, liberating small molecules from ingested food. Most absorption of these molecules (amino acids, monosaccharides and lipids) also occurs in the small intestine.

The wall of the small intestine produces a number of secretions. The duodenum secretes mucus, from Brunner's glands, embedded in the submucosa. Mucus is needed at this point to counteract the strong acidity which arrives with the stomach contents. Mucin glycoproteins possess unique gel-forming properties, creating a slippery, viscoelastic gel mucous layer that lubricates the inner mucosal lining of the duodenum.

The secretions from Brunner's glands also contain bicarbonate ions and bactericidal and growth factors. Thus, as well as providing a protective barrier against gastric acid and enzymes, Brunner's glands also provide some basic immunological defence mechanisms within the duodenum. The duodenum receives secretions from the pancreas and liver (Figures 10.8 and 10.9).

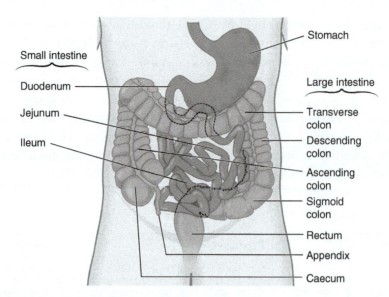

Figure 10.8 Anatomy of small and large intestines

Source: Image courtesy of *Nursing Times*

The pancreas

The pancreas is a compound gland, measuring between 12.5 and 15 cm. It is situated in close proximity to the duodenum, lying transversely across the posterior wall of the abdomen. Anatomically, the pancreas has a broad head end, with a tapering tail. The two ends are separated by the main portion of the organ, the body.

The pancreas has a major role in digestion. The bulk of the pancreas is composed of secretory cells (acini) and ducts. Collectively they secrete pancreatic juice, which is sent to the duodenum via the pancreatic duct.

Pancreatic juice is composed of a significant collection of enzymes and their precursors, of which four are critical for effective digestion.

1. Trypsin (secreted as a precursor – trypsinogen).
2. Chymotrypsin (secreted as a precursor – chymotrypsinogen).
3. Pancreatic amylase.
4. Pancreatic lipase.

Trypsin and chymotrypsin are pancreatic proteases that are synthesised and packaged as the inactive enzymes, trypsinogen and chymotrypsinogen, which, once released into the duodenum, must be converted into their active forms. This conversion is initiated by an enzyme, enterokinase (enteropeptidase), which is released from the intestinal mucosa and acts to convert trypsinogen into trypsin. Trypsin then activates chymotrypsinogen to form chymotrypsin. Thus, these two potent proteases can now act on proteins and peptides present in chyme in the duodenum.

Trypsin and chymotrypsin can digest proteins into very small peptides, but not into single amino acids (this is mainly the job of peptides from duodenal epithelial cells). Pancreatic amylase acts on starch, the major dietary carbohydrate. Amylase hydrolyses starch into the disaccharide maltose, and pancreatic lipase carries out hydrolysis of triglyceride (fat) molecules to release constituent glycerol and fatty acids, enabling digestion and absorption of dietary fat (Figure 10.1c). The pancreas also releases nucleases. These break down ingested nucleic acids (DNA and RNA) into their component nucleotides, which are further digested in the ileum into sugars, bases and phosphates.

Pancreatitis

Acute inflammation of the pancreas is usually mild but can progress into a severe inflammatory disease needing hospital care. Pancreatitis can develop because of disruption of the acini or ducts, which now allow pancreatic enzymes to leak into pancreatic tissue and commence auto-digestion. These proteases damage tissue and cell membranes, causing the release of numerous toxic enzymes and inflammatory mediators into the bloodstream. This may lead to further injury of other organs such as the lungs and kidneys and progress to multi-organ failure and mortality.

The most significant symptom of pancreatitis is epigastric or upper abdominal pain, which may radiate to the back. The two major causes of pancreatitis are chronic alcohol abuse and obstruction of the pancreatic duct by gallstones which can cause a backing-up of pancreatic juice.

The liver and bile

The liver is an organ vital to life. It is the largest internal organ, weighing 1.2–1.5 kg. It is approximately 15 cm thick and located in the right-upper abdomen, well protected by the rib cage. The major cells of the liver, the hepatocytes, are metabolically active cells that perform an astonishing range of functions. These include metabolism of ingested nutrients, storage (e.g. iron, vitamins), synthesis (e.g. plasma proteins), detoxification (e.g. drugs, alcohol) and bile production. The latter is the main digestive function of the liver. Each day, the hepatocytes produce between 500 and 1000 ml of bile, a thick, greenish-yellow alkaline fluid of pH 8.1.

Bile is a complex fluid, consisting mainly of water, bile salts (such as sodium taurocholate and sodium glycocholate), bile pigments (bilirubin and biliverdin) and lipids (cholesterol). Bile salts are of great importance to the digestive process, particularly for the digestion of fats. The bile salts, derivatives of cholesterol (cholic acid), carry out the emulsification of lipid aggregates in the duodenum. Emulsification breaks down large fat globules into much smaller droplets, thus making it easier for fat-digesting enzymes (lipases) to gain access to, and act on, the lipid droplets.

A second role of bile in terms of digestion is the presence of sodium hydrogen bicarbonate. This ion helps create a pH in the duodenum of 7–8 (the stomach contents enter the duodenum at pH 2.0). This elevated pH is necessary for optimal functioning of enzymes from the pancreas and duodenum itself.

After production by the liver cells, bile drains into the common hepatic duct. About 50 per cent of it enters the gallbladder, a small, pear-shaped organ situated directly below the liver (Figure 10.9), and is stored here until the gall bladder is stimulated to contract. The remaining 50 per cent enters the common bile duct and runs directly into the duodenum. The presence of food in the duodenum triggers the contraction of the gall bladder to further release bile into the duodenum.

The gall bladder and gall stones

Bile leaves the gall bladder via the cystic duct. The common hepatic duct joins with the cystic duct to form the common bile duct, which enters the duodenum. Bile drainage can be obstructed by the formation of gall stones lodging in these ducts (Figure 10.9). Since bile is an outlet for excess cholesterol, some types of gallstones form in the gall bladder when bile salts and cholesterol interact. Gall stones range in size but can be up to 4–5 cm long. Blockage of the gall bladder with stones is often the cause of acute pain (colic) following the ingestion of a meal rich in fats.

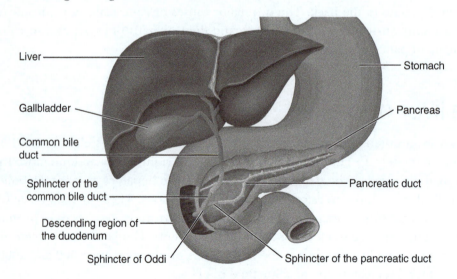

Figure 10.9 Stomach, liver, pancreas and duodenum

Source: Image courtesy of *Nursing Times*

Intestinal enzymes

Collectively, intestinal juice consists of mucus and an abundance of digestive enzymes such as enteropeptidases, lactase, maltase, sucrase and lipases. This clear, alkaline fluid is secreted into the lumen of the small intestine and works alongside secretions from the pancreas and gall bladder to enable complete digestion of ingested carbohydrates, proteins and fats. This intestinal juice is secreted by small pits that cover the entire surface of the small intestine. These pits are known as the crypts of Lieberkühn.

Control of secretion of pancreatic juice, bile and intestinal enzymes

The secretions entering the small intestine are under neural and hormonal control. The main hormones involved are secretin and cholecystokinin (CCK), but gastrin (from the stomach mucosa) also aids intestinal secretions. Secretin and CCK are both produced by endocrinocytes in the epithelium of the duodenum.

Secretin is released in response to the presence of acid chyme in the duodenum. It has several effects, including stimulating and increasing bile secretion to the duodenum and suppressing the secretion of gastric juices. The predominant effect of secretin, however, is on the pancreas, where it stimulates pancreatic duct cells to secrete water and bicarbonate, flushing enzymes out of the exocrine cells through the pancreatic duct into the duodenum. Secretin also increases small intestinal secretion, as does cholecystokinin.

Cholecystokinin release is stimulated by the presence of fat in the duodenum, and causes the contraction of the gall bladder and bile duct, enabling bile to be delivered to the duodenum. This hormone also stimulates the secretion of vast quantities of digestive enzymes from the pancreatic cells (by binding to receptors on the surface of these cells). Gastrin also stimulates the exocrine (secretory) cells of the pancreas.

Mechanical digestion

Even though the release and actions of the various hormones and enzymes discussed above are critical in the digestion of ingested macro-molecules, chemical digestion is aided by mechanical, muscular movements within the small intestine. These movements can be divided into mixing contractions and propulsive contractions. The former are also known as segmentation contractions, and result in a 'chopping action' of chyme, enabling greater mixing of solid food particles with secretions in the small intestine. Propulsive contractions, or peristaltic waves, propel chyme (quite weakly) towards the rectum through the small intestine.

As a result of both chemical and mechanical digestion, chyme leaves the duodenum to enter the jejunum and ileum as fine micro-molecules in their simplest form, ready to be absorbed.

Absorption by the small intestine

Each day, approximately 8–9 litres of water (from dietary ingestion, saliva and other GI tract secretions and juices), and several hundred grams of carbohydrates, fats, amino acids and ions, pass across the wall of the small intestine, from the lumen into the blood.

The walls of the small intestine are structurally adapted for the absorption of nutrient molecules to occur efficiently. Transport of nutrients occurs across folds (folds of Kerckring) in the mucosal layer of the intestinal wall. These folds triple the surface area of the absorptive mucosa. There is an intimate association between the walls of the intestine and underlying blood capillaries (Figure 10.10). Finger-like projections known as villi project approximately 1 mm into the intestinal lumen. Villi increase in the surface area of the mucosa ten-fold. Within each villus is a central lacteal, which contains lymph and empties into the lymphatic system.

This lacteal is surrounded by a capillary network into which most nutrients are absorbed. Intestinal epithelial cells, which surround each protruding villus, have tiny projections themselves, about 1 micrometre in length, jutting out into the intestinal lumen. These projections, known as microvilli (Figure 10.10), form a velvety brush border and primarily serve to increase the absorptive area of the mucosal lining by a further 20 times. Thus, the total surface area available for the absorption of nutrients is vast, estimated to be about the surface area of a tennis court!

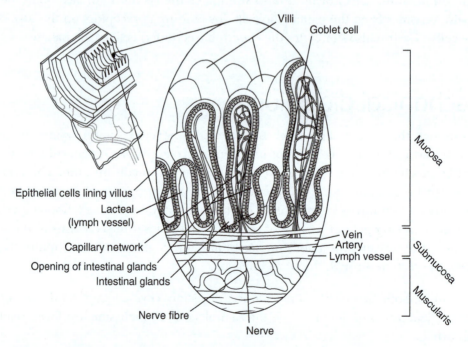

Figure 10.10   Villi of the small intestine

In addition to its absorptive role, the brush border also has an important digestive function. Tethered into the plasma membrane of the border microvilli are a series of digestive enzymes including lactase, intestinal lipases and peptidases. These enzymes participate in carrying out the final stages of digestion of ingested carbohydrate and proteins.

The transport of nutrients across the cell membranes of small intestinal epithelial cells, into the villi and from there into blood capillaries or lacteals, occurs either actively or passively. Active transport requires energy, often to pull molecules out of the lumen against a concentration gradient. Most molecules that come over actively require carrier molecules to take them across, for example glucose, galactose, amino acids and sodium ions. Passive transport requires no energy and usually involves the diffusion of simple molecules, along a concentration gradient, either into the blood or into lacteals. Water, lipids and some vitamins can cross the gut wall passively.

Absorption of carbohydrates

Almost all ingested carbohydrates are absorbed as monosaccharides; 80 per cent as glucose. The remaining 20 per cent of monosaccharides are galactose (from the disaccharide lactose in milk) and fructose (from fruit and digested sucrose). Glucose absorption occurs actively as a sodium co-transport mechanism. Absorbed carbohydrates enter the blood capillary system underlying each villus.

Absorption of proteins

Most peptide and amino acid molecules are absorbed in a similar way to glucose; that is, via an active sodium co-transport mechanism. Proteins also enter the blood capillary system of each villus.

Absorption of fats

Digested fats, in the form of glycerol and fatty acids, are dissolved in bile acid micelles. The micelles ferry these fat molecules across the gut wall cells. Once in the cells, the free molecules are reconstituted into larger glycerides and aggregated into fat globules called chylomicrons. Chylomicrons are taken into the central lacteals of villi and are then taken with lymph up to the thoracic duct, to be emptied where the lymphatic ducts drain into the blood supply at the subclavian veins near the neck, and eventually transported by the blood.

Absorption of ions

Ions (electrolytes), such as sodium (Na^+), potassium (K^+) and chloride (Cl^-), are also mainly handled and absorbed by the small intestine. Some, however, are absorbed by the colon or lost in faeces. Most of these ions need to be actively absorbed across the GI tract wall.

Absorption of vitamins

Vitamins are essential for growth and development and are vitally involved in numerous metabolic processes. Since we cannot synthesise most vitamins, we rely on dietary intake of these. Intestinal transport of many ingested water-soluble vitamins is aided by carriers and transporters such as sodium across the gut membrane. Transport of fat-soluble vitamins such as vitamin A and D occurs by simple, passive diffusion.

Malabsorption

Malabsorption syndrome is the name given to a range of disorders that result when nutrients cannot be absorbed properly from the small intestine. Malabsorption can occur either if food is not being digested completely, or because there is a direct interference with nutrient absorption. Either way, malabsorption can cause deficiencies of selective or all nutrients (proteins, fats, vitamins or carbohydrates), and the resulting symptoms will vary accordingly. If protein malabsorption occurs, symptoms such as tissue swelling or peripheral oedema may be seen. Malabsorption of fats will result in pale, bulky and foul-smelling stools (steatorrhea). Malabsorption of vitamins is associated with a wide range of symptoms including anaemia, weakness and pins-and-needles sensations.

Carbohydrate malabsorption, for example with lactase deficiency, can result in a range of symptoms including explosive diarrhoea, abdominal bloating and flatulence after drinking milk.

Normally, enzymes (carbohydrases) such as lactase, sucrase and maltase break down complex sugars into simple ones such as glucose, which can then be absorbed through the intestinal wall. If any of these enzymes are missing (i.e. not produced by the body), the corresponding sugar will not be digested, and will remain in the small intestine. This high concentration of indigested sugar causes an osmotic pull, resulting in drawing of fluid into the small intestine, causing diarrhoea.

The indigested, unabsorbed sugar will then travel to the large intestine, and will be fermented by bacteria present there (see later), producing acidic stool and flatulence. The most common form of sugar intolerance is due to the lack of lactase. People without this enzyme usually cannot tolerate milk or other dairy products that contain lactose. Non-infectious diarrhoea may also be caused by intolerance to gluten proteins in wheat products such as bread, and inflammatory conditions such as Crohn's disease. To further your understanding of Crohn's disease, read through Michael's case study below.

Case study: Michael – Crohn's disease

Michael is a 15-year-old who is small for his age. Periodically, he has experienced episodes of watery diarrhoea and abdominal pain. During these episodes, he didn't want to eat much as food made the symptoms worse and he lost weight. His mum was quite concerned because he wasn't growing as fast as his friends. Initially, Michael was embarrassed to mention the diarrhoea but eventually he told his mother as the symptoms were becoming more frequent and more severe. After visiting his GP, Michael was referred to a gastroenterologist who diagnosed Crohn's disease.

Crohn's disease in teenagers and young adults commonly affects the ileum. Ulcers develop in the deep layer of the bowel and result in the inability to absorb nutrients. Fistulas may develop from one part of the bowel to another or nearby tissues.

Unfortunately, there is no cure for Crohn's disease and treatment is concerned with managing the symptoms. Initially Michael was treated with a combination of steroids and immunosuppressant therapy. Michael will visit his consultant regularly and his progress will be monitored, as will potential side effects of treatment which may include weight gain, indigestion, problems sleeping, an increased risk of infections and slower growth.

If Michael doesn't respond to first-line treatment, biological medicines including adalimumab, infliximab, vedolizumab and ustekinumab may be offered. Surgery is also an option, which may include resection of the affected area or possibly an ileostomy.

Now that you have a good understanding of digestion and absorption and have had the opportunity of exploring some examples of food intolerances, we need to move on and explore the role of the final sections of the GI tract.

The large intestine

A vast quantity of chyme (approximately 1.5 litres daily), which has not been absorbed by the time it has left the ileum of the small intestine, enters the large intestine through a small valve, the ileocaecal valve, at the junction between the two intestines. The large intestine comprises the caecum, colon, rectum and anal canal and is approximately 1.5 metres long (Figure 10.11).

The caecum is a blind-ended sac which carries a small extension, the appendix. The histological structure of the small and large intestines is very similar, except that the mucosa of the large intestine is completely devoid of villi.

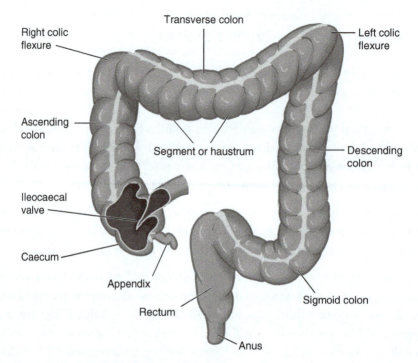

Figure 10.11   Anatomy of the large intestine

Source: Image courtesy of *Nursing Times*

Appendicitis

Appendicitis is the inflammation of the appendix, accompanied by the classical symptom of acute pain in the right side of the abdomen, beginning at the umbilicus and spreading and intensifying in the region of the right iliac fossa. Often nausea, vomiting and fever are associated symptoms. The initiating event of appendicitis is not always known; some causes include obstruction of the caecum by hardened, calcified, faecal material or a collection of thread or pinworms (*Enterobius vermicularis*). Such obstructions cause a pressure build-up, which may affect the blood supply to the appendix, resulting in ischaemic injury and infection.

If this condition remains untreated, the appendix could rupture and perforate, leading to severe peritonitis and possibly death within hours. Appendicitis represents one of the most common abdominal medical emergencies. Read through Tom's case study for a typical clinical presentation of this common pathology.

Tom's case study reveals the importance of thorough clinical assessment when patients present with abdominal pain.

The colon is by far the longest portion of the large intestine, and is subclassified into ascending, transverse, descending and sigmoid portions. Most distally, the large intestine expands into the rectum, which becomes continuous with the anal canal (Figure 10.11).

The large intestine has several functions, which can be categorised into three major groups: absorption (and secretion), transport of faeces and microbial activity.

Case study: Tom – appendicitis

Tom is a 19-year-old student who experienced nausea and vague central abdominal pain for several hours, which later became more severe and localised to the right iliac fossa in an area known as McBurney's point. Tom then vomited twice before calling his GP, who sent him to his local Emergency Department. On admission, Tom was found to have rebound tenderness over his right iliac fossa, a temperature of 38.2°C and a slightly elevated white cell count. A diagnosis of acute appendicitis was made. Tom was taken to theatre, where he had a laparoscopic removal of an inflamed appendix and made an uneventful recovery.

Absorption and secretion by the large intestine

Most of the 1.5 litres of fluid entering the large intestine is absorbed, leaving less than 100 millilitres to pass out with the faeces. The large intestine absorbs water and electrolytes (salts). The active absorption of most ingested sodium also occurs here, since colonic epithelial cells are more capable of sodium absorption than those of the small intestine. Water is absorbed by osmosis but this is absolutely dependent on the absorption of sodium ions.

Sodium absorption is increased when the hormone aldosterone is released, since aldosterone greatly enhances sodium absorption in the colon (see Chapters 3 and 11). Aldosterone also affects the blood concentration of K^+ ions, promoting their excretion in urine. The mucosal wall secretes bicarbonate ions, while it simultaneously absorbs chloride ions. Mucus is also produced by the large intestine and acts as a very important lubricant, helping to bind dehydrated chyme, and converting it into faeces.

Transport of faeces in the large intestine

Peristaltic (mass movements) and segmentation (haustral) contractions propagate this dehydrated matter along the colon towards the rectum and anus (although some anti-peristaltic contractions also occur, serving to slow down movement of waste through the colon, allowing a prolonged opportunity for water and electrolyte absorption).

Despite all the absorption of water and electrolytes that occurs, faeces, once formed, are usually 75 per cent water and 25 per cent solid matter. The solid matter is composed mainly of bacteria (30 per cent), fat (10–20 per cent), protein (2–3 per cent), inorganic waste (10–20 per cent) and undigested organic matter and fibre (30 per cent).

Microbial activity in the large intestine

Many microbes are resident in the large intestine. Here, they coexist with and benefit humans. They are invaluable in the metabolism of carbohydrates, proteins and amino acids that have escaped enzymatic breakdown. They also contribute to other essential gastrointestinal functions such as maturation of immune cells, fermentation and synthesis of certain vitamins. The diversity of microbes in the gut is established early in life with the introduction of a varied diet. The microbes have two major functions: fermentation and synthesis of vitamins.

Fermentation

Some of the ingested food matter that enters the small and large intestines is indigestible by the chemical and mechanical means described earlier. However, bacteria present in the colon are capable of producing enzymes that can ferment some of the remaining carbohydrates. In doing so, the bacteria release various gases into the intestine, e.g. hydrogen, carbon dioxide and methane. Fermentation by microbes is thus the major source of intestinal gas and flatulence. In addition, some bacteria can act on remaining proteins and amino acids.

These are converted to sulphurous substances including odorous ones such as indole, skatole and hydrogen sulphide. The nature of these malodorous substances, and the gas produced, depends on the type of food eaten. Some high-fibre diets, e.g. beans and cruciferous vegetables like cabbage and cauliflower, will produce a lot of gas. The importance of the intake of dietary fibre in maintaining a healthy digestive system is well established. In addition, fermentation of dietary fibre produces a fatty acid called butyrate that has been shown to protect against some forms of colonic cancer.

Colonic bacteria also provide a natural defence mechanism that protects the intestine from invasion of potentially harmful bacteria. In addition to diet, medications adversely affect gut microbiota. In particular, broad-spectrum antibiotics can shift the microbial balance in favour of pathogenic bacteria. Other drugs, such as proton pump inhibitors, NSAIDS and opioids, may change the pH of the GI tract and lead to pathogen colonisation, reduction in transit time or damage to the gut tissue. In Activity 10.3 we invite you to research an increasingly common microbial gut disturbance seen in hospitals throughout the world.

Activity 10.3   Evidence-based practice and research

Marjorie is an 80-year-old lady who developed a chest infection postoperatively. She was successfully treated with broad-spectrum antibiotics but within a week developed profuse foul-smelling diarrhoea, abdominal pain and a distended abdomen. Marjorie was subsequently identified as having *Clostridoides* or *Clostridium difficile* associated diarrhoea (CDAD).

Consider the role of the normal gut flora in protecting patients from *C. difficile* infection and the role of antibiotics in CDAD.

Although bacteria such as *C. difficile* examined in Activity 10.3 cause an immense amount of discomfort and suffering, other bacteria play key roles that are crucial to human health and well-being.

Vitamin synthesis by gut

Bacteria residing in the colon are capable of synthesising several B vitamins and vitamin K. The latter is a very important precursor in the formation of blood-clotting factors (see Chapter 8); this 'in-house' synthesis makes clinical vitamin K deficiency rare. However, prolonged, long-term intake of certain antibiotics can disrupt the colonies of synthesising, colonic bacteria, and lead to a deficiency in vitamin K production. This may result in serious effects in terms of blood-clotting ability.

The rectum and anus

The characteristic brown colour of faeces is caused by two derivatives of bile pigments, stercobilin and urobilin (which are breakdown products of haemoglobin from aged red blood cells). Faeces are not usually stored in the rectum for long; indeed, most of the time the rectum is usually empty of faeces. When a mass movement ejects faeces from the sigmoid colon into the rectum, this initiates the desire to defecate.

Following a meal, colonic motility increases significantly. As faeces enter the rectum, the rectal wall distends, sending impulses to centres in the spinal cord, and triggering reflex rectal contraction via the peripheral nervous system. This stimulates a (spinal) defecation reflex, which results in the relaxation of the internal anal sphincter, followed by voluntary relaxation of the external anal sphincter (Figure 10.12), and defecation.

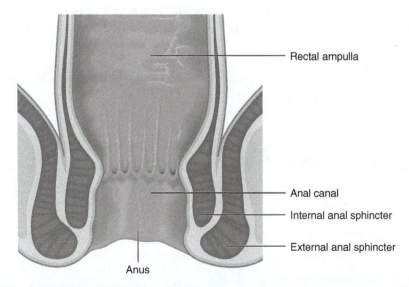

Rectal ampulla

Anal canal

Internal anal sphincter

External anal sphincter

Anus

Figure 10.12 Anatomy of the anal canal

Source: Image courtesy of *Nursing Times*

Diarrhoea and constipation

If the intestines are not absorbing fluids, there is potential for the body to lose several (7–9) litres of fluid a day. The consequences of diarrhoea can become serious, especially if fluid loss is not addressed or re-balanced by fluid intake. Complications such as dehydration, increased risk of clotting and loss of vital electrolytes (potassium, bicarbonate and sodium ions) may ensue. It is also possible for large losses of potassium ions to result in severe cardiac events. Severe diarrhoea may lead to so much water loss that patients may even slip into hypovolaemic shock.

Constipation is the slow movement of often hard, dehydrated faeces along the large intestine. It can be caused by many different conditions including a poor diet low in fibre, irritable bowel syndrome (IBS), medications such as iron supplements, mechanical obstruction of the intestines, e.g. tumours, or poor irregular bowel habits developed throughout life. Constipation can lead to complications, such as development of haemorrhoids or fissures, developed because of extreme straining and passing of hard faeces.

Faecal incontinence

Normally, defecation can be prevented by voluntary constriction of the external anal sphincter which, since it is composed of skeletal muscle, is under conscious control. However, in infants and some patients, as a result of a wide range of possible causes (e.g. injured or diseased spinal cord, injuries to rectum or anus, diabetes, severe dementia, surgical operations or childbirth), the inability to exercise voluntary control over the external anal sphincter, or lack of rectal sensation, can result in embarrassing and inconvenient defecation. Severe faecal incontinence (the accidental loss of solid or liquid stool at least once a week) can unfortunately prevent many patients undertaking everyday activities.

Now that you have completed the chapter, attempt the multiple-choice questions in Activity 10.4 to assess your understanding of the subject material.

Activity 10.4   Multiple-choice questions

1.   The acid produced in the stomach is

   a)   Acetic acid

   b)   Hydrochloric acid

   c)   Sulphuric acid

   d)   Nitric acid

2. Which cranial nerves promote the continuous secretion of saliva?

   a) I and II
   b) IV and V
   c) V and VI
   d) VII and IX

3. Which region of the brain controls swallowing?

   a) Hypothalamus
   b) Medulla oblongata
   c) Temporal lobe
   d) Sensory cortex

4. Which of these digestive enzymes is responsible for breaking down fat?

   a) Carbohydrases
   b) Proteases
   c) Lipases
   d) Salivary amylase

5. Which of these is not a region of the stomach?

   a) Fundus
   b) Body
   c) Atrium
   d) Ileum

6. Which of these pancreatic enzymes acts on starch?

   a) Trypsin
   b) Chymotrypsin
   c) Pancreatic amylase
   d) Pancreatic lipase

7. Bile salts are responsible for

   a) Emulsification of fat globules
   b) Digestion of protein
   c) Absorption of vitamins
   d) Breakdown of carbohydrates

(Continued)

(Continued)

8. Malabsorption of fat will result in

    a) Tissue swelling

    b) Steatorrhea

    c) Anaemia

    d) Constipation

9. The function of ghrelin is to

    a) Increase appetite

    b) Suppress appetite

    c) Increase thirst

    d) Inhibit hunger

10. Which of these is not a function of the large intestine?

    a) Re-absorption of water

    b) Absorption of fat

    c) Transport of faeces

    d) Re-absorption of electrolytes (salts)

Chapter summary

Digestion is the mechanical and chemical breakdown of food into simple components that can be absorbed and utilised by the body. The process of digestion begins in the mouth with mechanical chewing of food (mastication). The tongue helps to mix chewed food with saliva which begins the process of chemical digestion of carbohydrates and fats (lipids).

Following deglutition (swallowing), food is propelled along the oesophagus into the stomach where it is mixed with the acidic gastric secretions, which sterilise ingested food and initiate the chemical digestion of proteins. Food leaves the stomach in small portions and enters the duodenum, where it is mixed with pancreatic juice and bile. These continue the process of chemical digestion which is then completed in the jejunum and ileum.

The ileum is the largest section of the small intestine and is the primary site of nutrient absorption. Undigested components of food pass into the colon (large intestine), where water and electrolytes are re-absorbed into the blood. Faecal material is stored in the rectum before being eliminated through the anus during defecation.

Activities: Brief outline answers

Activity 10.1: Reflection (page 273)

Patients should be encouraged to take oral fluids regularly. The mouth should be kept clean. Dentures should be removed and all traces of food and debris should be removed. The patient's teeth and gums should be gently brushed twice a day with a soft toothbrush and toothpaste. Artificial saliva can be applied to the tongue to improve patient comfort.

Activity 10.2: Evidence-based practice and research (page 279)

Helicobacter pylori (*H. pylori*) is a bacterium which can live in the digestive tract of otherwise healthy individuals. According to the Centers for Disease Control and Prevention (CDC), two thirds of the population carry *H. pylori* but, for reasons not yet understood, most people will suffer no ill-effects. However, some people can develop ulcers, gastritis or stomach cancer from an *H. pylori* infection. In fact, the majority of gastric ulcers are caused by *H. pylori* infection.

In rare cases, an infection can cause stomach cancer. *H. pylori* damages the stomach lining, meaning that both the bacteria and acid can penetrate the lining and cause ulceration, leading to abdominal pain (described as either dull or burning). The pain is most commonly experienced between meals and overnight and may be alleviated by antacids, eating or drinking milk. *H. pylori* is spread by person to person through direct contact with saliva, faeces or untreated water.

Diagnosis of *H. pylori* infection can be through detecting antibodies in the blood, a carbon urea breath test, tests for antigen in stool or endoscopy and biopsy. *H. pylori* infection is treated by a combination of two or more antibiotics with a proton pump inhibitor.

Activity 10.3: Evidence-based practice and research (page 292)

C. difficile is a Gram-positive, spore-forming bacillus which often resides in the gut of elderly people with no ill-effects until antibiotics are administered. Antibiotics, particularly broad-spectrum antibiotics, reduce the number of resident organisms in the gut, allowing *C. difficile*, which is resistant to these drugs, to proliferate to the extent where it becomes pathogenic and causes symptoms such as those experienced by Marjorie.

Activity 10.4: Multiple-choice questions (pages 294–6)

1) b, 2) d, 3) b, 4) c, 5) d, 6) c, 7) a, 8) b, 9) a, 10) b

Further reading

Boore J et al. (2016) Chapter 8: The digestive system – Nutrient supply and waste elimination, in *Essentials of Anatomy and Physiology for Nursing Practice*. London: SAGE Publications Ltd.

A textbook to develop your knowledge of human anatomy and physiology that is aimed specifically at nurses.

Tortora G and Derrickson B (2017) Chapter 24: The digestive system, in *Tortora's Principles of Anatomy and Physiology* (15th edition). New York: John Wiley & Sons.

In-depth coverage of human anatomy and physiology.

Useful website

www.webmd.com/heartburn-gerd/your-digestive-system#1

A simple overview of the digestive system.

Chapter 11　The urinary system

Co-authored by Maria Andrade

Chapter aims

After reading this chapter, you will be able to:

- highlight the major functions of the urinary system;
- describe the anatomy of the kidneys, ureters, bladder and urethra;
- explain the physiological processes involved in urine production;
- explain how hormones interact with the kidneys;
- describe how the composition of urine can be used to screen for disease.

Introduction

Case study: Zubeyde – kidney stones

For the last two weeks, Zubeyde has been experiencing sporadic pain in her back, which she initially assumed was due to muscle strain after painting her child's bedroom. However, the last episode two days ago was so intense that she was doubled over in pain and experiencing chills and intense nausea. Gradually the pain subsided, and Zubeyde arranged to visit her GP who found fresh (non-haemolysed) blood in her urine, which also appeared cloudy with prominent sediment.

Zubeyde was referred to her local hospital where a computed tomography of kidneys, ureters and bladder (CT KUB) revealed renal calculi (kidney stones) in both kidneys. Since the stones appeared to be large, she underwent lithotripsy to help break up the stones and was sent home with instructions to increase her water intake to promote diuresis to help flush out the resultant debris.

Overview of the urinary system

The urinary tract consists of the kidneys, ureters, bladder and urethra (Figure 11.1). It is intimately involved in maintaining homeostatic balance throughout the body, working together in synergy with many of the other organ systems. The kidneys are responsible for removing a variety of waste materials from the blood and eliminating them in a pale, amber-coloured fluid termed urine. This fluid is carried away from the kidneys via two ureters and stored in a distensible bladder prior to elimination through the urethra.

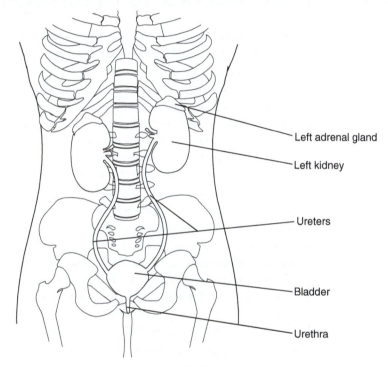

Figure 11.1   The components of the urinary system

An efficient urinary system is essential to health and survival. Renal function does decline with age, but in the absence of pathology it has evolved a built-in redundancy that will allow homeostasis to be effectively maintained well into old age. Unfortunately, the urinary system is prone to a diverse range of pathologies, from simple mechanical injuries such as that caused by Zubeyde's kidney stones, through to acute and chronic renal failure and common cancers that affect the kidney and bladder.

This chapter will begin by describing the major functions of the urinary system before examining the structure of the kidneys and the nature of their blood supply. We will then explore the physiology of the kidney, describing the process of urine formation. Since the composition of the blood is continually changing, the role played by key hormones in fine-tuning urine composition will be explored, together with the importance of the kidneys in maintaining homeostasis. To reinforce the key points, the reader will explore the nature of some of the renal pathologies that nurses routinely encounter in clinical practice.

The major functions of the urinary system

The urinary system has a multitude of diverse functions which are summarised in Table 11.1.

Table 11.1 Functions of the urinary system

Excretion of waste metabolites	Excretion is the process of eliminating metabolic waste products or other materials that are of no use to the body. Urine contains high concentrations of the toxic nitrogenous waste products, urea and uric acid. Unlike fat and carbohydrate, the body has no mechanism for storing excess proteins or amino acids. Therefore, following protein digestion, amino acids that are not of immediate use are quickly deaminated (have their nitrogenous amino groups removed) in the liver and converted to glucose for storage. Deamination produces potentially toxic nitrogenous waste products such as ammonia, which is subsequently converted into less toxic urea and released into the blood for elimination by the kidneys. Since the human diet is based around consuming plant and animal tissues, large amounts of nucleotides (the building blocks of DNA and RNA) are absorbed into the blood. Excess nucleotides are metabolised in the liver, producing uric acid, which is released into the blood. If uric acid is not eliminated efficiently by the kidneys, or excess dietary nucleotides are consumed in the diet, this molecule can build up and crystallise in the joints, leading to gout. Skeletal muscles are continually releasing creatinine from the metabolic breakdown of creatine phosphate (a high-energy phosphate molecule utilised by muscle cells). Creatinine is cleared from the blood at a consistent rate and provides a useful marker molecule for measuring renal function
Elimination of toxins	These include synthetic chemicals that may have been ingested in food and water such as pesticide residues, chemicals released from plastic containers such as phthalates and the breakdown metabolites of many commonly prescribed medications such as antibiotics
Regulation of blood volume and pressure	Hormones such as antidiuretic hormone (vasopressin) and atrial natriuretic peptide (ANP) effectively control the volume of urine produced, allowing blood volume and pressure to be regulated. Additionally, when the blood pressure is low, the kidneys produce the enzyme renin which activates the renin-angiotensin aldosterone pathway, which acts to restore blood pressure
Regulation of the ionic composition of the blood	The kidneys are responsible for retaining or eliminating many of the major ions (electrolytes) in the blood; in particular, sodium (Na^+) and potassium (K^+), which are intimately involved in nerve conduction, and calcium (Ca^{++}), which plays an important role in muscle contraction and synaptic transmission

Regulation of the osmotic potential of the blood	Since the kidneys are able to control both the blood volume and ionic composition, they provide the major mechanism for regulating plasma osmolarity. The ability to control the re-absorption of Na^+ ions via the hormone aldosterone is particularly important in this process. In health, the kidneys maintain the osmolarity of the blood within a tight range of between 275 and 299 milliosmoles per kilogram body weight
Regulation of blood pH	In addition to eliminating the ions Na^+, K^+, Ca^{++} and Cl^-, the kidneys have the ability to excrete hydrogen ions (H^+) when the blood is too acidic (acidosis) or retain H^+ ions when the blood becomes too alkaline (alkalosis). This process of regulating the blood pH is further enhanced by the ability to excrete a variety of acidic metabolites such as ketones and the ability to retain buffering bicarbonate ions (HCO_3^-) in the blood
Regulation of erythropoiesis (production of red blood cells)	The kidneys control the number of circulating erythrocytes, which directly affects the viscosity and oxygen-carrying capabilities of the blood. When the blood oxygen saturation is consistently low, the kidneys release the hormone erythropoietin. This directly stimulates the red bone marrow to produce and release more red blood cells. In diseased kidneys, the amount of erythropoietin synthesised and released may be significantly reduced, leading to anaemia and an observable drop in blood oxygen saturation (often revealed in the readings recorded on pulse oximeters)
Conservation of nutrients and bioactive molecules	The kidneys reclaim materials that are of use to the body such as glucose and amino acids as well as a variety of useful hormones, cytokines and other signalling molecules
Regulating blood glucose	The kidneys have the ability to take up and convert the amino acid glutamine into glucose via gluconeogenesis; this newly converted glucose can then be directly released into the blood to boost blood sugar levels
Biosynthesis of vitamin D	Together with the skin and liver, the kidneys play a major role in the production of vitamin D, which is essential for calcium homeostasis. Diseased kidneys play a less efficient role in this process, leading to reductions in calcium and phosphate absorption in the gut and potentially precipitating bone disorders such as osteoporosis

In health, the kidneys maintain a relatively stable internal environment which is close to optimal for cells and tissues to function. Any pathology that interferes with normal renal function can have major systemic effects by upsetting this optimal internal environment. For this reason, kidney disorders often result in systemic effects.

External kidney anatomy

The kidneys are bean-shaped organs positioned laterally, one on each side of the vertebral column, between vertebrae T12 and L3. Unlike most internal organs, they are positioned retroperitoneally (behind the peritoneal membrane), with the left kidney positioned slightly superior to the right (Figure 11.1).

Each kidney typically weighs between 115 and 175 grams and is around 12 cm long and 6 cm wide (as with the heart, in the average person the kidneys are roughly equivalent in size to the individual's clenched fist). The renal blood vessels, nerves, lymphatics and ureter enter and leave through a medial indentation termed the hilum.

Renal blood supply

Renal arteries

The renal arteries branch off the abdominal aorta and supply the kidneys with around one quarter of the total cardiac output. Although the kidneys are relatively small in terms of total mass and only account for about 1 per cent of the total body weight, they are metabolically very active and receive between 20 and 25 per cent of the cardiac output, which equates to between 1 and 1.1 litres of blood per minute (Kaufman et al., 2019). Blood arriving in the renal arteries is rich in oxygen and contains relatively high concentrations of the major nitrogenous waste products. The right renal artery is usually slightly longer in length than the left because of the more inferior position of the right kidney. The kidneys are such vascular organs that any mechanical damage (e.g. renal calculi or tumours) usually leads to the presence of blood in the urine.

Renal vein

The renal veins drain blood from the kidneys. The composition of the blood will have changed significantly from that of the renal artery. The levels of oxygen and nitrogenous waste products will be reduced, while levels of carbon dioxide will be much higher. The renal veins connect directly to the inferior vena cava, which is located on the right side of the body. For this reason, the left renal vein is longer than the right.

Protection of the kidneys

The kidneys are relatively fragile organs and are protected from mechanical trauma by being embedded in a thick layer of adipose tissue termed the renal fat pads. When patients experience sudden weight loss (e.g. anorexia nervosa or the cachexia often experienced in cancer), the support offered by the perirenal fat is diminished, and the kidneys may slip to a lower position (renal ptosis). This can potentially lead to post-renal failure if the ureters develop kinks or torsions, which impede the drainage of urine from the kidneys.

Other conditions that might cause obstruction leading to post-renal failure include tumours, stones and an enlarged prostate gland either due to prostatic cancer or benign prostatic hyperplasia. To understand how prostatic hyperplasia typically presents in clinical practice, read through Ali's case study.

Case study: Ali – benign prostatic hyperplasia

Ali is a 69-year-old man who has experienced difficulty with urination for several months. He often has to wait for several minutes before he can start urinating and has a poor stream. After urinating, Ali often feels that his bladder isn't completely empty, and as a result of this, he finds himself feeling the urge to urinate more frequently than before. He is otherwise fit and well.

At first, Ali tolerated this situation, assuming that it was an inevitable part of ageing, until one day he found that he could not urinate at all and throughout the day he became increasingly uncomfortable and developed severe abdominal pain. When catheterised, 900 ml of clear urine drained, and he was diagnosed with benign prostatic hyperplasia.

Internal kidney anatomy and histology

Each kidney is afforded further protection by a thin layer of fibrous connective tissue termed the renal capsule. This is a transparent membrane that surrounds each kidney and delineates the organ from its surrounding structures (Figure 11.2). In addition to affording mechanical protection, the renal capsule forms a physical barrier that helps to ensure that any pathogens causing kidney infections do not spread easily into the neighbouring tissues.

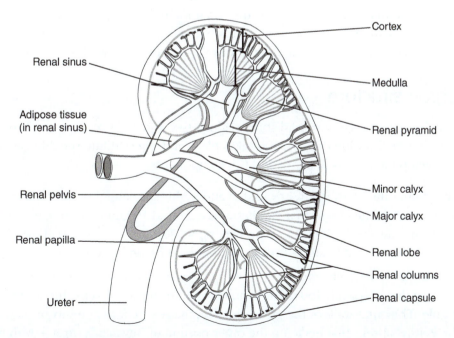

Figure 11.2 Gross renal structure

Beneath the renal capsule, each kidney has three distinct regions. The renal cortex forms the outer region of the kidney and is typically a pale-red colour and often has an uneven, grainy appearance (due mainly to the high density of renal corpuscles located in this region). The renal medulla forms the middle of the kidney. It has a darker rusty-brown appearance and is lobular in nature with prominent triangular cones referred to as renal pyramids; this area of the kidney corresponds to the positions of the densely packed loops of Henle of each nephron.

The renal pelvis is the innermost portion of the kidney where urine collects. It is a hollow branching chamber that is continuous with the ureters. The visible branches are formed by two or more major calyces, which themselves subdivide into minor calyces which continually drain urine from the proximity of the collecting ducts.

The nephron

Nephrons are the basic structural and functional units of the kidney that are responsible for the production of urine. The term nephron comes from the Greek word 'nephros', meaning kidney. In a healthy young adult, it has been estimated that there are on average around 800,000 of these functional units in each kidney (Charlton and Abitbol, 2016), although their numbers decline significantly with age.

There are two major types of nephron. The vast majority (around 80–85 per cent) are termed cortical nephrons because most of their structure is located within the renal cortex. These produce the bulk of the filtrate within the kidneys. The remaining nephrons (15–20 per cent) are termed juxtamedullary nephrons because of their location at the border of the renal cortex and medulla. Juxtamedullary nephrons have loops of Henle that extend deep into the renal medulla and play an essential role in maintaining a high osmotic potential in this region, which facilitates the re-absorption of water and concentration of filtrate in the cortical nephrons (see below).

Nephron structure

Each nephron consists of several distinct regions (see Figure 11.3). The renal corpuscle is the site where filtration of the blood takes place and where dilute renal filtrate is produced. Each renal corpuscle consists of two components:

The glomerulus: This is a tightly folded and highly specialised blood capillary cluster (tuft). The glomerular capillaries are around 100 times more permeable to water and dissolved solutes than capillary networks found in other regions of the body; this ensures efficient filtration and minimal frictional resistance.

Bowman's capsule: The glomerulus sits in a cup-shaped structure termed Bowman's capsule; this is typically 150 nm in diameter and forms the first portion of the renal tubule. The outer walls of the glomerular capillaries are intimately associated with the epithelial cells that make up the outer portion of Bowman's capsule with the two separated by a thin basement membrane.

Bowman's capsule narrows into the proximal convoluted tubule which consists of 12–24 mm of tightly folded tubule. The walls are composed of cuboidal epithelial cells with densely packed microvilli on their inner (luminal) surface. These serve to greatly increase the surface area available for the re-absorption of solutes and concentration of the filtrate.

The loop of Henle is the U-shaped segment of the nephron. It extends directly from the proximal convoluted tubule and is typically around 20 mm long. It consists of a descending limb which extends into the renal medulla before there is a sharp (hairpin) bend, whereupon an ascending limb emerges from the region of the renal cortex. The walls of this portion of the renal tubule are again composed of cuboidal epithelial cells but display reduced numbers of microvilli compared to the proximal convoluted tubule.

The distal convoluted tubule forms the final region of the nephron and follows on directly from the ascending limb of the loop of Henle, typically spanning a distance of 4–8 mm before connecting directly to a collecting duct. The distal convoluted tubule is again composed predominantly of cuboidal epithelial cells, except at the point where the tubule comes into the proximity of the glomerulus. Here the cells have a columnar appearance and form a structure termed the macula densa, which is part of the juxtaglomerular apparatus (see below). Collecting ducts collect concentrated filtrate from several nephrons before draining into the renal calices.

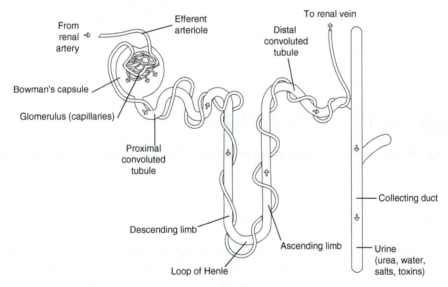

Figure 11.3   Nephron structure and peritubular blood vessels

Blood supply to the nephron

Each glomerulus is supplied with blood under high pressure from an afferent renal arteriole (see Figure 11.3). Following the process of filtration, the blood leaving the glomerulus via the efferent arterioles will be more concentrated and exert a strong osmotic pull, which aids the concentration of filtrate in subsequent portions of the nephron. The efferent arterioles branch to form a peritubular capillary network which surrounds and envelopes the proximal and distal convoluted tubules.

These peritubular capillaries branch further and extend down into the renal medulla, forming the vasa recta, which surrounds the loop of Henle. The peritubular capillaries and vasa recta connect to small venules which eventually connect up with interlobular veins to drain filtered blood into the renal veins.

The formation of urine

The initial filtrate formed in the renal corpuscle is virtually identical in chemical composition to the plasma, with the exception that it normally will not contain any of the large, high-molecular-weight plasma proteins. The presence of proteins in the filtrate in any more than trace amounts is usually the result of physical damage to the filtration membranes and is seen in a variety of kidney diseases and renal failure. The crude filtrate produced within the renal corpuscle is very dilute, and a healthy adult will produce about 180 litres per day (Kaufman et al., 2019).

The remaining regions of the nephron are dedicated to concentrating the filtrate and adjusting its chemical composition. An adult would normally produce between 1 and 2 litres of this concentrated filtrate per day, indicating that the nephrons can concentrate this crude filtrate by a factor of over 100. When this concentrated filtrate drains away from the nephron into the collecting ducts and on into the renal pelvis, it is referred to as urine.

Stages of urine production

Urine is formed by three physiological processes: filtration, tubular re-absorption, and secretion.

Filtration

Blood arrives at the glomerulus with a pressure of around 55 mmHg. The capillary walls that make up the glomerulus are fenestrated (they contain prominent pores), and fluid that is driven out under hydrostatic pressure through these pores collects in Bowman's capsule. The blood that has undergone filtration then passes into the efferent arterioles and into the peritubular capillaries and vasa recta that envelope the remaining portions of the nephron.

During the process of filtration small molecules such as water, sugars, hormones and nitrogenous wastes such as urea and uric acid pass freely into Bowman's capsule, but the size of the fenestrations and nature of the filtration membrane limit the passage of molecules larger than 5 nm, and exclude completely the passage of molecules larger than 8 nm. For this reason, in the absence of pathology, large molecules such as albumin and other plasma proteins are not usually observed in the urine.

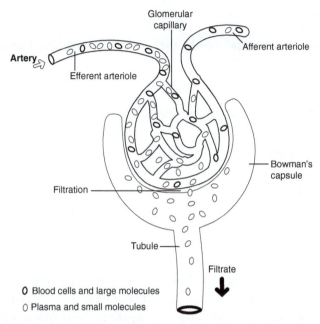

Figure 11.4 The renal corpuscle and glomerular filtration

Glomerular filtration rate (GFR)

This is the volume of filtrate formed per minute by both kidneys. In health, a typical adult has a GFR of 120–125 ml/minute. The kidneys have evolved elaborate mechanisms for maintaining a relatively constant GFR (see juxtaglomerular apparatus below).

The GFR is a very useful diagnostic tool in medicine as it can be affected by many clinically significant factors including dehydration, diabetes, recurring urinary tract infections, hypertension, heart disease, kidney stones, polycystic kidney disease, kidney failure and some medications. For more information on the use of GFR in assessing renal function, please visit the kidney.org website as indicated at the end of this chapter.

Tubular re-absorption and secretion

Following the production of the crude filtrate within the renal corpuscle, the remaining portions of the nephron are dedicated to concentrating the filtrate down to around 1 per cent of its original volume and modifying its chemical composition (see Figure 11.4).

Re-absorption in the proximal convoluted tubule

The filtrate passes directly from Bowman's capsule into the proximal convoluted tubule. Here the abundance of microvilli on the luminal surface affords a vastly increased surface area for the re-absorption of useful materials from the filtrate; for this reason, the proximal convoluted tubule is the region where most tubular re-absorption takes place.

Materials re-absorbed from the crude filtrate in the proximal convoluted tubule include:

- 65 per cent water content;
- 65 per cent sodium (Na^+) and potassium (K^+);
- 100 per cent glucose;
- 100 per cent amino acids;
- 50 per cent chloride (Cl^-);
- 85 per cent bicarbonate (HCO_3^-);
- variable amounts of calcium (Ca^{++}), magnesium (Mg^+), phosphate (HPO_4^-) and hydrogen ions (H^+);
- variable amounts of peptide and steroid hormones.

It is the re-absorption of the major solutes above that facilitates the re-absorption of water and progressive concentration of the filtrate. Along the length of the proximal convoluted tubule ions such as sodium and potassium are re-absorbed by active transport. This increases the osmotic potential of the blood in the peritubular capillaries and vasa recta, inducing the movement of water from the tubule back into the blood by osmosis. This type of water re-absorption is often referred to as obligatory water re-absorption because the increased concentration of solutes in the peritubular capillaries and vasa recta obliges the movement of water by osmosis.

Fructose, galactose and a variety of low-molecular-weight peptides are also re-absorbed back into the peritubular circulation via a combination of facilitated diffusion and active transport. These also contribute to increasing the osmotic potential of the blood, inducing further obligatory water re-absorption.

Re-absorption in the loop of Henle

The descending limb of the loop of Henle is highly permeable to water. The peritubular capillaries and the interstitial fluid within the renal medulla contain very high concentrations of sodium, chloride and urea. As the descending limb passes down into the medulla, further water is obligated to leave the tubule by osmosis. By the time the filtrate begins to travel up the ascending limb, typically a further 15 per cent of its water volume will have been re-absorbed and the filtrate will be isotonic to the concentrated interstitial fluid of the renal medulla.

Unlike the descending limb, the ascending limb is impermeable to water. It is primarily a region where salts (electrolytes) can be re-absorbed from the filtrate back into the blood. Here, positively charged sodium ions are actively pumped out of the tubule into the interstitial fluid and the capillaries of the vasa recta. Chloride ions that are negatively charged will follow via secondary active transport.

This movement ensures that the high concentration of electrolytes in the renal medulla is always maintained, ensuring efficient water re-absorption in the descending limb. Since the fluid travels up the ascending limb in the opposite direction to the descending limb, this is often referred to as a countercurrent mechanism. The removal of large amounts of sodium and chloride actually serves to dilute the filtrate, so by the time it arrives at the distal convoluted tubule, its concentration is below that of the interstitial fluid within the renal cortex.

Re-absorption in the distal convoluted tubule and collecting duct

The distal convoluted tubule and collecting duct are the locations where, under the control of hormones (see below), the composition and volume of the filtrate (and hence the blood plasma) are fine-tuned to meet the current physiological requirements of the body.

Typically, a further 19 per cent of the filtrate volume is re-absorbed within the distal tubule and collecting duct, leaving around 1 per cent of the original volume of the crude filtrate. Additionally, varying amounts of sodium and chloride are re-absorbed within the distal tubule.

Fine-tuning of urine volume, concentration and composition

Antidiuretic hormone (ADH)

As we have examined in Chapter 5, ADH is produced in the hypothalamus and stored and concentrated in the posterior pituitary gland. Any drop in blood pressure is detected by the aortic arch and carotid sinus baroreceptors (Chapter 3), which signal the rapid release of ADH into the blood. ADH is also released when the osmoreceptors of the hypothalamus detect an increase in blood concentration (osmolarity).

A common example of this is when a patient is dehydrated. Again, this is a perfect physiological adaptation since increased water re-absorption in the kidney will help dilute the blood and normalise the blood concentration.

ADH mechanism of action

The distal convoluted tubule and collecting duct are the regions of the nephron that ultimately determine the volume and concentration of urine produced. The tubular cells of these regions contain a group of specialised water-transporting proteins termed aquaporins. As the name implies, aquaporins function as simple water channels which allow water to flood out of these regions of the nephron back into the blood (Brown, 2017).

When ADH is released, it binds to receptors on the surface of the cells of the distal convoluted tubule and collecting duct, increasing the number of aquaporins within these regions. This increases the permeability of the distal convoluted tubule and allows more water to move out of the filtrate into the peritubular capillaries. ADH therefore has the effect of reducing the amount of urine produced (hence the term antidiuretic), and leads to a smaller volume of more concentrated urine.

Conversely, because more water is moving back into the blood, the concentration of the blood is diluted and the blood volume increases, which leads to an increase in mean arterial pressure. Effectively, ADH increases blood volume and pressure at the expense of urine volume. The effects of ADH are often noted in the different seasons.

In the summer months, when the weather is often hot, more water is lost through evaporation of sweat from the skin. This leads to an increase in plasma osmolarity, which stimulates the release of ADH and the production of darker, more concentrated urine. The opposite is often seen in the colder months of winter where sweating is reduced, and more dilute urine can be produced without risk of dehydration.

Atrial natriuretic peptide (ANP)

ANP is released by the cardiac muscle cells of the atria when there is an increased return of blood to the heart. In many ways, ANP can be regarded as the natural antagonist of ADH because, as its name implies, its major function is to induce diuresis, which reduces blood volume and pressure.

ANP achieves this via three major mechanisms: (1) inducing vasodilation in the kidney, increasing renal blood flow to the glomeruli and elevating the glomerular filtration rate; (2) inhibiting the release of ADH secretion by the posterior pituitary gland; (3) inhibiting the release of aldosterone by the adrenal cortex, which reduces the amount of blood sodium and the osmotic potential of the blood.

The juxtaglomerular apparatus

The juxtaglomerular apparatus is a specialised area of the nephron, which plays a vital role in regulating blood pressure and the glomerular filtration rate. It consists of two major regions. At the point where the distal convoluted tubule comes into the close proximity of the glomerulus, the cuboidal cells, which form the wall of the tubule, elongate and take on a columnar appearance. This area is termed the macula densa (dense spot) and is extremely sensitive to changes in the concentration of sodium chloride within the filtrate.

When the glomerular filtration rate drops, the filtrate inside the tubule travels more slowly, allowing more sodium chloride to be re-absorbed into the peritubular blood vessels. The reduced concentration of sodium chloride within the filtrate is detected by the cells of the macula densa, which release paracrine (locally acting) signalling molecules such as prostaglandins and nitric oxide. These dilate the afferent arterioles supplying each glomerulus, increasing blood flow and the glomerular filtration rate.

The afferent arterioles that supply blood to each glomerulus contain granular cells which synthesise and store the enzyme renin. When blood pressure falls, these cells release their renin stores, activating the renin-angiotensin aldosterone system to restore blood pressure.

The renin-angiotensin aldosterone system (RAAS)

Often referred to as the renin-angiotensin aldosterone cascade or mechanism, the RAAS provides a powerful mechanism for regulating blood pressure and fluid balance within the human body. The RAAS is triggered when there is a drop in blood pressure. The granular cells of the juxtaglomerular apparatus continually synthesise and accumulate the enzyme renin.

When blood pressure within the afferent and efferent arterioles of the glomerulus falls, the pressure-sensitive granular cells release their stored renin into the blood (see Chapter 3 for a full overview of this pathway).

Tubular secretion

Some potentially toxic substances can be removed directly from the blood within the peritubular circulation by secretion into the kidney tubules. These include nitrogenous wastes such as ammonia which diffuses rapidly across the walls of the kidney tubules. Other molecules actively excreted include potassium, creatinine and many toxic metabolites produced by the liver during drug metabolism.

The tubular secretion of hydrogen ions provides an important mechanism for controlling the pH of the blood. Although the respiratory system can influence the pH of the blood by controlling the amount of carbon dioxide in the blood, only the kidneys can excrete acids directly and are ultimately the most important organs in acid/base balance.

Because of its complex physiology, the urinary system is one of the areas that many nursing students struggle with during assessments and in clinical practice. To help consolidate and reinforce what you have learnt so far in this chapter, attempt Activity 11.1.

Activity 11.1   Evidence-based practice and research

On a piece of blank paper, draw a simple diagram of a nephron and label the major regions.

On this diagram, identify:

- the location where filtration takes place;
- the region where glucose and amino acids are re-absorbed back into the blood;
- the regions where the hormone ADH exerts its effects.

There are some possible answers to all activities at the end of the chapter, unless otherwise indicated.

Now that you have examined the production of urine in some detail, we will examine how urine is stored and eliminated from the body.

The collecting ducts and renal pelvis

Each distal convoluted tubule connects up with a collecting duct which drains several neighbouring nephrons. The collecting ducts are also sensitive to the effects of ADH and aldosterone, allowing final adjustments to the filtrate composition and volume to take place. When filtrate leaves the collecting ducts, its chemical composition and volume cannot be further altered, and at this stage the fluid is referred to as urine. Each collecting duct drains via the branching renal calices into the renal pelvis of each kidney, which are continuous with the ureters.

Ureters

Each renal pelvis has a smooth muscle component which undergoes rhythmical contractions (under the control of the autonomic nervous system). These contractions aid the flow of urine into the ureters and ensure continual drainage of the collecting ducts. The ureters are muscular tubes approximately 20–30 cm long, connecting the renal pelvis of each kidney to the urinary bladder (Figure 11.1).

Each ureter is lined by transitional epithelium (identical to that found lining the bladder). This stratified epithelium is elastic, allowing expansion of each ureter to accommodate increased urine flow and allowing contraction of the muscular wall. The smooth muscle of the renal pelvis is continuous along the length of each ureter and contracts in peristaltic waves, ensuring urine is drained away from the kidneys even when the body is in a supine position.

The urinary bladder

Each ureter opens directly into the urinary bladder (Figure 11.5). The urinary bladder is positioned inside the pelvic cavity beneath the peritoneal membrane. It is roughly a spherical distensible sac composed predominantly of a thick layer of smooth muscle lined by an elastic transitional epithelium. In addition to providing a stretchable inner lining, the transitional epithelium that lines the bladder is impermeable to salts and water, ensuring that the stored urine undergoes no further modification in terms of composition or volume prior to elimination.

The outer portion of the bladder is covered by a serous membrane which secretes a thin, watery (serous) fluid that reduces any friction between a replete bladder and the surrounding organs and tissues. The human bladder varies in size but typically has a capacity of 400–600 ml (Hoffman, 2018). The wall of the bladder is lined by sensitive stretch receptors which continually monitor the current volume of urine stored. These receptors are not activated by small amounts of urine, but when the volume reaches around 150 ml, the receptors are stimulated, and action potentials are generated and travel via pelvic nerves to the base of the spinal cord.

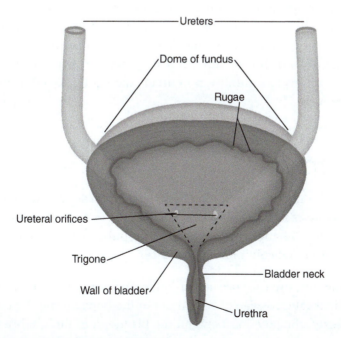

Figure 11.5 The ureters and urinary bladder

These nerve impulses are relayed to the conscious areas of the brain and are perceived as a sensation of fullness, which elicits the urge to micturate (pass urine). When the volume approaches around 80 per cent of the maximal bladder volume, the urge to micturate becomes urgent and is often perceived as an unpleasant, even painful sensation.

Micturition

The process of micturition is normally under conscious control. The opening of the bladder leading to the urethra is surrounded by two ring-like sphincter muscles. The internal urinary sphincter is actually a continuation of the smooth muscle wall of the bladder and is not under direct conscious control. This internal sphincter is innervated with nerves of the parasympathetic branch of the autonomic nervous system.

The external urinary sphincter is composed of striated (skeletal) muscle and is innervated by somatic motor nerves. As with all striated muscles, this outer sphincter is under direct conscious control. When a person becomes aware of a full bladder, the outer urinary sphincter can be relaxed to initiate the process of micturition. The dilation of the external urinary sphincter induces waves of contraction within the walls of the bladder, increasing the pressure within and opening the internal urinary sphincter. This initiates a flow of urine out of the bladder through the urethra. Although the process of micturition is normally under conscious control, if a person chooses (perhaps because of a lack of available facilities or social constraints) to hold onto their urine volume, the bladder will continue to fill.

If the urine volume increases towards the maximum capacity of the bladder, the urge to micturate will become irresistible, and the contents of the bladder will be voided. This is a safety mechanism that has evolved to prevent structural damage to the lining and walls of the bladder and ultimately to prevent the bladder from rupturing. It also serves to minimise potentially damaging backflow of urine up the ureters to the kidneys.

The urethra

The urethra is a thin muscular tube that connects the bladder to the external environment. Its lining consists of transitional epithelium in the portion immediately adjacent to the bladder before changing appearance at around the mid-point, whereupon it takes on a classic stratified columnar appearance.

In women, its sole purpose is to provide an outlet for urine. In men, in addition to this role, it also facilitates the passage of semen out of the body during the process of ejaculation. In both sexes, the junction between the bladder and the urethra is marked by a thin ring of smooth muscle termed the urethral sphincter. Unless micturition is taking place, this sphincter is kept tightly closed to prevent urine leaking from the bladder as the internal pressure builds up between episodes of micturition. Prior to entering the urethra, urine is usually a sterile fluid that is relatively odourless.

The urethra is colonised by a variety of microorganisms, particularly Gram-negative facultative anaerobic bacteria such as various species of proteus. These microorganisms can rapidly metabolise urea, leading to the release of pungent ammonia gas and a variety of other odours associated with urine.

The female urethra

In females, the urethra is a relatively short structure between 3 and 4 cm in length. This opens out into the vestibule through the external urethral opening which is typically located midway between the clitoris and the opening of the vagina. The relatively short length of the female urethra predisposes women to more frequent urinary tract infections compared to men. For a common clinical presentation, read through Diane's case study.

Case study: Diane – urinary tract infection (UTI)

Diane is a 23-year-old, sexually active woman who had a 24-hour history of urinary frequency, burning, urgency and lower back pain. She noticed some blood in her urine which alarmed her so much that she attended her local Emergency Department. On admission, Diane's pulse and blood pressure were normal, although her temperature was slightly raised at 37.7°C. The triage nurse suspected a urinary tract infection and so asked Diane for a specimen of urine. Routine urinalysis revealed protein+, leukocytes++ and blood++, and a pH of 5.6. A mid-stream urine (MSU) was requested for microscopy, culture and sensitivity.

Microscopy confirmed the presence of Gram-negative bacteria, which in conjunction with the presenting symptoms confirmed the diagnosis of urinary tract infection. Diane was prescribed a course of trimethoprim and discharged home. Two days later, the bacterium in Diane's urine was identified as *Escherichia coli* (*E. coli*), which was found to be sensitive to trimethoprim. No further action was required.

As we have just seen with Diane, the relatively short length of the female urethra can allow motile bacteria such as *E. coli* access to the bladder. We will now examine the structure of the male urethra.

The male urethra

The urethra is a much longer structure in men at around 18–20 cm long. It has three recognisable regions. The first portion is termed the prostatic urethra because it passes through and is surrounded by the prostate gland.

In many men, as they pass into their 40s and beyond, there is a gradual increase in the size of the prostate gland. This is referred to as benign prostatic hyperplasia and while (as the name implies) it is generally a harmless condition, the gradual increase in prostate mass can compress the prostatic urethra, diminishing its diameter and reducing the urine stream. This can make passing urine difficult and elicit symptoms that are almost identical to the early symptoms of prostate cancer.

The second portion of the male urethra is termed the membranous urethra and passes through the muscular floor of the pelvic cavity (the urogenital diaphragm) into the superior portion of the penis. The remaining portion of the male urethra is termed the spongy or penile urethra and extends the length of the penis before exiting through the external urethral opening at the tip of the glans penis. Hospitalised patients, particularly those who are confined to bed, often have to be catheterised. To help you reflect on why this may be necessary, attempt Activity 11.2.

Activity 11.2   Reflection

Urinary tract infection is the most common complication of urethral catheterisation. Reflect on an occasion when you have cared for a patient with an indwelling urinary catheter and consider why this is the case.

Now that we have examined how urine is produced and eliminated from the body, we can examine the composition of this body fluid and highlight its use in clinical diagnosis.

Normal urine composition

Urine is normally a sterile aqueous solution with water accounting for roughly 95 per cent of its volume.

The solutes dissolved in this water account for the remaining 5 per cent of urine volume and include:

- urea, 9.3 g per litre;
- chloride, 1.87 g per litre;
- sodium, 1.7 g per litre;
- potassium, 0.75 g per litre;
- creatinine, 0.67 g per litre.

Unlike taking blood, which is an invasive process, analysis of urine samples using chemically reactive diagnostic strips (urinalysis strips) allows a multitude of diagnostic criteria to be gathered quickly (see Table 11.2 for common urine abnormalities). Patients such as those with diabetes mellitus can also check their renal health at home following minimal training.

Table 11.2 Common urine abnormalities

Abnormality	Potential cause
Glycosuria (presence of sugar/glucose in the urine)	Since most glucose is re-absorbed from the urine in the proximal convoluted tubule, a healthy urine sample should not contain more than 0.1–0.3 g per litre. The presence of larger amounts is referred to as glycosuria and usually indicates very high levels of glucose in the blood. This is commonly seen in patients with diabetes where a lack of insulin or an insensitivity to the effects of insulin prevents cells and tissues absorbing glucose from the blood. The filtrate produced in the nephrons of patients with diabetes is therefore extremely rich in glucose, overburdening the normal mechanisms of glucose re-absorption in the proximal convoluted tubule. This glucose-rich filtrate exerts a strong osmotic pull on the blood in the surrounding peritubular capillaries and vasa recta, resulting in large volumes of water moving into the nephrons by osmosis. For this reason, patients with diabetes often experience polyuria (production of large amounts of urine) and glycosuria together. If a healthy individual eats a large amount of refined carbohydrate (for example, a large bar of chocolate in a single sitting), the blood sugar level will rise dramatically. If plasma glucose exceeds the normal renal threshold of between 10 and 12 mmol, so much glucose will appear in the filtrate that the re-absorption mechanisms of the proximal tubule are overwhelmed, resulting in some of this glucose over-spilling and appearing in the urine. Some individuals have a low renal threshold for glucose and will show glycosuria even when normal amounts of carbohydrates are consumed. Positive urine glucose tests in these patients are followed up by a blood glucose test, which will confirm whether they have diabetes
Haematuria (presence of blood in urine)	The filtration membranes within the renal corpuscle do not permit the passage of blood cells into the filtrate. Haematuria commonly follows any kind of mechanical damage to the kidney. This includes trauma (e.g. from road traffic collisions or sporting injury), the presence and growth of renal calculi (kidney stones) or tumours. The kidneys are such vascular organs that even minor disruptions to the kidney structure caused by the early stages of tumour formation will lead to detectable haematuria and thus provide an early indication of potential renal malignancies. Similarly, blood is often detected in the urine when malignancies affect other areas of the urogenital tract, including the ureters, bladder and prostate gland. Often leukocytes (white blood cells) are found without the presence of erythrocytes (red cells). This often indicates the presence of pus in the urine (pyuria), which is commonly observed in a variety of urinary tract infections
Ketonuria (presence of ketone bodies in the urine)	Ketone bodies are produced during the metabolism of fatty acids and include aromatic molecules such as acetone. These rapidly cross the filtration membranes and often give the urine a characteristic fruity aroma (often described as smelling like pear drops or nail varnish remover). Ketonuria indicates that relatively large amounts of fat are being mobilised and utilised within the body and is commonly seen in patients with type I diabetes who, because of a lack of insulin, can no longer utilise the preferred energy substrate glucose. In such patients, these ketones often cannot be removed from the body quickly enough and accumulate in the blood, leading to potentially fatal ketoacidosis. Ketonuria can be present in the absence of any pathology and is commonly seen in individuals who follow low-calorie or low-carbohydrate-type diets (e.g. the Atkins diet). Similarly, eating disorders such as anorexia nervosa or bulimia often lead to ketonuria

(Continued)

Table 11.2 (Continued)

Abnormality	Potential cause
Proteinuria (presence of protein in the urine)	Proteins are such large molecules that they do not usually cross the filtration membranes of the renal corpuscle. However, many diseases such as hypertension and diabetic nephropathies damage these delicate membranes, allowing the passage of even large proteins into the filtrate and urine. Some urinary tract infections, particularly kidney infections, also lead to the presence of detectable amounts of protein in the urine. False positives for proteinuria are often seen in menstruating women and in both women and men following sexual intercourse (semen is very rich in protein). These false positives can be reduced by ensuring urine samples are collected mid-stream

Now that you have completed the chapter, attempt the multiple-choice questions in Activity 11.3 to assess your understanding of the subject material.

Activity 11.3   Multiple-choice questions

1. What proportion of the cardiac output is directed to the kidneys?

   a) 5–10 per cent
   b) 10–15 per cent
   c) 30–40 per cent
   d) 20–25 per cent

2. The left renal vein is longer than the right because

   a) It is located at the base of the kidney
   b) It connects to the inferior vena cava
   c) It connects to the superior vena cava
   d) It allows absorption of additional water

3. The outer region of the kidney is the

   a) Renal cortex
   b) Renal medulla
   c) Renal pelvis
   d) Nephron

4. Which of these is not a stage in urine formation?

   a) Filtration

   b) Tubular re-absorption

   c) Secretion

   d) Egestion

5. What proportion of water is re-absorbed in the proximal convoluted tubule?

   a) 45 per cent

   b) 55 per cent

   c) 65 per cent

   d) 75 per cent

6. The renal corpuscle consists of

   a) The glomerulus and proximal convoluted tubule

   b) The proximal convoluted tubule and collecting duct

   c) The loop of Henle and collecting duct

   d) The glomerulus and Bowman's capsule

7. The juxtaglomerular apparatus is responsible for regulating

   a) Blood pressure and GFR

   b) GFR and concentrations of Cl^- ions

   c) Plasma glucose concentrations

   d) Plasma pH

8. The tubular secretion of what ion is responsible for controlling the pH of blood?

   a) Na^+

   b) Cl^-

   c) K^+

   d) H^+

(Continued)

(Continued)

9. Which of these statements about the urethra is incorrect?

    a) The function of the urethra in both sexes is solely to provide an outlet for urine

    b) The junction between the bladder and urethra is marked by the urethral sphincter

    c) Prior to entering the urethra, urine is sterile

    d) The urethra is colonised by a variety of microorganisms

10. The presence of pus in urine is called

    a) Pyrexia

    b) Pyuria

    c) Pyaemia

    d) Pyometra

Chapter summary

The urinary system is primarily responsible for the elimination of metabolic waste products, particularly nitrogenous wastes such as urea. The kidneys contain filtration units called nephrons in which a dilute filtrate is produced and then concentrated into an amber-coloured fluid termed urine. The production and composition of urine is regulated by several hormones including antidiuretic hormone, atrial natriuretic peptide and aldosterone.

Urine leaves the kidneys via tubes termed ureters and is collected into a distensible urinary bladder prior to elimination through the urethra. The kidneys also play an important role in regulating the pH of the blood (acid-base balance), controlling blood pressure, producing vitamin D and regulating the production of erythrocytes.

Activities: Brief outline answers

Activity 11.1: Evidence-based practice and research (page 312)

You should have drawn a simple diagram of a nephron in line with Figure 11.3 in this book, ideally labelling the glomerulus, Bowman's capsule, the proximal tubule, the loop of Henle, the distal tubule and the collecting duct.

The glomerulus and Bowman's capsule (renal corpuscle) should have been identified as the region where filtration takes place. The proximal tubule should have been identified as the region where glucose and amino acids are re-absorbed and the distal tubule and collecting duct identified as the sites where ADH exerts its effects.

Activity 11.2: Reflection (page 316)

Microorganisms in the lower urethra are flushed away during micturition before they can ascend into the bladder, ureters and kidneys, thereby reducing the risk of urinary tract infection. This flushing action does not take place when an indwelling catheter is present, and it is common for organisms to either ascend the catheter into the bladder or adhere to the surface of the catheter.

Organisms that are capable of producing biofilms, e.g. *Proteus sp.*, easily colonise the catheter surface and commonly cause urine infections. The biofilms protect the organisms from antibiotics, making infections difficult to treat. The perineal area should be kept clean. However, no special meatal care is recommended. The size of the catheter can also influence the occurrence of infection. A catheter with a large lumen is likely to result in a more traumatic insertion than a narrower catheter, predisposing the patient to infection.

Catheterisation should only be undertaken if absolutely necessary, and catheters should be inserted under aseptic conditions. The balloon securing the catheter in place should be as small as possible to both retain the catheter and minimise the volume of residual urine in the bladder. The holes in the catheter that allow urine to drain are situated above the balloon. The larger the balloon, the larger the volume of urine that cannot drain out of the bladder. This residual urine frequently becomes contaminated, resulting in infection. The connection between the catheter and the drainage tubing must be secure, and the drainage port of the catheter bag must not be excessively handled.

Bags should be emptied only when necessary. Good hand hygiene techniques should be employed whenever the system is handled. The catheter should be removed as soon as possible.

Activity 11.3: Multiple-choice questions (pages 318–20)

1) d, 2) b, 3) a, 4) d, 5) c, 6) d, 7) a, 8) d, 9) a, 10) b

Further reading

Boore J et al. (2016) Chapter 11: The renal system – Fluid, electrolyte and acid-base balance, in *Essentials of Anatomy and Physiology for Nursing Practice.* London: SAGE Publications Ltd.

A textbook to develop your knowledge of human anatomy and physiology that is aimed specifically at nurses.

Tortora G and Derrickson B (2017) *Tortora's Principles of Anatomy and Physiology* (15th edition). New York: John Wiley & Sons.

In-depth coverage of human anatomy and physiology.

Useful websites

www.kidney.org/news/kidneyCare/summer09/gfr

An overview of glomerular filtration rate (GFR).

www.nhs.uk/conditions/kidney-disease

An overview of renal disease.

www.nhs.uk/conditions/kidney-stones

An overview of the nature of kidney stones.

Chapter 12 The reproductive systems

Chapter aims

After reading this chapter, you will be able to:

- describe the major anatomical structures of the male and female reproductive tracts;
- explain the processes of spermatogenesis and oogenesis;
- describe the stages of the menstrual cycle;
- highlight the role of the major sex hormones on human physiology;
- provide an overview of some of the common pathologies that affect the reproductive systems.

Introduction

Case study: Ahmed – prostate cancer

Ahmed visited his GP a month ago on the insistence of his wife, who had been worried about his constant visits to the toilet. Ahmed has noticed for the last couple of years that it has become increasingly difficult to urinate and has noticed a weakening in his urine stream which has progressively reduced to a trickle. More worryingly, for the last few weeks passing urine has become painful with a burning sensation, and Ahmed is having to strain to produce a urine stream.

During a digital rectal exam, Ahmed's GP noted a hard, palpable, nodular mass and arranged for a blood sample to be collected which revealed elevated levels of prostate-specific antigen (PSA). Ahmed was referred to the urology clinic and, following an endorectal ultrasound scan and 12-core needle biopsy, received a diagnosis of stage II prostate cancer for which he is currently receiving treatment.

Introduction

As well as facilitating the process of human reproduction, the male and female reproductive tracts produce a variety of sex hormones including testosterone, oestrogen and progesterone, which play diverse roles in human physiology. This chapter will begin by exploring the anatomy and physiology of the male reproductive tract, including the role of the testes in spermatogenesis (production of sperm) and testosterone synthesis.

We will then explore the anatomy and physiology of the female reproductive tract, including the processes of oogenesis (production of ova) and the synthesis of oestrogen and progesterone within the ovaries. Finally, we will examine the phases of the menstrual cycle and its influences on female physiology. Throughout the chapter, some common examples of pathologies that affect the reproductive tracts will be explored.

The male reproductive tract

The male reproductive tract (Figure 12.1) consists of several organs and glands and is intimately associated with the urinary tract. The primary male reproductive organs are the testes which are located outside the major body cavities and therefore lack the protection afforded most other major organs. During prenatal development the testes descend from the abdominopelvic cavity along the inguinal canal into a specialised pouch of skin called the scrotum.

This external location of the testes is essential since, for efficient spermatogenesis, the testes need to be maintained at around 2°C cooler than the core body temperature. Several accessory glands including the prostate and seminal vesicles produce secretions that form an aqueous medium called semen in which the sperm are suspended. The penis is the male erectile organ of copulation that facilitates the delivery of mature sperm into the female reproductive tract during sexual intercourse.

Structure of the testes

The testes are oval-shaped organs with an internal lobular structure (Figure 12.2). Each lobule is densely packed with highly folded seminiferous tubules which are the site of spermatogenesis. Within the seminiferous tubules are located three major populations of cells dedicated to the production of spermatozoa and the major male sex hormone testosterone (Table 12.1). The seminiferous tubules connect to an outer region of tubes called the epididymis which functions primarily as a region of sperm storage and maturation before ejaculation.

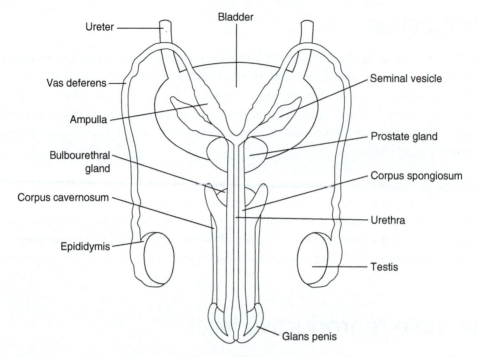

Figure 12.1   Overview of the male reproductive tract

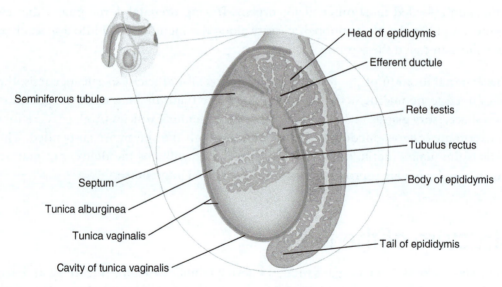

Figure 12.2   Testicular structure

The epididymis of each testicle is connected to the vas deferens, the sperm duct into which sperm are released (Figure 12.1). Each testicle is surrounded by an outer protective capsule of collagen-rich connective tissue called the tunica albuginea.

Table 12.1   Cells of the seminiferous tubules

Cell type	Function
Spermatogonia	The round/oval germinal cells of the testes which are continually dividing by meiosis (Chapter 13) to produce haploid spermatozoa with 23 chromosomes
Sertoli cells (nurse cells)	Large cells that extend into the lumen (interior) of the seminiferous tubule and release nutrients and growth factors which allow differentiation of haploid cells into recognisable spermatozoa
Interstitial cells (cells of Leydig)	Synthesise the major male sex hormone testosterone, which is an anabolic steroid that promotes the development of male secondary sexual characteristics during puberty, promotes muscle growth and helps maintain bone density throughout life. The biosynthesis of testosterone and activity of the interstitial cells is regulated by the hypothalamus and anterior pituitary

The spermatic cords and testicular blood supply

The testes are suspended from the body on string-like structures called spermatic cords. A testicular artery and vein run longitudinally through each cord, forming the blood supply to each testicle. Each cord also contains the vas deferens and a highly sensitive testicular nerve. Running the length of each spermatic cord and enclosing the internal structures is a layer of smooth muscle termed the cremaster. The cremaster muscles play an important role in regulating testicular temperature (see below).

Case study: William – testicular torsion

William is 16 years old and a keen rugby player. One morning, the day after a rugby match, he woke early in the morning with a severe pain in his right testicle. His scrotum was slightly swollen and his right testis seemed to be positioned higher than normal. He felt sick but had no discharge and his temperature was normal. William was subsequently diagnosed on ultrasound examination as having an intravaginal testicular torsion in which the testis (and attached epididymis) was twisted around the spermatic cord. Testicular torsion is an emergency and requires urgent surgery to untwist the affected testis and spermatic cord.

(Continued)

(Continued)

Testicular torsion is often due to a congenital abnormality such as 'bell clapper defor-
mity' in which the testes are not adequately attached to the scrotum, and the chance
of developing a further torsion is higher than average in those who have experienced
the problem before. Therefore, both of William's testes were stitched to the scrotum to
prevent torsion happening again. Fortunately, William's recovery was uneventful but if
torsion is prolonged, i.e. over 6–8 hours, it may not be possible to save the testis. If surgery is not performed within 12 hours of the onset of pain, there is only a 50 per cent
chance of saving the testicle. This drops to 10 per cent after 24 hours.

In William's case study we saw that he experienced testicular pain, but there are many
causes of pain in the pelvic and groin region. Activity 12.1 invites you to explore other
potential causes.

Activity 12.1   Evidence-based practice and research

Before exposing a patient to the risks of surgery, it is important to be as
sure as possible of the diagnosis. What other possible diagnoses should be
excluded before confirming testicular torsion?

*There are some possible answers to all activities at the end of the chapter, unless otherwise
indicated.*

Now that we have explored the susceptibility of the spermatic cords to torsion, we will
examine how they participate in maintaining optimal testicular temperature.

Thermoregulation of the testes

For optimal spermatogenesis to take place, the testes need to be maintained between
32°C and 35°C, which is significantly cooler than core temperature (Durairajanayagam
et al., 2014). The scrotum is formed from a pouch of skin which is lined by a layer of
smooth muscle called the dartos. In a cold environment the dartos muscle contracts,
bunching and gathering the scrotum; simultaneously the cremaster muscles of the
spermatic cords contract. Both these events pull the testes closer to the heat source
provided by the trunk of the body, thereby warming the testes.

In a warm environment the opposite happens: the dartos and cremaster muscles relax,
allowing the scrotum to become flaccid and loose and the testes to drop further away

from the trunk and to cool. These mechanisms are generally very effective at keeping the testicular temperature close to optimum, although the wearing of tight-fitting underwear or outer garments can interfere with these mechanisms.

Although tight clothing may reduce the sperm count, other environmental factors have a much more dramatic effect on male fertility. Explore this further by attempting Activity 12.2.

Activity 12.2   Evidence-based practice and research

Using textbooks or online resources, research the potential causes of the declining male sperm count.

Now that we have explored the role of the testes in spermatogenesis and researched declining male fertility, we will examine the role of the testes as endocrine glands.

Testosterone

Testosterone is the dominant male sex hormone; it is an anabolic steroid which, in addition to regulating spermatogenesis and the male sex drive, is also responsible for the development of secondary male sexual characteristics.

Biosynthesis of testosterone

Testosterone is predominantly produced by the interstitial cells of the testes. As with all steroids, it is synthesised from cholesterol with the rate and quantity of production tightly regulated by negative feedback (Figure 12.3). The hypothalamus is continually monitoring the plasma concentration of testosterone, and as this begins to fall, it releases gonadotropin-releasing hormone (GTRH) which stimulates the anterior pituitary gland to release luteinising hormone (LH). LH is a key hormone in both male and female physiology; in females, it stimulates ovulation and the production of progesterone (see below), while in males its release stimulates the biosynthesis and secretion of testosterone.

Biological roles of testosterone

Testosterone has multiple, diverse effects throughout the human body. Even before birth, testosterone plays a role in the foetus, ensuring that the rudimentary sex organs adopt the characteristic male appearance. When boys reach puberty (typically around the age of

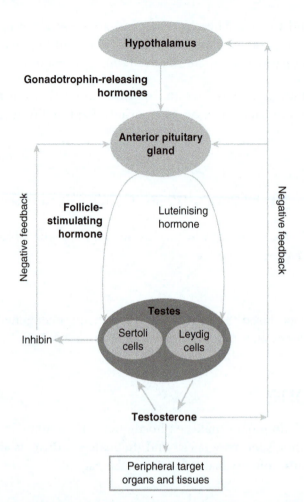

Figure 12.3 Control of testosterone synthesis and release

12 in the UK), testosterone levels increase significantly, resulting in the dramatic physical changes characteristic of adolescence. Testosterone promotes maturation of the testes and penis, which increase in size while driving the process of spermatogenesis.

During puberty, testosterone promotes the expansion of the larynx, resulting in deepening (breaking) of the voice and stimulating the growth of pubic, axial (armpit) and facial hair. Progressive increases in testosterone throughout puberty trigger major structural changes within the brain, with rewiring and development of new neural pathways frequently associated with noticeable changes in behaviour and mood.

Testosterone is also largely responsible for the male libido (sex drive) which is greatest in the teenage years. As the dominant anabolic (to build up) steroid, testosterone is responsible for increasing muscle mass and strength during adolescence and is the major reason why males typically have a higher lean muscle mass and greater physical strength than females. Additionally, testosterone increases bone density and strength, which is essential to cope with increased forces exerted on bones during muscle contraction and to support the increased weight of the average male body.

The andropause

Testosterone levels reach a peak in the teenage years and gradually decrease with age. As testosterone levels fall, testicular mass and rate of spermatogenesis decrease along with libido; together, these effects progressively reduce male fertility. Decreased production of this key anabolic steroid leads to reduced muscle mass and strength and decreases in bone density, which can increase the risk of fracture.

The progressive decrease in testosterone seen in most men as they grow older is frequently referred to as the 'male menopause'. This is an inaccurate term since men cannot experience menopause since they have never had a menstrual cycle, and so the term andropause was introduced to describe this age-related decline in testosterone secretion and its effects.

Testosterone-based hormone replacement therapy (TRT) is available for older males with significant symptoms to help offset some of the effects of the andropause. TRT is available in the form of pills or dermal patches and has been demonstrated to improve reduced libido, fatigue and depression, which are common features of the andropause. However, TRT can have significant side effects including testicular shrinkage, growth of breast tissue and increased risk of heart disease.

Accessory glands of the male reproductive tract: production of semen

The spermatozoa produced by the testes are motile and during the process of ejaculation are released in a fluid medium termed semen. As with most bodily fluids, semen is an aqueous-based medium that is rich in proteins such as albumin, sugars (particularly fructose), mucus and electrolytes. This complex mixture is produced by three major glands (Table 12.2).

Table 12.2 Accessory glands of the male reproductive tract

Gland	Function
Seminal vesicles	The two seminal vesicles are oval-shaped glands located close to the prostate. Each is around 5 cm in length and releases its secretions into the urethra during ejaculation. The seminal vesicles are responsible for around 60 per cent of the semen volume with secretions rich in a variety of proteins, the monosaccharide sugar fructose and prostaglandins. The seminal vesicles also secrete large amounts of the protein semenogelin which causes semen to coalesce into a gel-like mass following ejaculation

(Continued)

Table 12.2   (Continued)

Gland	Function
Prostate gland	In young adults this gland is typically the size and shape of a walnut. The prostate surrounds the urethra and has multiple ducts which carry the prostatic secretions away from the gland. The prostate contributes around 30 per cent of the total semen volume, with prostatic secretions typically thin and watery and containing prostaglandins and the enzyme prostate-specific antigen (PSA), which helps maintain semen fluidity by breaking down the semenogelin produced by the seminal vesicles
Bulbourethral glands (Cowper's glands)	The two bulbourethral glands are roughly pea-sized and located beneath the prostate gland at the base of the penis. They secrete a mucus-rich fluid which functions to lubricate and protect the urethra. During arousal the secretions of the bulbourethral glands are discharged onto the tip of the penis, acting as a natural lubricant. The bulbourethral glands contribute around 5 per cent to the total semen volume, with the final 5 per cent comprising the sperm-rich fluid carried from the testes during ejaculation

Benign prostatic hyperplasia (BPH) and prostate cancer

In most men, there is a general benign increase in the size of the prostate gland with age. The once walnut-sized gland typically increases to the size of an apricot in the 40s and may reach the size of a small lemon in the 60s. Since the urethra runs through the centre of the prostate, this progressive enlargement can compress the urethra, making urination difficult.

Prostate cancer is the most common cancer in males in the UK, accounting for around 26 per cent of all cancers in men (Cancer Research UK, 2019b). Age is the major risk factor for prostate cancer with the vast majority of cases occurring in the over-50s, with the average age of diagnosis occurring between 65 and 69. Black males are at greater risk than either white or Asian men, while the inheritance of cancer-causing genes is thought to account for 5–9 per cent of prostate cancers. Recently, environmental and lifestyle risk factors for this disease have been identified, including exposure to certain pesticides, smoking and obesity.

Unfortunately, symptoms of prostate cancer usually do not manifest until the condition is fairly advanced. The most common problem, as with BPH, is progressive difficulty in urination, which indicates that the tumour mass is beginning to compress the urethra. Progressively, urination may become more and more difficult and painful, and patients will often find that their sleeping patterns are being disturbed as a result of frequent visits to the toilet during the night. As with Ahmed's case study at the beginning of this chapter, a palpable mass may be detectable during digital rectal examination, and levels of prostate-specific antigen may be elevated.

When prostate cancer is suspected, a biopsy is usually required to confirm the diagnosis and to help grade the cancer. Since many cancers are detected in older men, a watchful, waiting approach is often adopted. When required, surgery can be performed to remove the prostate, but this type of surgery may result in impotence or even urinary incontinence. Prostate cancer is typically driven by testosterone and may be treated through the use of testosterone-blocking drugs. During its later stages, prostate cancer frequently undergoes metastasis to distant regions including the bone, liver and lungs.

The penis

The penis is the male organ of copulation and also facilitates the elimination of urine from the body via the urethra. It consists of an outer sheath of skin and connective tissue, beneath which run two parallel longitudinal bands of erectile tissue called the corpora cavernosa (Figure 12.4). The urethra runs the length of the penis, exiting at the external urethral meatus. The glans penis forms the tip of the organ and is the location of densely arranged sensory neurons.

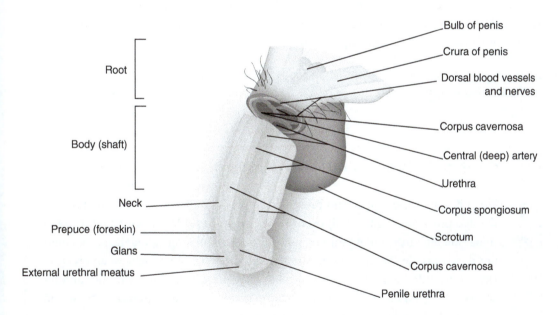

Figure 12.4   Structure of the penis

Physiology of erection and ejaculation

The process of erection is driven by the parasympathetic nervous system (Chapter 6). This branch of the autonomic nervous system is most active when in a relaxed, calm state; for this reason, erections frequently occur at night and early morning, with most occurring when asleep. During erection blood vessels at the base of the penis rapidly dilate, allowing blood to rush into the corpora cavernosa, which become engorged and press on the outer sheath of the skin and connective tissue. Stimulation of the penis during sexual intercourse or other forms of sex help maintain penile blood flow.

Eventually, repeated stimulation, particularly to the nerve endings at the glans, will trigger an orgasm and ejaculation. During ejaculation the muscular walls of the sperm ducts contract rhythmically, forcing fluid rich in sperm from the epididymis up through the vas deferens where this fluid is mixed with the secretions of the prostate, seminal vesicles and bulbourethral glands. During a typical ejaculation between 1.5 and 6 ml of semen is ejected, containing up to 200 million sperm per ml. A sperm count below 15 million sperm per ml is termed oligospermia and is often associated with reduced fertility and difficulties in conceiving naturally.

There are many causes of a reduced sperm count, including chromosomal disorders such as Klinefelter's syndrome, low testosterone levels, undescended testicles or certain sexually transmitted diseases such as chlamydia and gonorrhoea. Recently it has been established that obesity can also be associated with reduced sperm counts (NHS, 2019d). Men with low sperm counts may still be able to conceive naturally by lifestyle modifications (e.g. losing weight, reducing alcohol consumption and smoking or, when required, via testosterone replacement therapy). Where sperm counts remain very low, in vitro fertilisation (IVF) techniques can allow conception.

As men grow older, problems achieving an erection frequently occur; this is explored in David's case study.

Case study: David – erectile dysfunction

David is a 53-year-old man who presented to his GP with a loss of erectile function that has progressed significantly over the past year. Originally, he attributed the occasional inability to maintain an erection to tiredness or overindulgence in alcohol, but these episodes became more common and he now cannot achieve an erection. Despite his wife being supportive, this has caused extreme distress to him and has adversely affected his marital life, and he now avoids any type of intimacy with his wife in case he feels under pressure to perform sexually.

David has a three-year history of hypertension and is obese at 120 kg (178 cm tall). He smokes 15 cigarettes a day and drinks alcohol occasionally. He has a sedentary occupation and other than taking his elderly dog for gentle walks, leads a sedentary lifestyle with no exercise.

Initially David was reluctant to seek help but at the insistence of his wife, he visited his GP who prescribed Viagra, and more importantly referred him to the practice nurse for support in changing his lifestyle.

The female reproductive tract

The female reproductive tract consists of the ovaries, fallopian tubes, uterus and vagina (Figure 12.5). In addition to producing ova and the sex hormones oestrogen and progesterone, it provides an optimal environment to allow successful fertilisation, implantation and development of a foetus. Following gestation, the female reproductive tract facilitates parturition, allowing delivery of new offspring.

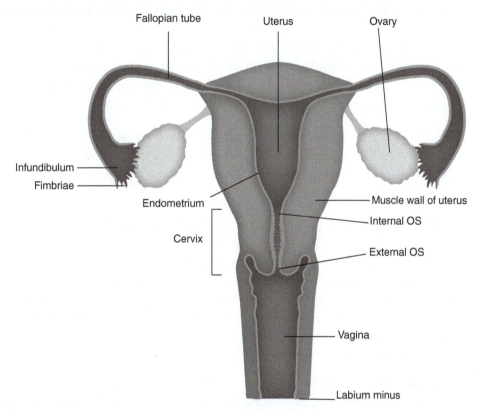

Figure 12.5   Overview of the female reproductive tract

Structure of the ovaries

The ovaries are small, greyish-white, oval-shaped organs around 2.5–3.5 cm in length with a slightly lumpy outer surface. It is a common misconception that the ovaries are fused to the fallopian tubes, and indeed many diagrams in textbooks can foster this misconception. As can be seen from Figure 12.5, the ovaries are suspended on ligaments within the funnel-shaped openings of the fallopian tubes.

As with spermatozoa, the ova (eggs) or oocytes are formed by meiosis (Chapter 13), which ensures that each mature ovum is a haploid cell containing 23 chromosomes. Each ovum develops within a fluid-filled sac termed a follicle which, as it expands, can distort the outer wall of the ovary, giving the ovaries their lumpy, irregular appearance.

The fallopian tubes

The fallopian tubes are also frequently referred to as the uterine tubes; nurses should familiarise themselves with both terms since they are used interchangeably in clinical practice. Each fallopian tube is typically around 10 cm in length and extends from the uterus before widening at the distal end into a funnel-shaped region termed the infundibulum, which has long, thin extensions termed fimbriae.

Each ovary is positioned in close proximity to the infundibulum, with the fimbriae surrounding the ovary where they serve to guide ova into the fallopian tube following ovulation. Internally the fallopian tubes are lined by a motile, ciliated columnar epithelium. The cilia beat in rhythmic waves which propel the ovum along and into the uterus. If the ovum has been fertilised, this ensures that the zygote is eventually transported to the organ of gestation where implantation can take place.

Sometimes this ciliated transporting mechanism may be damaged and a fertilised ovum can become stuck and begin to develop within the narrow confines of the fallopian tube. This is known as an ectopic pregnancy and is explored in Sarah's case study.

Case study: Sarah – chlamydia and ectopic pregnancy

Sarah was delighted to be seven weeks pregnant and was coping well with her pregnancy until she noticed some light bleeding, which she was reassured was quite normal in early pregnancy. However, over a period of several days, she developed pain in the right side of her abdomen which was worse when she passed urine. She also had some diarrhoea and initially she thought she had a stomach bug, but then developed some pain in her right shoulder tip.

One day, the pain became significantly worse and she felt dizzy and was pale in colour. Her partner called an ambulance and Sarah was taken to the local Emergency Department, where she was diagnosed as having a ruptured fallopian tube as a result of an ectopic pregnancy. When talking to a counsellor after she had recovered from emergency surgery to remove the affected fallopian tube, Sarah revealed that she had suffered from a chlamydia infection a few years before the pregnancy.

Chlamydia trachomatis is a common cause of pelvic infection including pelvic inflammatory disease, pelvic sepsis and salpingitis, which can be spread by unprotected intercourse. It is the most common of the sexually transmitted diseases seen in the UK. Chlamydia is a major public health concern. Infection in women can spread from the cervix to the womb and fallopian tubes, causing infertility and increasing the risk of ectopic pregnancy.

The presenting symptoms are usually lower abdominal pains, abnormal or heavy periods, painful sexual intercourse, change in vaginal discharge or painful urination. More than two thirds of women may have very mild symptoms or may be asymptomatic and are unaware that they are infected.

Sarah's case study highlights the importance of thoroughly investigating abdominal pain. In most pregnancies the ciliated transporting mechanism of the fallopian tubes functions well and the fertilised ovum will be delivered into the uterus, which is examined next.

The uterus

The uterus is composed predominantly of smooth muscle and functions as the organ of gestation. Structurally, it is composed of three distinct layers, which are summarised in Table 12.3.

Table 12.3   Layers of the uterus

Layer	Function
Endometrium (inner layer composed of a mucous membrane)	The endometrium is the inner layer of the uterus. Its outer layer is termed the functional layer which is formed from a single layer of columnar epithelial cells, supported by a thicker connective tissue that is rich in mucus-producing glands. This functional layer breaks down and is shed every month (menstruation) before being rebuilt from below
	The inner layer of the endometrium is called the basal layer and is continuous with the myometrium below. This is a constant layer, and unlike the functional layer, is never shed. Following menstruation, the functional layer is regenerated from this basal layer
Myometrium (middle muscle layer)	The myometrium is composed almost entirely from smooth muscle fibres and is recognised as the thickest and most powerful layer of smooth muscle in the human body. The myometrium contracts in response to hormones such as oxytocin and locally produced chemicals (autacoids) such as prostaglandins. Contraction of the myometrium facilitates the delivery of babies during parturition (labour)
Perimetrium (outer serous layer)	The outer layer of the uterus is a serous membrane formed from a single layer of squamous epithelial cells. These secrete a watery serous fluid which acts as a lubricant on the outer surface of the uterus. This fluid is particularly important to prevent abrasion in the final trimester of pregnancy when the uterus is greatly expanded and pressing on other surrounding structures

The cervix

The cervix is the inferior 2–3 cm portion of the uterus, frequently referred to as the neck of the womb (the word cervical is Latin for neck). It separates the uterus from the vagina below (Figure 12.5). It has a sphincter-like structure with a central cervical canal which opens into the uterine cavity above and the vagina below. The inferior aperture of the cervical canal is termed the external os, and this is usually obstructed by a small plug of mucus to seal off the uterus from the vagina. It used to be thought that this plug of mucus acted as a barrier to prevent the resident bacteria of the vagina extending into the uterine cavity, but recent research suggests that vaginal bacteria also typically colonise the uterus.

The mucus plug usually dissolves away midway through the menstrual cycle to allow transit of spermatozoa and fertilisation to occur. As with the uterus, the cervix has three distinct layers: a mucosal layer, a muscular layer and a serous layer. The mucosal layer of the cervical canal is called endocervix and is composed of columnar epithelial cells and mucous glands which continually secrete alkaline mucus which contributes to the formation of the resident mucus plug. The endocervical mucosa is folded and forms small pockets which trap semen in small reservoirs following intercourse. The outer portion of the cervix which bulges into the vagina is covered by stratified, non-keratinised, squamous epithelial cells which are continuous with the walls of the vagina.

These cells are vulnerable to infection from the human papillomavirus (HPV), which is thought to be carried by around one in three people. Over 100 strains of HPV have been identified and many cause no issues in reproductive health; however, strains HPV16 and HPV18 are known to be the major causes of cervical cancer. Like all viruses, HPV injects its genetic material into cells and uses them as factories to make copies of new viral particles. With strains 16 and 18, infected cervical cells are transformed into precancerous cells (cervical dysplasia), which can subsequently develop into cervical cancer.

Fortunately, regular cervical screening (pap smears) allows these dysplasic cells to be detected and removed before cervical cancer can progress. The cervix plays a key role throughout pregnancy, ensuring that the developing foetus is retained in the uterus. The cervix usually remains closed throughout pregnancy before beginning to dilate in the early stages of labour to facilitate delivery.

Since cervical cancer is so common, it is frequently encountered in clinical practice. Samia's case study highlights a common scenario.

Case study: Samia – cervical cancer

Samia is a 54-year-old post-menopausal woman with five children. Samia began to notice that she had slight bleeding following sexual intercourse. Initially, because of embarrassment, she ignored it until she also began to experience some discomfort during sex. Samia had never attended any cervical screening (smear test) appointments. Samia's GP sent her to the colposcopy clinic at the local hospital where a biopsy of her cervix and the surrounding tissue was taken, following which stage II cervical cancer was diagnosed.

Samia underwent a radical hysterectomy in which the cervix, uterus, top of the vagina, surrounding tissue, lymph nodes, fallopian tubes and ovaries were removed. This was followed by a six-week course of radiotherapy.

Samia's case study highlights the importance of regular cervical smears, since early detection of dysplasic cells will usually allow successful treatment without the need for hysterectomy. To develop your knowledge of cervical cancer further, now attempt Activity 12.3.

Activity 12.3   Evidence-based practice and research

What are the risk factors associated with cervical cancer and what health promotion advice would you give to reduce the risk of acquiring cervical cancer?

Now that we have explored the role of the cervix and its susceptibility to infection from HPV, which may lead to malignancy, we will explore the role of the vagina and external female genitalia.

The vagina

The vagina is the female organ of copulation and is a simple muscular tube lined by a mucous membrane. It extends from the cervix to the outer female genitalia (vulva) and is typically 7–9 cm in length. The walls of the vagina are lined with a stratified, non-keratinised, squamous epithelium. There is no glandular tissue present here, with the lubricating secretions which help keep the vagina moist and provide lubrication for intercourse primarily originating from specialised glands present within the vulva.

In health, the vagina is colonised by a lactobacillus-rich microbiota which generates copious amounts of lactic acid, ensuring the vagina has an acidic pH of around 3.8–4.5. The presence of a healthy vaginal microbiota and a low pH ensures that other potentially pathogenic bacteria and fungi cannot thrive, helping to maintain vaginal health.

Unfortunately, broad-spectrum antibiotics have a bactericidal or bacteriostatic effect on the healthy microbiota, thereby reducing their number, which results in less lactic acid being produced and a corresponding rise in pH. This can lead to opportunistic infections, for example thrush, which is caused by a yeast known as *Candida albicans*.

The vulva

The vulva is the collective name for the external female genitalia and consists of several distinct regions (Figure 12.6). Anatomical knowledge of the vulva is essential to nurses to allow the female urethra to be located for catheterisation. The outer region of the vulva consists of fleshy folds of skin termed the labia majora; the labia majora enclose and protect the inner more delicate regions of the vulva. The labia minora are found inside and running parallel to the labia majora. These inner lip-like structures (labia is Latin for lip) are covered by a mucous membrane and lead into the opening of the vagina.

The labia minora extend upwards before fusing at a point just below the clitoris. The clitoris develops from the same embryonic tissue as the penis in men and, like the penis, contains erectile tissue which can become engorged with blood during sexual arousal. The clitoris is rich in sensory nerve endings which, when stimulated during sexual activity, can result in female orgasm. During orgasm, rhythmic contractions of the pelvic floor muscles help ensure aspiration of semen into the cervical aperture, where it can saturate the folds of the cervical mucosa that act as semen reservoirs.

The prostaglandins present in semen (see above) also aid the process of conception by triggering uterine contractions, which further aid semen aspiration and transit through the cervical canal. Like the penis, the clitoral head is covered by a thin layer of skin called the prepuce, which is analogous to the male foreskin. The female urethral opening is found inferiorly to the clitoris and superiorly to the vaginal opening; in some women this opening may be very difficult to locate, and so during training nurses often find it useful to practise catheterisation of females using anatomically correct models.

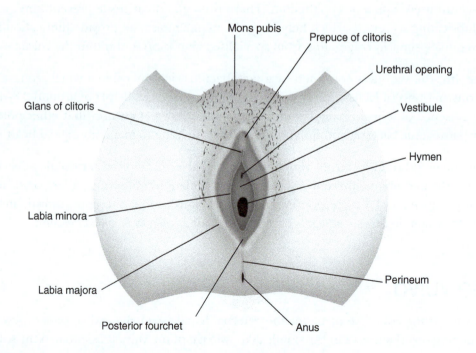

Figure 12.6 Anatomy of female external genitalia: the vulva

The menstrual cycle

The word menstrual derives from the Latin for monthly, and so the menstrual cycle literally translates into the monthly cycle. In most women, the menstrual cycle is close to 28 days, although there is much variation in length. Puberty is marked in females by the first episode of menstrual bleeding which is termed the menarche. In the UK the average age for the menarche and therefore puberty is 11. During the fertile years, if adequate nutrition is maintained and in the absence of pathology, the menstrual cycle is usually fairly regular and predictable.

It is essential that nurses understand that changes to the length and frequency of the menstrual cycle in women of child-bearing years should always be thoroughly investigated, as variations may be caused by diseases such as ovarian cancer or anaemia or by eating disorders. The absence of a menstrual cycle in fertile women is termed amenorrhea, with most cases associated with poor nutrition and particularly with the eating disorder anorexia nervosa. At the time of puberty and as the menopause approaches (perimenopause), the monthly cycle tends to be far more irregular and less predictable. In reality the monthly cycle that women experience actually consists of two interrelated cycles: the ovarian cycle and the uterine cycle.

The ovarian cycle

Each month within the ovaries, a new ovarian follicle containing a mature ovum develops before rupturing, expelling the ovum into a fallopian tube during the process of ovulation. The ovarian cycle consists of three distinct phases (Figure 12.7).

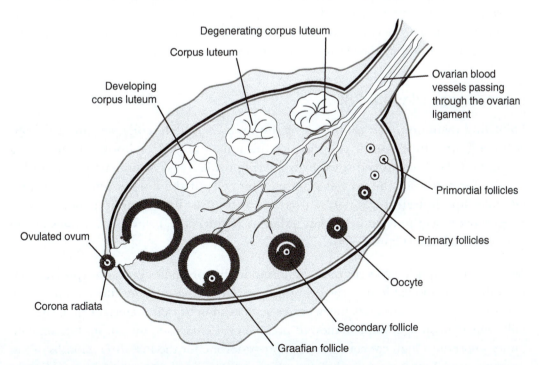

Figure 12.7   Ovarian structure and follicular development

The follicular phase (day 1–14)

The anterior pituitary gland progressively releases greater amounts of follicle-stimulating hormone (FSH), which encourages the growth of immature primary follicles. Growing ovarian follicles utilise cholesterol to synthesise the major female sex hormone oestrogen, which encourages rebuilding and thickening of the endometrium (see below).

As the follicles enlarge, they begin to accumulate a watery fluid which collects in a chamber called the antrum. Gradually the pressure within the follicle begins to build up, and the enlarged follicle may begin to deform the outer wall of the ovary. This enlarged mature follicle is called a Graafian follicle, and with further pressure rises, it becomes more and more unstable.

Ovulation (typically around day 14)

In addition to producing FSH, the anterior pituitary gland releases luteinising hormone (LH); this reaches a peak midway through the ovarian cycle around day 14 (Figure 12.8), triggering ovulation (Figure 12.7). During ovulation the wall of the Graafian follicle and outer wall of the ovary rupture, releasing the ovum into the distal portion of the fallopian tube.

Ovulation is an explosive event reliant on the progressive build-up of pressure within the follicle, and some women experience a twinge of pain termed mittelschmerz (pain mid-cycle) at the time of ovulation, which corresponds to the rupturing of the ovarian wall. In most cases the expelled ovum will be gathered by the finger-like fimbriae, funnelled into the fallopian tube and begin its passage towards the uterus. If fertilisation takes place, it usually occurs at the distal end of the fallopian tube with the early conceptus taking around six days to reach the uterus.

Luteal phase (day 14–28)

Following ovulation, the remnants of the ovarian follicle collapse into a yellow-coloured structure called the corpus luteum (the yellow body). Luteinising hormone (LH) is so named since by triggering ovulation it is ultimately responsible for the formation of the corpus luteum. The cells of the corpus luteum continually take up cholesterol, which is used to synthesise the hormone progesterone. Progressively, as the corpus luteum enlarges (Figure 12.7), levels of progesterone gradually increase (Figure 12.8).

As the name implies, progesterone is a hormone that promotes gestation (pregnancy). Initially it is responsible for triggering the secretory phase of the uterine cycle (see below), where the endometrium secretes a sticky, mucus-rich material called uterine milk which encourages implantation. If pregnancy occurs, then the corpus luteum continues to produce high concentrations of progesterone for the first three months of the pregnancy until the placenta takes over this role. Progesterone is essential to maintain the pregnancy and functions primarily to stop degeneration of the endometrial lining and menses, which would result in a miscarriage.

At around the switchover in progesterone production from corpus luteum to placenta (at around 12 weeks), there is often a slight drop in progesterone production, which deprives the endometrium of its hormonal supports and may trigger 'spotting', where some endometrial breakdown occurs, and some blood is shed. If endometrial breakdown is significant, a miscarriage can occur, and indeed many miscarriages occur at this point in the switchover of progesterone production.

In most menstrual cycles a pregnancy will not occur, and the corpus luteum degenerates into a small area of scar tissue called the corpus albicans (white body). Throughout the fertile years these areas of scar tissue accumulate in the walls of the ovary, which progressively become tougher and may make ovulation more difficult. As the corpus luteum degenerates, the progesterone levels fall, depriving the endometrium of its hormonal support and triggering menstruation.

The uterine (menstrual) cycle

The endometrial lining of the uterus undergoes dramatic changes throughout the typical 28-day cycle. As with the ovarian cycle, three distinct phases of the uterine cycle are recognised, which correspond to changes in the levels of oestrogen and progesterone.

Menses (day 1–5)

When progesterone levels fall as a result of corpus luteum degeneration, the blood vessels of the endometrial lining go into spasm and the functional layer of the endometrium begins to die off and release intracellular enzymes that begin to autodigest the endometrial lining. Blood vessels beneath the functional layer then dilate, and the increased blood flow washes out the partially digested endometrial layer through the cervix during menses (Figure 12.8).

Proliferative phase (day 5–14)

Following menses, the functional layer of the endometrium lining the uterus has sloughed away, leaving the germinal tissue of the basal layer underneath. At this time the ovarian follicles are enlarging and secreting oestrogen (Figure 12.8), which stimulates cell division in the basal layer and the progressive regrowth, proliferation and maturation of the functional layer.

Secretory phase (day 14–28)

Following ovulation, at around day 14 the corpus luteum progressively secretes greater and greater amounts of progesterone. This hormone stimulates growth and activity of mucous glands within the endometrium, leading to the production of uterine milk. This modified form of mucus coats the outer layer of the endometrium, making it extremely tacky.

If an ovum is fertilised within the fallopian tube, the conceptus will take around six days to reach the uterine cavity, and the presence of sticky uterine milk will increase the chances of the conceptus attaching and implanting into the endometrial lining. Uterine milk also provides some nutrition to the early conceptus before it can fully implant and establish a blood supply.

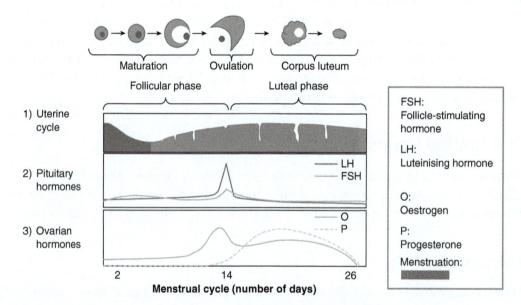

Figure 12.8 Hormonal control of the uterine (menstrual) cycle

Now that you have completed the chapter, attempt the multiple-choice questions in Activity 12.4 to assess your understanding of the subject material.

Activity 12.4   Multiple-choice questions

1. In the male reproductive tract what is the primary function of the interstitial cells (cells of Leydig)?

   a) To produce spermatozoa

   b) To synthesise testosterone

   c) To release nutrients and growth factors

   d) To produce fluid to support the growth of spermatozoa

2. Which of the following testicular temperatures will be most favourable to efficient spermatogenesis (sperm production)?

   a) 37°C

   b) 35°C

   c) 38°C

   d) 37.5°C

3. The andropause leads to

   a) An increase in male libido, fertility, muscle mass and bone density

   b) A decrease in male libido, fertility, muscle mass and bone density

   c) An end to male fertility

   d) An increased risk of testicular cancer

4. Semen is produced by

   a) The prostate gland, urethra and bladder

   b) The prostate gland, seminal vesicles and urethra

   c) The prostate gland, seminal vesicles and bulbourethral glands

   d) The seminal vesicles, bladder and bulbourethral glands

5. Which of these statements is *untrue?*

   a) Prostate cancer is more common in black males than Asian and white men

   b) 5–9 per cent of prostate cancer is thought to be inherited

   c) Prostate cancer is the least common cancer in men

   d) Environmental and lifestyle factors contribute to the incidence of prostate cancer

6. *Chlamydia trachomatis* is

   a) A common sexually transmitted disease in the UK

   b) Often asymptomatic and therefore harmless

   c) Only harmful to pregnant women

   d) An inevitable consequence of unprotected sexual intercourse

7. The acid environment inside the human vagina

   a) Provides an inhospitable environment for spermatozoa

   b) Contributes to lubrication during sexual intercourse

(Continued)

(Continued)

    c) Helps to ensure that potentially pathogenic microorganisms cannot thrive in the vagina

    d) Is a symptom of thrush

8. A major function of the endocervix is to

    a) Prevent microorganisms from entering the uterus

    b) Trap semen following sexual intercourse

    c) Protect the uterus from HPV

    d) Strengthen the entrance of the uterus

9. On which day of the ovarian cycle is ovulation most likely to occur?

    a) Day 1

    b) Day 14

    c) Day 21

    d) Day 28

10. A key role of progesterone during the uterine cycle is

    a) To prevent the implantation of a fertilised ovum

    b) To restrict blood loss during menstruation

    c) To stimulate growth and activity of the mucous glands within the epithelium leading to the production of uterine milk

    d) To ensure that a pregnancy results in a female foetus

Chapter summary

The major role of the male and female reproductive tracts is to facilitate the union of **gametes** during the process of fertilisation. The primary male reproductive organs are the testes, which produce spermatozoa and the male sex hormone testosterone. The testes are suspended on the spermatic cords and located within the scrotum; these jointly regulate testicular temperature for optimal spermatogenesis. The prostate gland, seminal vesicles and bulbourethral gland collectively produce secretions which form semen, which is the fluid medium in which sperm swim.

The penis is the erectile male organ of copulation which facilitates delivery of sperm into the female reproductive tract. In females the primary reproductive organs are the ovaries which produce ova and the female sex hormones oestrogen and progesterone. During ovulation, an ovum is released into the fallopian tube where a ciliated transport mechanism facilitates its transport into the uterus. The endometrium forms the inner lining of the uterus which is shed and rebuilt each month during the menstrual cycle.

The myometrium is the muscular layer of the uterus which contracts during labour, allowing delivery of the newborn. The cervix forms the neck of the womb and has a central aperture called the os which leads into the uterus. The vagina is the female organ of copulation and connects the uterus to the vulva, which is the collective term for the external female genitalia.

Activities: Brief outline answers

Activity 12.1: Evidence-based practice and research (page 326)

Testicular torsion differential diagnosis:

- epididymo-orchitis;
- testicular abscess;
- testicular tumours;
- torsion of the epididymal appendix;
- acute idiopathic scrotal oedema;
- testicular trauma;
- hernia complications.

Activity 12.2: Evidence-based practice and research (page 327)

Potential causes of declining male sperm counts are poorly understood but thought to be linked to:

- environmental pollutants, particularly hormone-disrupting organic molecules;
- smoking;
- alcohol consumption;
- certain prescription medications.

Activity 12.3: Evidence-based practice and research (page 337)

Risk factors for cervical cancer:

- smoking;
- having a weakened immune system;
- multiple sexual partners;
- infection with HPV (human papillomavirus) 16 and HPV18;
- long-term use of the oral contraceptive pill for more than five years;
- having more than five children, or having them at a young age;
- your mother taking the hormonal drug diethylstilboestrol (DES) while pregnant with you.

Health promotion advice to help reduce cervical cancer risk:

- HPV vaccination;
- use a condom;
- regular screening.

Activity 12.4: Multiple-choice questions (pages 342–4)

1) b, 2) b, 3) b, 4) c, 5) c, 6) a, 7) c, 8) b, 9) b, 10) c

Further reading

Boore J et al. (2016) Chapter 16: The reproductive systems, in *Essentials of Anatomy and Physiology for Nursing Practice*. London: SAGE Publications Ltd.

A textbook to develop your knowledge of human anatomy and physiology that is aimed specifically at nurses.

Useful websites

www.mayoclinic.org/healthy-lifestyle/womens-health/in-depth/menstrual-cycle/art-20047186

A useful overview of what is normal and what is not in relation to the menstrual cycle.

www.niddk.nih.gov/health-information/urologic-diseases/prostate-problems

An overview of prostate problems including BPH and prostate cancer.

www.nhs.uk/conditions/cervical-cancer

An overview of cervical cancer including treatment options.

Chapter 13 Genetics and inheritance

Introduction

Case study: Christopher – albinism

Christopher is 18 years old and was born with albinism, a genetic disease that is associated with a lack of the pigment melanin in the skin, eyes and hair. Throughout his life, Christopher has had to be careful to protect his skin and eyes from direct sunlight because of the damaging effects of ultraviolet (UV) light. Despite wearing glasses that block UV light and ensuring that his exposed skin was always covered by sunblock, Christopher has recently noted an unusual patch of raised skin on the tip of his nose.

Subsequent investigations and a skin biopsy revealed the lesion to be a squamous cell carcinoma which was excised under local anaesthetic the following week. Christopher was told that this type of skin cancer is prevalent in patients with albinism, and that because the lesion had been identified so quickly, the malignant tissue had been completely removed with minimal chance of scarring.

Genetic diseases such as the albinism that has affected Christopher are routinely encountered in nursing practice. To understand how genetic diseases arise and are inherited, knowledge of DNA and its role as our genetic blueprint is essential.

This chapter will begin by examining the nature of DNA and the processes of DNA replication and cell division.

We will then explore how information encoded in DNA is used to construct the proteins that build our bodies and drive our internal biochemistry. The nature of genes as the units of inheritance will be discussed, and we will conclude by exploring how genetic diseases such as cystic fibrosis (CF) and albinism are passed down the generations from parents to offspring.

Deoxyribonucleic acid (DNA)

The genetic blueprint used to construct the proteins that build our body is encoded in the form of deoxyribonucleic acid (DNA). DNA molecules have a characteristic shape, adopting the form of a double helix (double spiral). DNA molecules are synthesised from building blocks called nucleotides, while each nucleotide is itself constructed from a five-carbon sugar (deoxyribose), a phosphate group and a nitrogenous base (Figure 13.1).

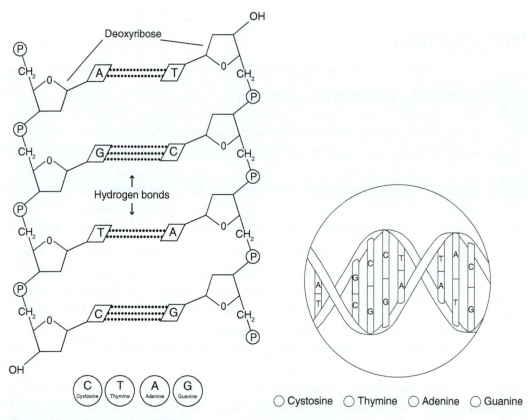

Figure 13.1   Structure of DNA

Complementary base pairing

There are four nitrogenous bases which pair up in a predictable manner, slotting together like pieces of a jigsaw puzzle. This process is called complementary base pairing (Figure 13.1).

- Adenine always pairs with Thymine (A-T).
- Cytosine always pairs with Guanine (C-G).

Adenine and guanine are referred to as purine bases and are found in high concentrations in certain foods including oily fish, offal and fermented beers. Some patients can find it difficult to metabolise purines from food, which can result in the build-up of damaging uric acid crystals in their joints, leading to the painful inflammatory joint condition known as gout (UK Gout Society, 2019).

Cell division

To allow for growth and repair, many cells retain the ability to divide. For cell division to take place our genetic blueprint needs to be copied before being passed on to new daughter cells. This involves the copying of DNA molecules by a process called DNA replication.

DNA replication and the role of DNA polymerase

Complementary base pairing forms the basis of DNA replication and involves two specialised enzymes. Helicase unzips a small section of the DNA double helix to expose the nucleotide bases, while a second enzyme called DNA polymerase fills in the gaps using the complementary base-pairing rule. The end result is two new daughter strands of DNA which are identical to the original parent strand (Figure 13.2).

To help you understand the nature of DNA base pairing, attempt Activity 13.1.

Activity 13.1 Consolidation of learning

Assuming an original DNA sequence on the parent strand shown below, using the base-pairing rule, indicate the sequence expected on the complementary strand.

ACCCGAATGATT

There are some possible answers to all activities at the end of the chapter, unless otherwise indicated.

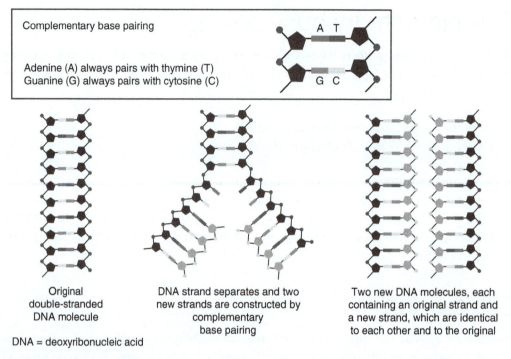

Original double-stranded DNA molecule	DNA strand separates and two new strands are constructed by complementary base pairing	Two new DNA molecules, each containing an original strand and a new strand, which are identical to each other and to the original

DNA = deoxyribonucleic acid

Figure 13.2 DNA synthesis

Types of cell division

Once DNA is copied, cell division can take place. There are two types of cell division that occur: the first is called mitosis and is the type of cell division necessary for normal growth repair and bodily maintenance. The second type is called meiosis and occurs only in the ovaries and testes to produce ova and spermatozoa (see Chapter 12).

Interphase

Cells spend most of their time in interphase, which can be defined as the time between cycles of cell division. Just prior to cell division, DNA replication is initiated, and a full copy of the cell's genetic material (its genome) is produced. To facilitate the segregation of the two genomic copies, enzymes begin to coil the thin strands of DNA into thicker coils, which gradually condense and become visible in the nucleus as chromosomes.

Mitosis

Mitosis occurs in four distinct phases (Figure 13.3).

Prophase

During prophase, the nuclear envelope (membrane) dissolves to leave the chromosomes suspended in the cytoplasm of the cell. Since our full complement of DNA has been copied during interphase, each of the 46 chromosomes is seen to consist of two identical sister chromatids joined at a central region termed the centromere.

Metaphase

Small cellular organelles called centrioles produce a network of thin contractile tubules which attach to the centromere of each chromosome. These fibres and their associated centrioles are collectively known as the spindle apparatus because they are spindle-shaped (resembling a diamond). During metaphase, coordinated contractions of the spindle tubules pull each chromosome into the equator (central region) of the cell.

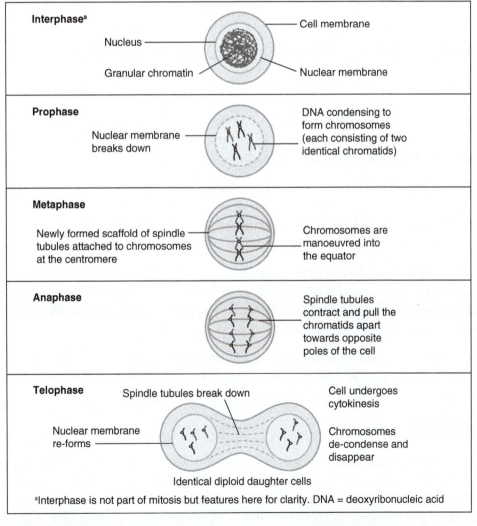

Figure 13.3 Mitosis

Source: Image courtesy of *Nursing Times*

Anaphase

During anaphase, further contractions of the spindle tubules pull the sister chromatids of each chromosome apart and towards opposite poles (ends) of the cell.

Telophase

Each pole of the cell now has a full diploid complement of 46 chromatids which, following separation, are now called chromosomes. A new nuclear envelope forms around each chromosome set, and the cytoplasm begins to cleave by a process termed cytokinesis. Cleavage ensures that each cell has sufficient cytoplasm to allow it to function as a discrete independent unit. Finally, the tightly wound DNA characteristic of chromosomes is progressively unwound, and the DNA adopts its looser, uncondensed configuration. During this process, the chromosomes become less distinct and eventually disappear, marking the point where the cell returns to interphase.

The dynamic nature of human tissues

The process of mitosis allows continual replacement of senescent (aged) cells throughout our lifespan, ensuring that our organs and tissues function efficiently as we grow older. It is essential that nurses are aware that the human body is a dynamic structure, with our organs and tissues in a continual state of flux as aged, senescent cells are replaced with new daughter cells originating from mitosis.

Cells have greatly varying lifespans, e.g. the most common leukocyte (neutrophil) lives 1–5 days, epidermal skin cells live 10–30 days and fat cells (adipocytes) live around 8 years, while cells in the lens of our eye and some neurones in our central nervous system are thought to last a lifespan (Bionumbers, 2019).

Clearly, cells with a short lifespan have to be replaced much more quickly than cells with a longer lifespan, and this requires a faster rate of cell division. Unfortunately, rapidly dividing cells are prone to malignancy, and many cancers arise in tissues where cell division occurs quickly such as bone marrow, skin and gut.

Now that we have examined mitosis, we will turn our attention to the second type of cell division that gives rise to the ova and sperm cells necessary for reproduction.

Meiosis

Mitosis results in daughter cells that are genetically identical to their parent cells, retaining the diploid number of 46 chromosomes. Meiosis differs since it requires that the diploid number of chromosomes is halved to ensure that ova and spermatozoa are haploid cells possessing 23 chromosomes. This is essential to ensure that during fertilisation (where the two haploid cells fuse) the resulting zygote will have the normal diploid number of 46 chromosomes restored.

Meiosis is also responsible for randomly reorganising genetic material to ensure variability in the offspring. This is the reason why siblings from the same parents have great variability in their physical and some of their behavioural characteristics. The only exception would be identical siblings which originate from the same fertilised ovum and therefore share the same genes.

As with mitosis, before meiosis is initiated, DNA must be replicated towards the end of interphase (see above). The process of meiosis is split into two distinct stages which are referred to as meiosis I (Figure 13.4a) and meiosis II (Figure 13.4b).

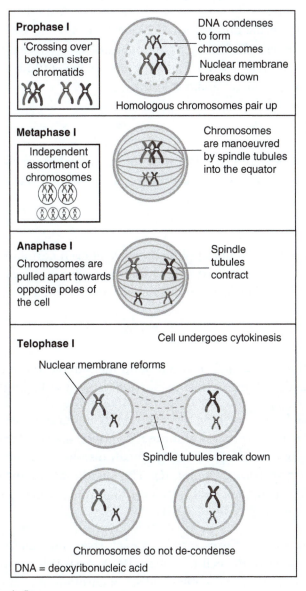

Figure 13.4a   Meiosis I

Source: Image courtesy of *Nursing Times*

There are four distinct phases of meiosis I.

Prophase I

The loosely arranged DNA condenses into visible chromosomes, and the nuclear envelope disappears, leaving the chromosomes suspended in the cytoplasm.

All diploid cells, including the germinal cells of the ovaries and testes (Chapter 12), have 23 pairs of chromosomes. One member of each pair is inherited from our mother via her ovum, and the other member is inherited from our father via his spermatozoan.

These maternal and paternal chromosomes pair up during prophase I, allowing segments of chromosomes to be exchanged via a process called 'crossing over'. This involves pieces of maternal and paternal chromosomes being cut and exchanged to form new chromosomes, which have a random assortment of maternal and paternal genes. This process is often described as being similar to shuffling a deck of cards and is essential to ensure genetic variability in offspring.

Metaphase I

The spindle apparatus begins to form, with contractile **microtubules** attaching to the centromeres. The chromosome pairs are moved to the equator region of the cell.

Anaphase I

Contraction of the spindle tubules pulls a member of each chromosome pair to opposite poles of the cell, effectively halving the number of chromosomes at each end of the cell from the diploid number of 46 to the haploid number of 23.

Telophase I

A new nuclear envelope gradually forms around the haploid set of chromosomes and cytokinesis is initiated, with the cytoplasm cleaving to give two haploid daughter cells.

Each of the two haploid daughter cells now rapidly undergoes a second cell division which is very similar to the process of mitosis described above. During meiosis II, the nuclear membrane of each daughter cell gradually dissolves, leaving the chromosomes suspended in the cytoplasm (prophase II). The spindle apparatus forms and microtubules attach to the centromeres of each chromosome, which are shifted into the equatorial region of the cell (metaphase II).

Contraction of the spindle fibres separates each sister chromatid, which are then moved to opposite poles of the cell (anaphase II). Meiosis II is completed when a new nuclear envelope forms around each haploid set of chromosomes and cytokinesis takes place, resulting in two new haploid daughter cells (telophase II).

It is important to note that during meiosis, each original diploid germinal cell in the ovaries and testes gives rise to four haploid daughter cells.

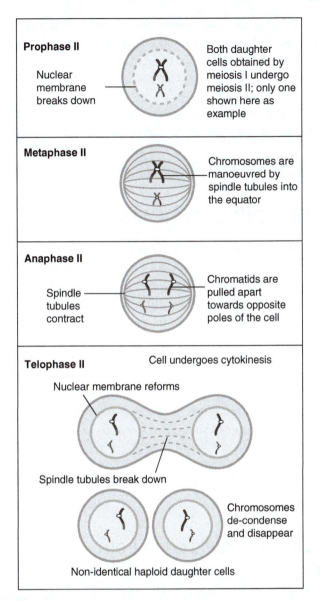

Figure 13.4b   Meiosis II

Source: Image courtesy of *Nursing Times*

Gametes and non-disjunction

The key feature of meiosis is that it gives rise to haploid daughter cells containing 23 chromosomes. Unfortunately, with age, the separation of chromosomal pairs via the contractile microtubules of the spindle apparatus becomes less efficient, and extra chromosomes can be carried over into ova and spermatozoa. This poor separation of chromosomes is known as non-disjunction and may lead to common chromosomal diseases where missing or extra chromosomes are present. Any deviation from the diploid number of chromosomes is known as aneuploidy.

The aneuploid chromosome disorder most frequently encountered by nurses is Down syndrome, which is seen in around 1 in 800 live births; here cells usually have an extra copy of chromosome 21 (trisomy 21), so instead of 46 chromosomes, the cells of individuals with Down syndrome usually have 47 (see Chapter 1 for further details).

Now that we have an understanding of how cells divide, we need to turn our attention back to DNA and examine how this molecule is used as the genetic blueprint to construct our body.

DNA and protein synthesis

The set of instructions for building the human body is encoded in sequences of DNA called genes. Many genes contain information for producing structural proteins such as keratin, actin and myosin that are used to build elements of the body such as skin and muscle, while other genes contain information for synthesising the enzymes that are essential to catalyse the chemical reactions that keep us alive.

Proteins are constructed from 20 naturally occurring amino acids, and the order in which these are joined together is determined by the nucleotide sequences in our DNA. As we have seen in Chapter 1, within the cytoplasm we have a region called the rough endoplasmic reticulum (rough ER), which has organelles termed ribosomes covering its surface. It is the ribosomes that build proteins by linking amino acids together by peptide bonds.

The production of proteins involves two major stages called transcription and translation.

Transcription of the genetic code from DNA into RNA

Since DNA is a huge molecule (macromolecule), it is physically too large to pass through the nuclear envelope and deliver information directly to the ribosomes to enable protein synthesis. To get around this problem, the information stored in genes is copied into a much smaller molecule called ribonucleic acid (RNA). Unlike DNA which is double-stranded (a double helix), RNA is single-stranded, and since this molecule is carrying information to the ribosomes to build proteins, it is called messenger RNA (mRNA). The process of copying genes from DNA into RNA is called transcription (Figure 13.5).

Like DNA, mRNA is also constructed from the nucleotide bases adenine, cytosine and guanine, but RNA lacks the base thymine which is replaced by its RNA equivalent; a base called uracil.

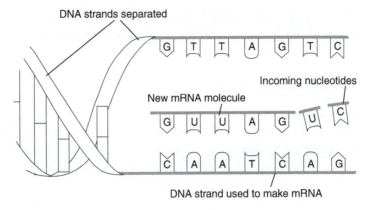

DNA strands separated

Incoming nucleotides

New mRNA molecule

DNA strand used to make mRNA

DNA gene sequence is transcribed into messenger RNA,
DNA base Thymine is replaced by Uracil

Figure 13.5   Transcription

The process of transcription again makes use of complementary base pairing to transcribe a gene coding for a protein (e.g. keratin) into its mRNA sequence. This process occurs in several distinct stages which are summarised below:

The enzyme RNA polymerase binds to the beginning of the DNA gene sequence

↓

RNA polymerase unwinds a small section of the DNA, exposing its bases (genetic code of the gene). This small area of unwound DNA is called a transcription bubble

↓

RNA polymerase synthesises a complementary mRNA strand using the base-pairing rule to fill in the complementary bases

This process results in the generation of a strand of mRNA, which holds the genetic information necessary to construct a protein.

For example, if the original DNA sequence for a gene is as indicated below:

TCAGCATGC

Using the base-pairing rule, the corresponding mRNA sequence would be as follows:

TCAGCATGC – DNA sequence
AGUCGUACG – mRNA sequence

Since mRNA molecules are single-stranded, they can pass freely through the nuclear envelope and associate with a ribosome in the rough ER of the cytoplasm.

The nature of the genetic code

In Chapter 10, we examined the digestion of dietary protein into its component amino acids; these can be used by our cells to produce our own proteins. The human body can synthesise 11 of the 20 amino acids; these are referred to as non-essential amino acids. However, the remaining nine cannot be synthesised and must be obtained through our diet; these are termed essential amino acids.

The genetic code uses three bases to code for each amino acid. With only 20 naturally occurring amino acids, three bases are more than sufficient to represent each amino acid; indeed, some are represented more than once (Figure 13.6).

	U		C		A		G		
U	UUU UUC	Phenylalanine	UCU UCC	Serine	UAU UAC	Tyrosine	UGU UGC	Cysteine	U C
	UUA UUG	Leucine	UCA UCG		UAA** Stop Codon UAG** Stop Codon		UGA** Stop Codon UGG Tryptophan		A G
C	CUU CUC CUA CUG	Leucine	CCU CCC CCA CCG	Proline	CAU CAC CAA CAG	Histidine Glutamine	CGU CGC CGA CGG	Arginine*	U C A G
A	AUU AUC AUA	Isoleucine	ACU ACC ACA	Threonine	AAU AAC AAA	Asparagine Lysine	AGU AGC AGA	Serine	U C A
	AUG	Methionine (start codon)	ACG		AAG		AGG	Arginine	G
G	GUU GUC GUA GUG	Valine	GCU GCC GCA GCG	Alanine	GAU GAC GAA GAG	Aspartate Glutamate	GGU GGC GGA GGG	Glycine	U C A G

Figure 13.6 The genetic code

Translation of the genetic code into proteins

When mRNA leaves the nucleus, it attaches to a ribosome, and the process of translating the genetic code into a physical protein begins (Figure 13.7). Since each amino acid is represented by three nucleotide bases, the genetic code is referred to as a triplet code, and each group of three bases is referred to as a codon.

Transfer RNA (tRNA)

Transfer RNA (tRNA) facilitates the delivery of amino acids to the ribosomal site for incorporation into a protein in accordance with the instructions encoded in the transcribed mRNA strand. Every one of the 20 amino acids has a unique complementary tRNA molecule which attaches to its amino acid in the cytoplasm and transfers it to the ribosome.

tRNA effectively functions as a shuttle vehicle, ensuring a steady supply of amino acids for incorporation into the growing protein molecule (Figure 13.7). Each tRNA molecule that binds to its corresponding amino acid has its own triplet base sequence. Since this will be complementary to the codons on the mRNA molecule, it is referred to as an anticodon.

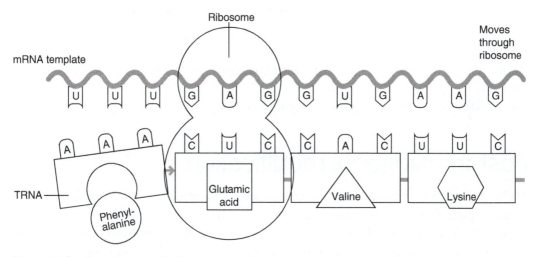

Figure 13.7   Protein translation

The process of translation involves several steps which are summarised below.

A strand of mRNA travels from the nucleus and attaches to a ribosome

↓

A single codon (three bases) on the mRNA strand is positioned on the ribosome

↓

tRNA delivers the corresponding amino acid to the ribosome. In Figure 13.6 the codon GAG is exposed on the ribosome.

Therefore, the corresponding anticodon is CUC which indicates that glutamic acid is the correct amino acid to be incorporated into the protein

↓

The mRNA strand is shifted along the ribosome by three bases exposing the next codon. A tRNA molecule with its complementary anticodon delivers the next amino acid

$$\downarrow$$

Peptide bonds are created between each adjacent amino acid, and the process repeats, progressively elongating the protein molecule

Now that we have examined the processes of transcription and translation, attempt Activity 13.2.

Activity 13.2   Consolidation of learning

Assuming an mRNA sequence of GUACCACAA, using the genetic code in Figure 13.6, identify which three amino acids would be joined together.

We have now examined how amino acid sequences are created using the information stored in the genetic code; however, these initial proteins usually require further chemical modification, and this process is examined below.

Post-translational modification

At the end of protein translation, a crude protein consisting of a chain of amino acids linked together in the sequence specified within the original gene is created. At this stage, the protein may not have the correct shape or configuration and may need to be refined. Crude proteins are moved to the Golgi apparatus, where they can be refined by the addition of carbohydrate and lipid components (Chapter 1). Refined proteins will have the correct three-dimensional configuration and function fully in their designated roles, potentially as structural proteins or enzymes.

Mutations

Errors in the genetic code can lead to proteins having missing, extra or wrong amino acids, which can affect their three-dimensional configuration and render the protein useless. With over 3 billion base pairs in the human, genome errors are inevitable and frequently arise during incorrect DNA replication. Errors in our DNA are termed mutations, and while many will have no noticeable effects, others may result in serious genetic diseases. Mutations may be triggered by environmental pollutants, certain medications and infections or through exposure to radiation, including ultraviolet light. Anything that can cause a mutation is referred to as a mutagen. Some mutagens are also known to cause cancer, and these are termed carcinogens.

DNA and inheritance

We have just explored how the information stored in our genes is used as a blueprint to construct the proteins that are used to build our body. Genes are arranged linearly along the length of chromosome like beads on a string. Earlier in the chapter, we described how chromosomes are found in pairs, with one member of each pair inherited from our mother and one from our father. As a consequence, we have two copies of each gene, one of which will be maternal in origin and one paternal.

Genes are responsible for most of our physical characteristics, including relatively simple attributes such as our hair and skin colour through to more complex traits such as body size and shape. It is also becoming apparent that some of our mental characteristics and personality traits are also heavily influenced by genes that we inherit from our parents.

Single-gene defects

Gene mutations can lead to single-gene defects which are responsible for a wide variety of genetic diseases. In many of these, the abnormal disease-causing genes are passed down the generations in a predictable manner. A good example is cystic fibrosis which is particularly common in European races, with around 1 in 2,000 to 1 in 3,000 babies currently born with this disease.

Inheritance of cystic fibrosis

In genetics, genes can be represented by letters of the alphabet. Some genes are dominant in nature, with their effects usually expressed in the individual; dominant traits are traditionally represented by capital letters. Recessive traits tend to be masked by the presence of dominant genes and are represented by lower-case letters.

The combination of genes that we inherit from our parents is called our genotype, while the physical effect exerted by those genes is known as our phenotype.

The abnormal cystic fibrosis gene is found on chromosome 7 and is recessive in nature. Since we inherit two genes (one from each parent), there are three possible gene combinations or genotypes:

CC – Normal

Cc – Carrier

cc – Sufferer of cystic fibrosis

Clearly, the CC genotype will be free of CF since two normal genes have been inherited. However, it is important to note that the genotype Cc also results in a normal, healthy, disease-free phenotype. This is because the effects of the recessive, disease-causing gene (c) are masked by the presence of the dominant healthy gene (C). Although these people are healthy, they are referred to as carriers because they carry a single copy of the disease-causing CF gene. Only those individuals that inherit two copies of the defective gene (cc) will develop the disease.

In the UK, around 1 in 25 people are carriers of the CF gene (Cystic Fibrosis Trust, 2018). If two people who are carriers have children, a simple tool called a Punnett square can be used to calculate their chances of having a child with CF (Figure 13.8). A Punnett square is a grid onto which the parent's genes can be added to the top (father) and side (mother). The parental genes are then added to the boxes inside the square to establish the possible genotypes of the offspring.

When two carriers of a single recessive cystic fibrosis gene have a child, there is a 1 in 4 risk that the child will inherit the two recessive genes and thus develop the disease		Father carrying one dominant and one recessive cystic fibrosis gene	
		C	**c**
Mother carrying one dominant and one recessive cystic fibrosis gene	**C**	CC	Cc
	c	Cc	CC

Figure 13.8   Inheritance of a recessive genetic disease: cystic fibrosis

The Punnett square illustrates that when two carriers of the CF gene have children, each child will have a one in four chance of inheriting both the disease-causing recessive genes and suffering from CF. This 3:1 ratio is a feature common to inherited single-gene recessive diseases and is referred to as a Mendelian ratio after the father of genetics, Gregor Mendel, who first noted it when studying inheritance in plants in the 1800s.

You have just seen above that Punnett squares provide a simple tool for predicting the genotypes and phenotypes of offspring. Now attempt Activity 13.3 to gain experience in their use.

Activity 13.3   Consolidation of learning

Draw a Punnett square and use it to predict the offspring of a father with CF (cc) and a carrier mother (Cc).

What is the proportion of children that are likely to suffer from CF? What proportion of children will be carriers of the disease-causing gene?

Now that you have an understanding of how the disease-causing cystic fibrosis gene is inherited, we will briefly examine the pathophysiological consequences of suffering from this disease.

CF patients have difficulty regulating the movement of electrolytes and water within their tissues. This can progressively lead to a build-up of thick, sticky mucus in the respiratory tract, pancreatic ducts and GI tract. As a result, CF patients experience difficulty in breathing and may also have problems with the movement and digestion of food in the gut. Patients will require medications to help thin the mucus and regular physiotherapy sessions to help shift the thickened mucus from the lungs to aid breathing and gas exchange. Unfortunately, nurses routinely encounter CF patients in hospital since the presence of thick mucus in the lungs increases the risk of respiratory tract infections.

Now that you have completed this chapter, attempt the multiple-choice questions in Activity 13.4 to assess your acquired understanding.

Activity 13.4   Multiple-choice questions

1. In DNA, which of the following bases is complementary to adenine?

    a) Cytosine
    b) Thymine
    c) Guanine
    d) Uracil

2. Which of the following statements concerning DNA is true?

    a) The letters DNA stand for deoxyribonucleic acid
    b) DNA is constructed from nucleotides
    c) DNA is a molecule with a characteristic double-helical shape
    d) All are true

3. The enzyme DNA polymerase

    a) Digests DNA molecules
    b) Converts DNA into RNA
    c) Is responsible for synthesising new strands of DNA during DNA replication
    d) Is responsible for synthesising the nuclear envelope

(Continued)

(Continued)

4. During mitosis

   a) The diploid number of chromosomes is maintained

   b) The diploid number of chromosomes is halved

   c) The haploid number of chromosomes is always doubled

   d) The haploid number of chromosomes is always halved

5. In both mitosis and meiosis DNA replication occurs during

   a) Interphase

   b) Prophase

   c) Metaphase

   d) Telophase

6. Transcription involves copying DNA gene sequences into

   a) mRNA

   b) tRNA

   c) rRNA

   d) mDNA

7. The cytoplasmic component responsible for linking amino acids together during protein synthesis is

   a) The Golgi apparatus

   b) Ribosomes

   c) Centrioles

   d) Lysosomes

8. A codon is a

   a) Name given to the information stored in a single DNA base

   b) Sequence of three bases on a tRNA molecule

   c) Sequence of four bases in DNA

   d) Sequence of three bases on an mRNA molecule

9. With recessive genetic diseases

   a) The disease only occurs if one disease-causing gene is inherited

   b) The disease only occurs if two disease-causing genes are inherited

   c) These diseases require the presence of at least one dominant gene

   d) These diseases cannot be passed down the generations

10. When two carriers of the cystic fibrosis gene have children, the ratio of healthy children to children suffering the disease would be expected to be

   a) 1:1

   b) 2:1

   c) 3:1

   d) 4:1

Chapter summary

The blueprint for building the human body is stored in DNA which is constructed from building blocks called nucleotides. The genetic code is encoded using four bases called adenine, cytosine, guanine and thymine. Mitosis is normal cell division and generates the new cells necessary for growth, maintenance and repair of the body.

The daughter cells produced during mitosis are genetically identical to their parent cells and retain the diploid number of 46 chromosomes. Meiosis only occurs in the testes and ovaries during the generation of ova and spermatozoa. Meiosis involves a halving of the diploid number of chromosomes so that resultant cells have the haploid number of 23. Protein synthesis occurs in two distinct phases. Transcription involves copying DNA gene sequences into the molecule mRNA.

Translation uses mRNA as a template to assemble amino acids into the correct sequence to build a functioning protein. Genes are subject to mutations that may lead to genetic diseases, many of which are passed down the generations in a predictable manner.

Activities: Brief outline answers

Activity 13.1: Consolidation of learning (page 349)

ACCCGAATGATT – Parent strand

TGGGCTTACTAA – Complementary strand

Remember, all you need to know is that A always pairs with T (A-T) and C always pars with G (C-G).

Activity 13.2: Consolidation of learning (page 360)

An mRNA sequence of GUACCACAA would indicate that Valine-Proline-Glutamine should be linked together.

Remember, every three bases in the mRNA strand make up a codon, and you can identify which amino acid is required using the base-pairing rule to identify the corresponding anticodon.

GUACCACAA – Codons on mRNA sequence

CAUGGUGUU – Anticodons on tRNAs (CAU = Valine: GGU = Proline: GUU = Glutamine)

Activity 13.3: Consolidation of learning (page 362)

Table 13.1   Punnett square

	c	c
C	Cc	Cc
c	cc	cc

The Punnett square shows offspring of a father (top) with CF (cc) and a mother (side) who is a carrier of the CF gene (Cc).

Half the children will develop CF and half will be carriers who show no symptoms of CF.

Activity 13.4: Multiple-choice questions (pages 363–5)

1) b, 2) d, 3) c, 4) a, 5) a, 6) a, 7) b, 8) d, 9) b, 10) c

Further reading

Boore J et al. (2016) Chapter 3: Genetic and epigenetic control of biological systems, in *Essentials of Anatomy and Physiology for Nursing Practice.* London: SAGE Publications Ltd.

A textbook to develop your knowledge of human anatomy and physiology that is aimed specifically at nurses.

Knight J and Andrade M (2018) Genes and chromosomes 1: Basic principles of genetics. *Nursing Times*, 114(7): 42–5.

A gentle overview of the nature of genes and chromosomes.

Knight J and Andrade M (2018) Genes and chromosomes 2: Cell division and genetic diversity. *Nursing Times*, 114(8): 40–7.

An illustrated overview of cell division.

Useful websites

www.youtube.com/watch?v=RNwJbMovnVQ

Animated overview of mitosis.

www.youtube.com/watch?v=5pvwIsDE6eg

Animated overview of meiosis.

www.youtube.com/watch?v=gG7uCskUOrA

Animated overview of protein synthesis, including transcription and translation.

Glossary

Active transport: Movement of solutes against their natural concentration gradient and requiring the expenditure of adenosine triphosphate.

Adenosine triphosphate (ATP): Simple energy-storage molecule generated by mitochondria during cellular respiration.

Anatomy: The study of bodily structure and the physical arrangement and relationship between different organs and tissues.

Antigen: A molecule that is complementary to an antibody which may be foreign (e.g. a component of pathogen) or self (e.g. a component of a human cell membrane).

Appendicular skeleton: Predominantly the bones of the arms and legs.

Arteries: Thick-walled muscular blood vessels that usually carry oxygenated blood away from the heart under high pressure.

Atria: Thin, elastic upper chambers of the heart (singular atrium).

Axial skeleton: Predominantly the bones of the skull and trunk of the body to which the bones of the appendicular skeleton attach.

Boyle's law: Law that states pressure is inversely proportional to volume.

Capillaries: The smallest blood vessels usually found in convoluted networks called capillary beds which connect arteries to the veins and act to distribute blood to organs and tissues.

Cardiac cycle: The sequence of five distinct physical phases occurring during each heartbeat.

Cardiac muscle: A branching type of involuntary muscle found in the myocardium of the heart and responsible for the muscular contractions which allow the heart to function as a pump.

Cardiac output (CO): Volume of blood pumped by the heart per minute.

Central nervous system (CNS): The brain and spinal cord.

Centrioles: Organelles associated with the spindle apparatus which is essential for chromosome segregation during cell division.

Cerebral cortex: The two cerebral hemispheres that form the largest portion of the human brain. Essential for sensory perception, motor control and higher thought functions.

Channel proteins: Small structural pores in the plasma membrane allowing the passage of water-soluble materials (e.g. sugars) into and out of the cell.

Chromosomes: Condensed strands of DNA only visible during cell division.

Cilia: Motile cellular extensions which move in coordinated waves to shift material (e.g. mucus).

Compact bone: Also called cortical bone, this is formed from concentric tubes of bone and forms the diaphysis of long bones and outer regions of flat bones. Its laminated structure imparts great strength.

Cones: Photoreceptor cells responsible for detecting colour; concentrated at the fovea centralis of the retina.

Coronary circulation: The crown of blood vessels that surround the heart and circulate blood to and from the myocardium.

Cranial nerves: The 12 pairs of peripheral nerves that originate from within the brain. Each has sensory or motor or both sensory and motor function.

Cytokinesis: Cleavage of the cytoplasm during cell division.

Cytoplasm: The central region of a cell found between the nucleus and the plasma membrane. Location of cellular organelles and a fluid intracellular medium termed the cytosol.

Dermis: The second and thickest layer of the skin where structural components such as blood vessels, hair follicles and sweat glands are located.

Diastole: Relaxation phase of the atria or ventricles.

Diencephalon: Central region of the brain connecting the cerebral cortex to the brain stem; location of the hypothalamus.

Diffusion: Passive movement of material from a region of higher concentration to a region of lower concentration.

Diploid number: The normal expected number of chromosomes in nucleated cells (except gametes).

DNA (deoxyribonucleic acid): Large heritable macromolecule built from nucleotides which is used to encode the 'genetic blueprint'; has a characteristic double-helical structure.

Dorsal: Anatomical term that indicates towards the back of the body (near the spinal column).

Endocrine gland: A ductless gland that secretes one or more hormones directly into the blood.

Endoplasmic reticulum (ER): Labyrinth-like series of stacked, flattened membranes in the cytoplasm. There are two types: rough ER has a rough appearance due to the presence of ribosomes and is a region of protein biosynthesis. Smooth ER has no ribosomes and hence a smooth appearance and is a region of lipid biosynthesis.

Enzymes: Biological catalysts that speed up chemical reactions. Anabolic enzymes are used to build molecules (e.g. glycogen or DNA), while catabolic enzymes break down molecules (e.g. digestive enzymes).

Epidermis: The tough outer layer of skin that is rich in keratin. Surface cells are dead and continually being shed. The location of pigment-producing cells called melanocytes, which are responsible for skin colour.

Epithalamus: Deep region of the brain and location of the pineal gland.

Epithelial tissue: The simplest human tissue which is found on outer surfaces of the body, lining internal organs and in glandular tissue; involved in absorption, protection and secretion. Simple epithelium consists of a single layer of cells, while stratified epithelium is multilayered.

Erythrocytes (red blood cells): The most abundant formed elements of blood; biconcave discs lacking a nucleus that transport oxygen and carbon dioxide.

Exocrine glands: Glands that release their secretions into a duct, e.g. sweat or digestive glands in the gastrointestinal tract.

Flagellum: A motile, whip-like cellular extension which facilitates propulsion of spermatozoa.

Formed elements of blood: The whole cells (leukocytes and erythrocytes) and platelets produced by red bone marrow that circulate suspended in plasma.

Gametes: The haploid sperm and ova which are capable of fusing to form a diploid zygote.

Golgi apparatus (Golgi body or Golgi complex): A specialised region of smooth endoplasmic reticulum involved in refining proteins and packaging material into secretory vesicles for export out of cells.

Haemostasis: Mechanisms that arrest blood loss through a combination of vascular spasm, platelet plug formation or activation of the blood-clotting cascade.

Haploid number: Half the diploid number of chromosomes, usually restricted to gametes (sex cells).

Heart rate (HR): Heart beats per minute commonly recorded by assessing the pulse.

Hematopoiesis: Production of blood cells; may be split into erythropoiesis (production of erythrocytes) and leukopoiesis (production of leukocytes).

Histology: Microscopic study of biological tissues, usually involving sectioning and staining of samples to clearly view their physical features.

Homeostasis: The ability to maintain a relatively stable internal environment. Most homeostatic mechanisms involve negative feedback control.

Hormone: A chemical signal transported in the blood to exert its effects on specific cells, tissues or organs, usually by binding to complementary receptors.

Hypodermis (subcutaneous layer): The layer of adipose tissue found immediately below the dermis; a common injection site.

Immunity: The ability to resist disease and infection; involves complex and interrelated barriers and responses including mechanical, chemical and cellular defences and the inflammatory response.

Interventricular septum: The thick band of myocardial tissue that separates the left and right ventricles.

Iris: The coloured region of the eye that regulates the aperture of the pupil.

Leukocytes (white blood cells): The formed elements of blood that form a key part of the cellular defences of the immune system and function to protect the body from foreign material and pathogens.

Limbic system: A primitive region of the brain consisting primarily of the hypothalamus, the amygdala, the thalamus and the hippocampus; involved in arousal, emotional responses and formation and recall of memories.

Lipids: Family of molecules including triglyceride fats, cholesterol and phospholipids. Lipids are insoluble in water.

Lymph nodes: Bean-shaped collections of lymphoid tissue involved in trapping foreign and potentially pathogenic materials. Found in major clusters such as the cervical (neck), axial (armpit) and inguinal (groin) groupings. Palpation of swollen lymph nodes is of clinical use in the identification of sites of infection.

Lymphocytes: Leukocytes involved in specific immune responses; they generate antibodies or recognise cellular changes that are indicative of disease.

Lysosomes: Sacs of enzymes originating from the Golgi apparatus; involved in intracellular digestion (e.g. breaking down trapped bacteria in immune cells).

Macrophages: Cells that develop from monocytes when they leave the blood and enter the major organs and tissues. They act primarily as tissue-resident phagocytes.

Major histocompatibility complex (MHC): A group of 'self-proteins' found on the surface of most human cells that identify the cells as belonging to that individual; important in immune surveillance to allow differentiation between self- and non-self-material.

Mammary glands: Modified sweat glands found within breast tissue which produce milk.

Meiosis: The specialised type of cell division occurring in the primary reproductive organs (testes and ovaries) which facilitates the production of gametes (spermatozoa and ova). Meiosis results in a reduction in the diploid number of chromosomes (46) to the haploid number (23), thereby ensuring restoration of the diploid number when gametes fuse during fertilisation.

Melatonin: Hormone produced by the pineal gland of the brain that is involved in regulating the sleep/wake cycle and circadian rhythm.

Messenger RNA (mRNA): Single-stranded RNA gene sequence transcribed (copied) from DNA; allows the gene sequence to pass from the nucleus into the cytoplasm to be translated into a protein in the rough endoplasmic reticulum.

Metabolism: Biochemical processes that result in the breakdown of molecules and formation of new products, e.g. the use of glucose as a substrate within cells to release energy to synthesise adenosine triphosphate.

Microtubules: Contractile hollow filaments involved in intracellular movement such as segregation of chromosomes during cell division.

Mitochondria: Bean-shaped cytoplasmic organelles; primary location of cellular respiration and adenosine triphosphate formation. Mitochondria carry their own complement of DNA and are capable of independent replication within cells.

Mitosis: The process of normal cell division in which the diploid number of 46 is maintained and daughter cells are genetically identical.

Monosaccharides: The end products of carbohydrate digestion; single sugar units (glucose, fructose and galactose). Glucose is the primary energy source for most human cells.

Motor neurons: Conduct action potentials from the central nervous system to effector organs such as muscles or glands.

Negative feedback: The homeostatic mechanism where deviations from the ideal set point of a variable are resisted and minimised, usually ensuring that the variable fluctuates within its normal range.

Nephrons: The functional units of the kidney that produce urine.

Nerve: A bundle of neurons held together as a discrete unit by connective tissue.

Neuroglial cells: Specialised cells that provide support and protection for neurons and play a role in neural growth and formation of synapses.

Neurons: Cells of the nervous system that conduct action potentials (nerve impulses).

Nucleus: The region of the cell that contains the bulk of the cell's DNA. The nucleus is separated from the cytoplasm by a double-layered membrane called the nuclear envelope.

Olfaction: Sense of smell.

Oogenesis: Generation of haploid ova (oocytes) in females by meiosis.

Organelles: Small, discrete structures that perform a specific function, e.g. ribosomes produce proteins; mitochondria release energy during cellular respiration.

Osmosis: Diffusion of water molecules across a semi (selectively)-permeable membrane from a region of high water (low-solute) concentration to a region of low water (high-solute) concentration.

Parasympathetic nervous system: Division of autonomic nervous system responsible for vegetative functions (rest and digest); usually seen as antagonistic to the sympathetic nervous system.

Peripheral nervous system (PNS): The collective name for the nerves located outside the central nervous system; includes the cranial and spinal nerves.

Peristalsis: Waves of coordinated contraction of the muscular layer (muscularis) of the gut; responsible for transit of food along the gastrointestinal tract.

Phagocyte: A type of leukocyte or other cell capable of trapping material by phagocytosis.

Phagocytosis: The process by which cells take up solid particulate material (cell eating); important in immune reactions to allow phagocytic cells to trap and remove particulate pathogens.

Physiology: The study of the functions and activities of organs, tissues or cells, including their internal biochemistry.

Plasma: The straw-coloured, fluid portion of blood in which the formed elements of blood are suspended; consists predominantly of water, plasma proteins and electrolytes.

Plasma (cell) membrane: The outer membrane of a cell that separates the cytoplasm from the external cellular environment. Composed predominantly of a fluid phospholipid bilayer containing various types of glycoproteins.

Platelets (thrombocytes): Cellular fragments of megakaryocytes which play a key role in blood coagulation and thrombus (clot) formation.

Polysaccharides: Complex carbohydrates formed from linear or branching chains of monosaccharide sugars (usually glucose).

Positive feedback: Physiological responses where deviations from a variable's ideal set point are amplified and made larger.

Proteins: Large molecules (macromolecules) composed of sequences of amino acids which are joined together according to the genetic code.

Pulmonary circulation: Circulation of blood through the lungs.

Pupil: Aperture that controls entry of light into the eye; its diameter is regulated by dilation or constriction of the iris.

Receptors: Specialised sensory structures, e.g. touch or pain receptors or structures found on or in cells that respond to chemical signals, e.g. hormone receptors.

Retina: The photosensitive inner layer of the eye composed of rods and cones.

Rhesus blood grouping: Blood grouping determined by the presence (Rh +ve) or absence (Rh –ve) of the D antigen on the surface of erythrocytes.

Ribosomal RNA (rRNA): The form of RNA produced by the nucleolus before travelling into the rough endoplasmic reticulum to be assembled into a ribosome.

Rods: The most numerous of the photoreceptors in the retina; detect light intensity rather than colour.

Sensory neurons: Nerve cells that conduct action potentials from sensory organs/receptors to the central nervous system.

Skeletal muscle: Voluntary muscle with a striated (stripy) appearance, usually found attached to bone.

Smooth muscle: Involuntary muscle composed of diamond-shaped cells that are usually found in smooth sheets/layers lining the walls of hollow organs, e.g. the intestines, bladder and uterus.

Spermatogenesis: Production of haploid spermatozoa within the seminiferous tubules of the testes via meiosis.

Spinal cord: Portion of the central nervous system consisting of a cord-like extension of the brain stem that runs through the vertebral canal.

Spleen: Large and fragile lymphoid organ with multiple functions including removing foreign material, sequestering aged/damaged erythrocytes and acting as a blood reservoir.

Spongy bone (cancellous bone): Honeycombed soft type of bone found in the epiphyses of many long bones and in the centre of most flat bones; major location of red bone marrow.

Steroids: Molecules derived from cholesterol; includes sex hormones such as testosterone, oestrogen and progesterone, together with hormones produced by the adrenal cortex, e.g. cortisol and aldosterone.

Stroke volume (SV): Volume of blood ejected from each ventricle during ventricular systole.

Sympathetic nervous system: Division of the autonomic nervous system involved in preparing the body for action (fight or flight); usually seen as antagonistic to the parasympathetic nervous system.

Synapse: Connection between a neuron and another neuron or a neuron and an effector organ such as a muscle or gland.

Systemic circulation: Circulation of oxygenated blood via the left ventricle to the major organ systems of the body.

Systole: Contraction phase of the atria or ventricles.

Tissue: A group of one or more cell types that act together for a common purpose.

Veins: Thin-walled vessels that usually carry deoxygenated blood under low pressure towards the heart; most large and medium veins are equipped with valves to prevent backflow of blood.

Ventricles: The thick muscular lower chambers of the heart that function as the primary pumping chambers.

Vesicles: Membrane-bound sacs that allow material to be transported within cells, e.g. the secretory vesicles that bud from the Golgi apparatus.

Zygote: The diploid structure formed from the fusing of a haploid spermatozoon and a haploid ovum (oocyte).

References

Aronson D (2009) Cortisol: Its role in stress, inflammation, and indications for diet therapy. *Today's Dietitian*, 11(11): 38.

Azzam I, Gilad S, Limor R, Stern N and Greenman Y (2017) Ghrelin stimulation by hypothalamic–pituitary–adrenal axis activation depends on increasing cortisol levels. *Endocrine Connections*, 6(8): 847–55.

Bae Y, Shin E-C, Bae Y-S and Van Eden, W (2019) Editorial: Stress and immunity. *Frontiers in Immunology*, 10: 245. doi: 10.3389/fimmu.2019.00245

Bailey K and Hall A (2006) Angina: Management in the elderly. *Geriatric Medicine Journal*. www.gmjournal.co.uk/media/20105/may06p75.pdf

Benner P (1984) *From Novice to Expert: Excellence and Power in Clinical Nursing Practice.* Menlo Park, CA: Addison-Wesley Publishing Company.

Bilder G (2016) *Human Biological Aging: From Macromolecules to Organ-Systems.* Hoboken, NJ: John Wiley & Sons, Inc.

Bionumbers (2019) How quickly do different cells in the body replace themselves? http://book.bionumbers.org/how-quickly-do-different-cells-in-the-body-replace-themselves

Blundo C, Gerace C and Ricci M (2015) An overview on vitamin B12 and dementia with behavioral and executive disturbances, in Martin, CR and Preedy, VR (eds) *Diet and Nutrition in Dementia and Cognitive Decline* (pp. 649–62). London: Academic Press. https://doi.org/10.1016/B978-0-12-407824-6.00060-4

British Heart Foundation (2014) Cardiovascular Disease Statistics 2014. www.bhf.org.uk/informationsupport/publications/statistics/cardiovascular-disease-statistics-2014

Brown D (2017) The discovery of water channels (aquaporins). *Annals of Nutrition and Metabolism*, 70(suppl 1): 37–42.

Calsolaro V, Niccolai F, Pasqualetti G, Calabrese AM, Polini A, Okoye C, Magno S, Caraccio N and Monzani F (2019) Overt and subclinical hypothyroidism in the elderly: When to treat? *Frontiers in Endocrinology*, 10: 177.

Cancer Research UK (2016) Melanoma skin cancer. www.nhs.uk/conditions/melanoma-skin-cancer/causes/https://www.nhs.uk/conditions/melanoma-skin-cancer

Cancer Research UK (2019a) Lymphoedema after breast cancer treatment. www.cancerresearchuk.org/about-cancer/coping/physically/lymphoedema-and-cancer/infection-lymphoedema

Cancer Research UK (2019b) Prostate cancer statistics. www. cancerresearchuk.org/health-professional/cancer-statistics/statistics-by-cancer-type/prostate-cancer#heading-Zero

Carter A (2019) What is the link between prednisone and diabetes? www. medicalnews today.com/articles/317015.php

Chao AM, Jastreboff AM, White MA, Grilo CM and Sinha R. (2017) Stress, cortisol, and other appetite-related hormones: Prospective prediction of 6-month changes in food cravings and weight. *Obesity*, 25(4): 713–20.

Charlton JR and Abitbol CL (2016) Can renal biopsy be used to estimate total nephron number? *Clinical Journal of the American Society of Nephrology*, 12(4): 553–5.

Choi, Won-Il (2014) Pneumothorax. *Tuberculosis and Respiratory Diseases (Seoul)*, 76(3): 99–104.

Chu DH (2008) Overview of biology, development, and structure of skin, in Wolff, K, Goldsmith, LA, Katz, SI, Gilchrest, BA, Paller, AS and Leffell, DJ (eds) *Fitzpatrick's Dermatology in General Medicine* (7th ed., pp. 57–73). New York: McGraw-Hill.

Cystic Fibrosis Trust (2018) What are the causes of cystic fibrosis? www.cysticfibrosis.org.uk/what-is-cystic-fibrosis/what-causes-cystic-fibrosis

Devis P and Knuttinen MG (2017) Deep venous thrombosis in pregnancy: Incidence, pathogenesis and endovascular management. *Cardiovascular Diagnosis and Therapy*, 7(suppl 3): S309–S319. doi: 10.21037/cdt.2017.10.08

Diabetes UK (2019a) Blood sugar level ranges. www.diabetes.co.uk/diabetes_care/blood-sugar-level-ranges.html

Diabetes UK (2019b) Diabetes prevalence. www.diabetes.co.uk/diabetes-prevalence.html

Dinarello CA (2015) The history of fever, leukocytic pyrogen and interleukin-1. *Temperature (Austin)*, 2(1): 8–16.

Docherty JR (1990) Cardiovascular responses in ageing: A review. *Pharmacological Review*, 42: 103–25.

Drelich DA and Bray PF (2015) The traditional role of platelets in hemostasis, in Kerrigan, S and Moran, N (eds) *The Non-Thrombotic Role of Platelets in Health and Disease*. Rijeka, Croatia: InTech.

Druzd D, Matveeva O, Ince L, Harrison U, He W, Schmal C, Herzel H, Tsang AH, Kawakami N, Leliavski A, Uhl O, Yao L, Sander LE, Chen CS, Kraus K, de Juan A, Hergenhan SM, Ehlers M, Koletzko B, Haas R, Solbach W, Oster H and Scheiermann C (2017) Lymphocyte circadian clocks control lymph node trafficking and adaptive immune responses. *Immunity*, 46(1): 120–32. doi: 10.1016/j.immuni.2016.12.011

Durairajanayagam D, Sharma R, Du Plessis S and Agarwal A (2014) Testicular heat stress and sperm quality, in Smith, WB, Trost, LW, Chen, Y, Rosencrans, A and Hellstrom, WJG (eds) *Sexual Issues: Role of Sexually Transmitted Infections on Male Factor Fertility* (pp. 105–25) doi: 10.1007/978-1-4939-1040-3_8

Epel E, Lapidus R, McEwen B and Brownell K (2001) Stress may add bite to appetite in women: A laboratory study of stress-induced cortisol and eating behavior. *Psychoneuroendocrinology*, 26(1): 37–49.

Greenwald SE (2007) Ageing of the conduit arteries. *The Journal of Pathology*, 211: 157–72.

Growney Kalaf EA, Hixona KR, Kadakia PU, Dunn AJ and Sell SA (2017) Electrospun biomaterials for dermal regeneration, in Uyar, T and Kny, E (eds) *Electrospun Materials for Tissue Engineering and Biomedical Applications* (1st ed.). Cambridge: Woodhead Publishing.

Handel AC, Miot LD and Miot HA (2014) Melasma: A clinical and epidemiological review. *Brazilian Annals of Dermatology*, 89(5): 771–82.

Heidet M, Abdel Wahab A, Ebadi V, Cogne Y, Chollet-Xemard C and Khellaf M (2019) Severe hypoglycemia due to cryptic insulin use in a bodybuilder. *The Journal of Emergency Medicine*, 56(3): 279–81.

Hellebrekers P, Vrisekoop N and Koenderman L (2018) Neutrophil phenotypes in health and disease. *European Journal of Clinical Investigation*, 48(suppl 2): e12943.

Hoffman M (2018) Picture of the bladder. www.webmd.com/urinary-incontinence-oab/picture-of-the-bladder#1

Intriago M, Maldonado G, Cárdenas J and Ríos C (2019) Clinical characteristics in patients with rheumatoid arthritis: Differences between genders. *The Scientific World Journal*, Article ID 8103812. doi: 10.1155/2019/8103812

James WD, Berger TG, Elston DM and Neuhaus I (2015) *Andrews' Diseases of the Skin: Clinical Dermatology* (12th ed.). Philadelphia, PA: Elsevier Saunders.

Jørgensen N, Persson G and Hviid TVF (2019) The tolerogenic function of regulatory T cells in pregnancy and cancer. *Frontiers in Immunology*, 10: 911. doi: 10.3389/fimmu.2019.00911

Kaufman DP, Basit H and Knohl SJ (2019) Physiology, glomerular filtration rate (GFR). www.ncbi.nlm.nih.gov/books/NBK500032

Kiela PR and Ghishan FK (2016) Physiology of intestinal absorption and secretion: Best practice and research. *Clinical Gastroenterology*, 30(2): 145–59.

King CC, Piper ME, Gepner AD, Fiore MC, Baker TB and Stein JH (2017) Longitudinal impact of smoking and smoking cessation on inflammatory markers of cardiovascular disease risk. *Arteriosclerosis, Thrombosis, and Vascular Biology*, 37(2), 374–9. doi: 10.1161/ATVBAHA.116.308728

Knight J and Hore N (2018) Sepsis. *Standby CPD*, 8(6): 1–8.

Kolarsick PA, Kolarsick MA and Goodwin C (2011) Anatomy and physiology of the skin. *Journal of the Dermatology Nurses' Association*, 3(4): 203–13.

Komen MM, Breed WP, Smorenburg CH, van der Ploeg T, Goey SH, van der Hoeven JJ, Nortier JW and van den Hurk CJ (2016) Results of 20- versus 45-min post-infusion scalp cooling time in the prevention of docetaxel-induced alopecia. *Support Care Cancer*, 24(6): 2735–41. doi: 10.1007/s00520-016-3084-7

Kozier B, Erg G, Berman A, Snyder S, Harvey S and Morgan-Samuel H (2012) *Fundamentals of Nursing: Concepts, Process, and Practice.* Harrow: Pearson.

Legislation.gov.uk (2002) *The Nursing and Midwifery Order 2001.* www.legislation.gov.uk/uksi/2002/253/made

Maurer AH (2015) Gastrointestinal motility, part 1: Esophageal transit and gastric emptying. *The Journal of Nuclear Medicine,* 56: 1229–38. doi: 10.2967/jnumed.112.114314

Milner KA, Vaccarino V, Arnold AL, Funk M and Goldberg RJ (2004) Gender and age differences in chief complaints of acute myocardial infarction (Worcester Heart Attack Study). *The American Journal of Cardiology,* 93: 606–8.

Mitra R, Mishra N and Rath GP (2014) Blood groups systems. *Indian Journal of Anaesthesia,* 58(5): 524–8. doi: 10.4103/0019-5049.144645

Muddathir ARM, Abd Alla MI and Khabour OF (2018) Waterpipe smoking is associated with changes in fibrinogen, FVII, and FVIII levels. *Acta Haematologica,* 140: 159–65. doi: 10.1159/000492740

Nangia J, Wang T, Osborne C, Niravath P, Otte K, Papish S, Holmes F, Abraham J, Lacouture M, Courtright J, Paxman R, Rude M, Hilsenbeck S, Osborne CK and Rimawi M (2017) Effect of a scalp cooling device on alopecia in women undergoing chemotherapy for breast cancer: The SCALP Randomized Clinical Trial. *JAMA,* 317(6): 596–605. doi: 10.1001/jama.2016.20939

NHS (2017) Skin cancer (melanoma). www.nhs.uk/conditions/melanoma-skin-cancer

NHS (2018) Symptoms of heart attack. www.nhs.uk/conditions/heart-attack/symptoms

NHS (2019a) Preventing hypothermia. www.nhs.uk/conditions/hypothermia

NHS (2019b) Overactive thyroid (hyperthyroidism). www.nhs.uk/conditions/overactive-thyroid-hyperthyroidism/causes

NHS (2019c) Are pregnant women entitled to free NHS dental treatment? www.nhs.uk/common-health-questions/pregnancy/are-pregnant-women-entitled-to-free-nhs-dental-treatment

NHS (2019d) Low sperm count. www.nhs.uk/conditions/low-sperm-count

NICE (2015) Pressure Ulcers Quality Standard QS89. www.nice.org.uk/guidance/QS89

NICE (2018) Hypertension in adults: Diagnosis and management. www.nice.org.uk/guidance/CG127/chapter/1-Guidance#diagnosing-hypertension-2

NICE (2019a) Venous thromboembolism in over 16s: Reducing the risk of hospital-acquired deep vein thrombosis or pulmonary embolism. www.nice.org.uk/guidance/ng89/chapter/recommendations#lower-limb-immobilisation-2

NICE (2019b) Stroke and transient ischaemic attack in over 16s: Diagnosis and initial management. NICE Guideline, No. 128. www.ncbi.nlm.nih.gov/books/NBK546278/#lt90

NMC (2018a) Part 3 of Realising professionalism: Standards for education and training. www.nmc.org.uk/globalassets/sitedocuments/education-standards/programme-standards-nursing.pdf

NMC (2018b) Standards of proficiency for registered nurses. www.nmc.org.uk/standards/standards-for-nurses/standards-of-proficiency-for-registered-nurses

O'Driscoll BR, Howard LS, Earis J and Mak V (2017) BTS guideline for oxygen use in adults in healthcare and emergency settings. *Thorax*, 72(1): ii1–ii90. doi: 10.1136/thoraxjnl-2016-209729

Panarese A, D'Andrea V, Pironi D and Filippini A (2014) Thymectomy and systemic lupus erythematosus (SLE). *Annali Italiani di Chirurgia*, 85(6): 617–18.

Perello M and Dickson SL (2015) Ghrelin signalling on food reward: A salient link between the gut and the mesolimbic system. *Journal of Neuroendocrinology*, 27(6): 424–34.

Public Health England and Department of Health (2013) Immunisation against infectious disease. www.gov.uk/government/collections/immunisation-against-infectious-disease-the-green-book#the-green-book

Reuter S, Moser C and Baack M (2014) Respiratory distress in the newborn. *Pediatrics in Review*, 35(10): 417–29. doi: 10.1542/pir.35-10-417

Royal College of Physicians (2017) National Early Warning Score 2. www.rcplondon.ac.uk/projects/outputs/national-early-warning-score-news-2

Rugo HS, Klein P, Melin SA, Hurvitz SA, Melisko ME, Moore A, Park G, Mitchel J, Bageman E, D'Agostino RB Jr., Ver Hoeve ES, Esserman L and Cigler T (2017) Association between use of a scalp cooling device and alopecia after chemotherapy for breast cancer. *JAMA*, 317(6): 606–14. doi: 10.1001/jama.2016.21038

Sankaran VG and Orkin SH (2013) The switch from fetal to adult hemoglobin. *Cold Spring Harbor Perspectives in Medicine*, 3: a011643.

Sepsis Trust (2019) About sepsis. https://sepsistrust.org/about/about-sepsis

Shier D, Butler J and Lewis R (2018) *Hole's Human Anatomy and Physiology*. New York: McGraw-Hill Education.

Sözen T, Özışık L and Başaran NÇ (2017) An overview and management of osteoporosis. *European Journal of Rheumatology*, 4(1): 46–56.

Steenman M and Lande G (2017) Cardiac aging and heart disease in humans. *Biophysical Reviews*, 9(2): 131–7.

The UK Iodine Group (2019) How much iodine do you need? www.ukiodine.org/iodine-food-fact-sheet

UK Gout Society (2019) All about gout and diet. www.ukgoutsociety.org/docs/goutsociety-allaboutgoutanddiet-0113.pdf

Van Rossum EF (2017) Obesity and cortisol: New perspectives on an old theme. *Obesity*, 25(3): 500–1.

Walsh JS (2015) Normal bone physiology, remodelling and its hormonal regulation. *Surgery*, 33(1): 1–6.

Waterlow J (1985) The Waterlow Pressure Ulcer Prevention Manual. www.judy-waterlow.co.uk/the-waterlow-manual.htm

Williams JA (2014) Pancreatic polypeptide. *Pancreapedia: Exocrine Pancreas Knowledge Base.* doi: 10.3998/panc.2014.4

Wolf PA, Abbott RD and Kannel WB (1991) Atrial fibrillation as an independent risk factor for stroke: The Framingham Study. *Stroke,* 22, 983–8.

World Health Organization (2009) World Health Organization Guidelines on Hand Hygiene in Health Care. First Global Patient Safety Challenge. Clean Care is Safer Care. https://apps.who.int/iris/bitstream/handle/10665/44102/9789241597906_eng.pdf;js essionid=6A3362ADC28E7CAA294E46C2652C896D?sequence=1

Xue M and Jackson CJ (2015) Extracellular matrix reorganization during wound healing and its impact on abnormal scarring. *Advances in Wound Care,* 4(3): 119–36. doi: 10.1089/ wound.2013.0485

Yanez DA, Lacher RK, Vidyarthi A and Colegio OR (2017) The role of macrophages in skin homeostasis. *Pflugers Archiv: European Journal of Physiology,* 469(3–4): 455–63. doi: 10.1007/s00424-017-1953-7

Zdrojewicz Z, Pachura E and Pachura P (2016) The thymus: A forgotten, but very important organ. *Advances in Clinical and Experimental Medicine,* 25(2): 369–75.

Zimmerman A, Bai L and Ginty DD (2014) The gentle touch receptors of mammalian skin. *Science,* 346: 950–4.

Index

Note: References in *italics* are to figures, those in **bold** to tables; 'g' refers to the Glossary.